The Medical Library Association Guide to Data Management for Librarians

Medical Library Association Books

The Medical Library Association (MLA) features books that showcase the expertise of health sciences librarians for other librarians and professionals.

MLA Books are excellent resources for librarians in hospitals, medical research practice, and other settings. These volumes will provide health care professionals and patients with accurate information that can improve outcomes and save lives.

Each book in the series has been overseen editorially since conception by the Medical Library Association Books Panel, composed of MLA members with expertise spanning the breadth of health sciences librarianship.

About the Medical Library Association

Founded in 1898, MLA is a 501(c)(3) nonprofit, educational organization of 3,500 individual and institutional members in the health sciences information field that provides lifelong educational opportunities, supports a knowledge base of health information research, and works with a global network of partners to promote the importance of quality information for improved health to the health care community and the public.

Books in the Series:

The Medical Library Association Guide to Providing Consumer and Patient Health Information edited by Michele Spatz
Health Sciences Librarianship edited by M. Sandra Wood
Curriculum-Based Library Instruction: From Cultivating Faculty Relationships to Assessment edited by Amy Blevins and Megan Inman
Mobile Technologies for Every Library by Ann Whitney Gleason
Marketing for Special and Academic Libraries: A Planning and Best Practices Sourcebook by Patricia Higginbottom and Valerie Gordon
Translating Expertise: The Librarian's Role in Translational Research edited by Marisa L. Conte
Expert Searching in the Google Age by Terry Ann Jankowski
Digital Rights Management: The Librarian's Guide edited by Catherine A. Lemmer and Carla P. Wale
The Medical Library Association Guide to Data Management for Librarians edited by Lisa Federer

The Medical Library Association Guide to Data Management for Librarians

EDITED BY

Lisa Federer

ROWMAN & LITTLEFIELD
Lanham • Boulder • New York • London

Published by Rowman & Littlefield
A wholly owned subsidiary of The Rowman & Littlefield Publishing Group, Inc.
4501 Forbes Boulevard, Suite 200, Lanham, Maryland 20706
www.rowman.com

Unit A, Whitacre Mews, 26-34 Stannary Street, London SE11 4AB

British Library Cataloguing in Publication Information Available

Library of Congress Cataloging-in-Publication Data Available

ISBN 978-1-4422-6426-7 (cloth : alk. paper)
ISBN 978-1-4422-6427-4 (pbk : alk. paper)
ISBN 978-1-4422-6428-1 (ebook)

∞™ The paper used in this publication meets the minimum requirements of American National Standard for Information Sciences—Permanence of Paper for Printed Library Materials, ANSI/NISO Z39.48-1992.

Printed in the United States of America

Contents

Preface vii
Acknowledgments xi

Part I: Data Management: Theory and Foundations **1**

1 Research Data Management for the Biomedical Digital Research Enterprise: A Perspective from the National Institutes of Health 3
Valerie Florance

2 What Could Possibly Go Wrong?: The Impact of Poor Data Management 13
Chris Eaker

3 Research Data as Record 31
Bethany Myers

4 Raising Researchers' Awareness of Biomedical Data Journals to Promote Data Sharing 49
Katherine G. Akers

5 Data Science: New Librarian Roles for a New Field of Research 69
Lisa Federer

6 Data 101: Learning and Keeping Current in Data Management Skills 79
Abigail Goben and Rebecca Raszewski

Part II: Data Management across the Research Data Life Cycle **91**

7 Library Support for Data Management Plans 95
Carrie L. Iwema, Melissa A. Ratajeski, and Andrea M. Ketchum

8 Going Beyond the Data Management Plan: Services and Partnerships 109
Abigail Goben, Lisa Zilinski, and Kristen Briney

9 Library Infrastructures for Scholarship at Scale 123
Steven Braun

10 Contextualizing Visualization in Library Services 139
Marci D. Brandenburg and Justin Joque

Part III: Data Management in Practice **151**

11 Data Services at a Medium-Size Academic Library 155
Minglu Wang, Bonnie L. Fong, and Ann Vreeland Watkins

12 Data Information Literacy: Engaging with the Undergraduate Health Sciences Population 171
Yasmeen Shorish and Carolyn Schubert

13 Building Data Management Services at an Academic Medical Center: An Entrepreneurial Approach 187
Alisa Surkis and Kevin Read

14 Data Management in the Lab 203
Caitlin Bakker

15 Demystifying Data Management: Designing Services for Hospital-Based Researchers 215
Jeannine Cyr Gluck

Index 223

About the Authors 227

Preface

In the second decade of the twenty-first century, we are living in a culture that is obsessed with data. Data has been proclaimed "the new oil,"[1] and data scientist heralded as the "sexiest job of the twenty-first century."[2] We've been warned that the "data deluge" is upon us[3] and that we are "drowning in data but starving for insight."[4] Corporations now hire "chief data officers" to manage (and often monetize) business's ever-growing data.[5] Data have even invaded our everyday lives; the Quantified Self movement, which promises "self knowledge through numbers," is all about improving yourself through data analytics, self-monitoring, and crunching the numbers on steps walked, calories consumed, hours slept, or whatever your metric of interest might be.[6]

Scientific research and clinical medicine have also evolved with the rise of the digital data age. Clinicians now record patient data in electronic health records (EHRs), and their patients log in from the comfort of their home to view their latest test results, make appointments, and refill their prescriptions. Researchers can access millions of datasets online and make discoveries without ever setting foot in a laboratory. Intrepid scientists are even using social media data as fodder for their research, tracking drug abuse through Twitter[7] or using social media to deliver the intervention of interest.[8]

The ways that researchers are expected to share their research results have also evolved to frequently include the final research data as an essential component of research communication. It is no longer enough to just write an article for submission to a peer-reviewed journal; researchers are also expected to share the data they have gathered through the course of their research. Many major journals now require as a condition of publication that the supporting data be made available by the time the article is published. Many funders, as well, require that researchers share the data that arise from their funded research. Indeed, the United States Office of Science and Technology Policy (OSTP) issued a memorandum in 2013 directing federal agencies supporting research to create policies to increase access to the results of federally funded research, including research data.[9] Data sharing policies such as these are designed to enhance transparency and reproducibility of research, as well as increase the return on the research investment by allowing other researchers to reuse and reanalyze existing data.

As the practices of researchers and clinicians change, and as they find themselves subject to new expectations about scholarly communication and data sharing, their information needs are shifting and evolving. As librarians who serve and collaborate with these professionals, it is incumbent upon us to evolve as well. This book aims to provide librarians an introduction to the emerging field of data management.

Scope of This Book

While the term "data management" can be defined narrowly as the administration of data resources and their architectures, within this collection, we use the term broadly to refer to the set of practices and skills that are needed to work effectively and efficiently with data throughout the research cycle. These skills include not only managing and curating active research data, but also describing and organizing data based on accepted community standards, visualizing and analyzing data, sharing data and facilitating its discoverability, making decisions about data retention, and undertaking long-term preservation of valuable data, to name just a few.

The authors who have contributed to this collection are all working librarians, sharing their experiences with data management and how they support it in their libraries. They come from diverse academic and professional backgrounds and work in a variety of types of libraries, including general academic and academic health sciences libraries, hospital libraries, and government and special libraries. They also provide services to many different user groups, from undergraduates just getting started with research to later career researchers. As the varied backgrounds and experiences of these authors demonstrate, there is not just a single path to success in providing data management support, nor a single type of service that will be effective at every institution. Each of the chapters concludes with "pearls," take-home messages that the authors wish to highlight, as well as resources and additional readings the authors recommend for readers who wish to learn more.

This book is intended to be useful to librarians wherever they find themselves in their career, whether they have extensive experience working with research data or none at all. The chapters in this collection will provide useful background knowledge and examples for practicing librarians in all types of libraries, both those who are new to data management and those who already have experience in providing such services and are interested in exploring new techniques and services. This collection may also prove useful for library directors and administrators who are interested in developing a data services program, by helping them to understand programmatic considerations and to think strategically about how best to focus their services to meet the unique needs of their institution. This book is also intended to help students in master's-level library and information studies programs who are interested in pursuing a career in data librarianship. As more and more library and information studies programs begin to include classes on data management and related topics, students have opportunities to prepare themselves through study and practical experience to gain the skills they will need to be the next generation of data librarians.

Why Data, and Why Now?

We are living at an exciting time for scientific research; thanks to a variety of technological developments, researchers can gather data quickly, store it cheaply, and analyze it powerfully. Along with the incredible opportunities that come with the rise of the era of big data come new challenges. Data must be curated so that they can be used effectively, a task that is often as time-consuming as it is important, and as Howe et al. point out, "curation increasingly lags behind data generation in funding, development and recognition."[10] A 2013 study found that poor data management practices have led to a concerning loss of scientific research data, with 80 percent of data unavailable after twenty years.[11]

This significant loss of data is not without consequence. Critics have warned of a "reproducibility crisis" across many fields of science; *Nature* even dedicated a special issue to the problem of irreproducibility.[12] When research cannot be reproduced, it is difficult to trust the findings. The National Institutes of Health (NIH) has pointed to the importance of data availability and transparency in improving reproducibility, and has undertaken a variety of activities to increase access to data, including developing a data management and sharing policy and funding the creation of a "Data Discovery Index" that will make it easier for researchers to locate existing datasets.[13] Journals, too, have recognized that data availability is essential to reproducibility, and many have responded by developing data access policies that require researchers to make the research data underlying their results publicly available.[14]

As a result of these new policies and practices, the scientific research ecosystem has evolved significantly over the last ten years, and will likely continue to change as new technologies emerge and policies are updated. Researchers are now expected to write data management plans, share data that are well described and organized, and ensure that those data remain available and accessible on a long-term basis. These are new skills that most researchers have never had to use before and have likely never been taught; indeed, in a survey of NIH researchers that my colleagues and I conducted, fewer than a quarter of the respondents said they had ever had any training in data management.[15]

Many libraries have responded to these changes in the research ecosystem by developing data management and data services programs at their institutions. Librarians are especially qualified to provide support for data management. The skills and expertise that librarians bring to the management of information are often applicable to data management. Librarians know how to describe information using metadata standards, make information available and discoverable based on people's typical information-seeking behaviors, and preserve and ensure access to information over long periods—all skills that are essential for effective data management.

At the time of this writing, the job aggregation site Indeed.com lists 312 open positions matching the search "research data librarian." Many libraries have begun creating new positions and hiring librarians to focus specifically and exclusively on data services. Some librarians have even taken on highly specialized roles, such as data visualization librarian or digital curation librarian. A wealth of opportunities exists for librarians who have the expertise and skills to support research data management.

This collection explores this wealth of opportunities and some of the ways that librarians have responded to them. Part I lays the foundation for considering librarians' roles in data management, considering relevant theory and essential background. In part II, data management is approached in the context of the research data life cycle, which describes the activities and tasks of data management across all stages of the research process. In part III, librarians from a variety of different types of libraries describe how they have provided support in their specific settings, developing programs tailored to the unique needs of their users and institutions.

Notes

1. Pery Rotella, "Data Is the New Oil," *Forbes*, April 2, 2012, http://www.forbes.com/sites/perryrotella/2012/04/02/is-data-the-new-oil/#751b5ee877a9.
2. Thomas H. Davenport and D. J. Patil, "Data Scientist: The Sexiest Job of the 21st Century," *Harvard Business Review*, October 2012, https://hbr.org/2012/10/data-scientist-the-sexiest-job-of-the-21st-century/.
3. "The Data Deluge," *Economist*, February 25, 2010, http://www.economist.com/node/15579717.
4. Jeff Thomson, "Why CFOs Are Drowning in Data but Starving for Information," *Forbes*, October 30, 2013, http://www.forbes.com/sites/jeffthomson/2013/10/30/why-cfos-are-drowning-in-data-but-starving-for-information/#76fe0ed92623.
5. PricewaterhouseCoopers, "Great Expectations: The Evolution of the Chief Data Officer," 2015, https://www.pwc.com/us/en/financial-services/publications/viewpoints/assets/pwc-chief-data-officer-cdo.pdf.
6. Quantified Self Labs, "Quantified Self," http://quantifiedself.com/.
7. C. L. Hanson et al., "Tweaking and Tweeting: Exploring Twitter for Nonmedical Use of a Psychostimulant Drug (Adderall) among College Students," *J Med Internet Res* 15, no. 4 (2013).
8. S. M. Love et al., "Social Media and Gamification: Engaging Vulnerable Parents in an Online Evidence-Based Parenting Program," *Child Abuse Negl* (2016).
9. John P. Holdren, "Increasing Access to the Results of Federally Funded Scientific Research," 2013, https://www.whitehouse.gov/sites/default/files/microsites/ostp/ostp_public_access_memo_2013.pdf.
10. Doug Howe et al., "Big Data: The Future of Biocuration," *Nature* 455, no. 7209 (2008).
11. Elizabeth Howe and Richard Van Noorden, "Scientists Losing Data at a Rapid Rate," *Nature News*, December 19, 2013, http://www.nature.com/news/scientists-losing-data-at-a-rapid-rate-1.14416.
12. "Challenges in Irreproducible Research," *Nature*, Special issue, http://www.nature.com/news/reproducibility-1.17552.
13. Francis S. Collins and Lawrence A. Tabak, "Policy: NIH Plans to Enhance Reproducibility," *Nature*, January 27, 2014, http://www.nature.com/news/policy-nih-plans-to-enhance-reproducibility-1.14586.

14. "Data-Access Practices Strengthened," *Nature*, November 19, 2014, http://www.nature.com/news/data-access-practices-strengthened-1.16370.
15. Lisa M. Federer, Ya-Ling Lu, and Douglas J. Joubert, "Data Literacy Training Needs of Biomedical Researchers," *Journal of the Medical Library Association* 104, no. 1 (2016).

Bibliography

Collins, Francis S., and Lawrence A. Tabak. "Policy: NIH Plans to Enhance Reproducibility." *Nature*, January 27, 2014. http://www.nature.com/news/policy-nih-plans-to-enhance-reproducibility-1.14586.

Davenport, Thomas H., and D. J. Patil. "Data Scientist: The Sexiest Job of the 21st Century." *Harvard Business Review*, October 2012. https://hbr.org/2012/10/data-scientist-the-sexiest-job-of-the-21st-century/.

Economist. "The Data Deluge." February 25, 2010. http://www.economist.com/node/15579717.

Federer, Lisa M., Ya-Ling Lu, and Douglas J. Joubert. "Data Literacy Training Needs of Biomedical Researchers." *Journal of the Medical Library Association* 104, no. 1 (Jan 2016): 52–57.

Hanson, C. L., S. H. Burton, C. Giraud-Carrier, J. H. West, M. D. Barnes, and B. Hansen. "Tweaking and Tweeting: Exploring Twitter for Nonmedical Use of a Psychostimulant Drug (Adderall) among College Students." *J Med Internet Res* 15, no. 4 (2013): e62.

Holdren, John P. "Increasing Access to the Results of Federally Funded Scientific Research." (2013). https://www.whitehouse.gov/sites/default/files/microsites/ostp/ostp_public_access_memo_2013.pdf.

Howe, Doug, Maria Costanzo, Petra Fey, Takashi Gojobori, Linda Hannick, Winston Hide, David P. Hill, et al. "Big Data: The Future of Biocuration." *Nature* 455, no. 7209 (2008): 47–50.

Howe, Elizabeth, and Richard Van Noorden. "Scientists Losing Data at a Rapid Rate." *Nature News*, December 19, 2013. http://www.nature.com/news/scientists-losing-data-at-a-rapid-rate-1.14416.

Love, S. M., M. R. Sanders, K. M. Turner, M. Maurange, T. Knott, R. Prinz, C. Metzler, and A. T. Ainsworth. "Social Media and Gamification: Engaging Vulnerable Parents in an Online Evidence-Based Parenting Program." *Child Abuse Negl* (February 12, 2016).

Nature. "Data-Access Practices Strengthened," November 19, 2014. http://www.nature.com/news/data-access-practices-strengthened-1.16370.

———. "Challenges in Irreproducible Research." Special issue. http://www.nature.com/news/reproducibility-1.17552.

PricewaterhouseCoopers. "Great Expectations: The Evolution of the Chief Data Officer." 2015. https://www.pwc.com/us/en/financial-services/publications/viewpoints/assets/pwc-chief-data-officer-cdo.pdf.

Quantified Self Labs. "Quantified Self." http://quantifiedself.com/.

Rotella, Pery. "Data Is the New Oil." *Forbes*, April 2, 2012. http://www.forbes.com/sites/perryrotella/2012/04/02/is-data-the-new-oil/#751b5cc877a9.

Thomson, Jeff. "Why CFOs Are Drowning in Data but Starving for Information." *Forbes*, October 30, 2013. http://www.forbes.com/sites/jeffthomson/2013/10/30/why-cfos-are-drowning-in-data-but-starving-for-information/#76fe0ed92623.

Acknowledgments

This book would not have been possible without the work of many individuals. I am grateful for each of the authors who contributed for their willingness to share their insights in these chapters and for their patience with me as I worked through the process of pulling this collection together. In addition to providing her chapter, Jeannine Cyr Gluck indexed the final work.

I also thank everyone who supported me throughout the process of bringing this book together. I am grateful to the MLA Books Panel, in particular Karen McElfresh, for entrusting me with the responsibility to take on this project. Charles Harmon, my editor at Rowman and Littlefield, has been a great help at every step of the process, and with his guidance, I've learned a great deal about editing a book. Dr. Keith Cogdill, my director at the NIH Library, has always encouraged me to take on new challenges, and I appreciate his support of this project as well. I thank all the librarians who have provided friendship and mentorship along the way, especially my colleagues and friends at the NIH Library, the University of California–Los Angeles, the University of Southern California, and New York University.

Finally, I'd like to acknowledge my family and the friends who are like family, especially my parents and Ali Sabzevari, and of course, my four-legged best friend Ophelia. Without their love and support, I could not have made this book a reality.

Part I

Data Management: Theory and Foundations

Providing support for data management may seem overwhelming for librarians who have not had experience working with research data. Even librarians who have worked in this area have likely found that researchers' needs, policy requirements, and specific data management practices have changed over the last few years. Part I of this collection provides the background information that is essential for understanding the research data ecosystem and for providing effective services in a changing and emerging field.

Funders can play a significant role in driving change in the research community through policy measures; the National Science Foundation's (NSF) 2011 policy requiring researchers to submit a data management plan (DMP) with their grant proposals[1] exemplifies how policy leads to change in practice. In chapter 1, Valerie Florance provides an introduction to efforts currently underway at the National Institutes of Health (NIH) to support data science. NIH has started to address data sharing through several policies, and will continue to do so, in response to the 2013 OSTP memo. As Florance describes, the NIH has also highlighted the importance of data science by making it the focus of a major NIH initiative, Big Data to Knowledge (BD2K). With the participation of representatives of all twenty-seven of the NIH's institutes and centers, the BD2K initiative aims to develop the capacity of the biomedical research community to conduct data science and other data-intensive research.

Researchers sometimes find it cumbersome to do the additional work that comes with policies like the NSF's DMP requirement and the NIH's forthcoming data management and sharing policy.[2] However, thinking ahead about how data should be managed and curated throughout the research process is good practice regardless of whether a DMP is required. As Chris Eaker points out in chapter 2, lack of planning can have significant negative consequences. Writing a DMP (or at least thinking ahead about how data will be managed) is not just a requirement to check off the list for a grant proposal, but also an invaluable process for ensuring that data are not lost. Eaker provides advice and best practices that will help researchers avoid the kind of data disasters that can be the result of poor planning.

While the DMP requirement is new, and librarians may not have worked closely with research data before, many of the best practices for managing data are grounded in information management principles that are the foundations of libraries and archives. In chapter 3, Bethany Myers approaches research data through the lens of archival theory, providing an overview of the relevant background and exploring how these theories can be applied to research data. As librarians take on new roles working with research data, it is useful to remember that many of the skills we have brought to our work with other types of information are applicable in the management of data.

While information management and archival theory provide a helpful grounding for thinking about data management, scholarly communication can help drive thinking about how to share data. Data journals, which Katherine Akers describes in chapter 4, are one of the many methods for disseminating research data. Taking a new process, like sharing research data, and fitting it into a familiar practice, like journal publishing, can make new sharing requirements less burdensome. These types of incremental change, building upon the ways that researchers and librarians already think about and use information, make it possible to bring about significant enhancements to the ways that researchers work with data without, as the saying goes, having to "reinvent the wheel."

New requirements and methods for sharing research results are not the only drivers of change; the practice of research is evolving in nearly every field as new technologies allow researchers to collect new types of data at an unprecedented rate. In chapter 5, I describe how the age of "big data" has led to the emergence of a new scientific discipline: data science. Regardless of their field, most researchers are finding that their work is more data intensive and computationally driven in the twenty-first century than ever before, but data science is a distinct discipline that uses a set of specific processes for making sense out of large, complex datasets. I outline some of these processes and the tools used to accomplish them, as well as how librarians can get involved in supporting data science.

Working with researchers in new scientific disciplines often requires new knowledge. While librarians already have a great deal of relevant expertise for supporting research data management, retooling and learning new skills can make librarians even more invaluable. Drawing on adult learning theory, Abigail Goben and Rebecca Raszewski provide guidance in chapter 6 for librarians who would like to expand their skillset and learn new techniques that will help them provide the support for data management that many researchers so greatly need. As policies and technologies change, often at a rapid pace, librarians who work with research data must be willing to become lifelong learners who are capable of evolving with the field.

The world of research data management changes and evolves quickly. For example, as I write this chapter, the NIH's policy on data management and sharing plans is not yet in effect, but by the time this book is published and you are reading it, it's very likely that the specifics of this policy will have at least been announced, if not fully enacted. Having an understanding of the theory that grounds data management will help librarians be prepared to respond to the changing landscape and provide services that are timely and relevant to the researchers that they support.

Notes

1. National Science Foundation, "Dissemination and Sharing of Research Results," https://www.nsf.gov/bfa/dias/policy/dmp.jsp.
2. National Institutes of Health, "Plan for Increasing Access to Scientific Publications and Digital Scientific Data from NIH Funded Scientific Research," February 2015, http://grants.nih.gov/grants/NIH-Public-Access-Plan.pdf.

Bibliography

National Institutes of Health. "Plan for Increasing Access to Scientific Publications and Digital Scientific Data from NIH Funded Scientific Research," February 2015. http://grants.nih.gov/grants/NIH-Public-Access-Plan.pdf.

National Science Foundation. " Dissemination and Sharing of Research Results." https://www.nsf.gov/bfa/dias/policy/dmp.jsp.

Chapter 1

Research Data Management for the Biomedical Digital Research Enterprise

A PERSPECTIVE FROM THE NATIONAL INSTITUTES OF HEALTH

Valerie Florance, National Library of Medicine

There is worldwide interest in storing and sharing the raw data upon which biomedical research findings are based. Reuse of existing data to answer new questions can advance discovery and lower the cost of doing research by reducing duplication, supporting replication of findings, and expanding the number of researchers working on a problem. Bundling datatsets together provides scale and statistical power in research areas where data are sparse or difficult to obtain. In Europe and the United States, organizations are working to develop standard approaches and practices that simplify finding, characterizing, matching, and integrating data whose sources, structure, and focus are related but not identical.

Improving Coordination of Research Data Management at NIH

For decades, the individual Institutes and Centers (ICs) of the National Institutes of Health (NIH) have supported the development of large biomedical datasets, including the Database of Genotypes and Phenotypes (dbGAP),[1] the National Autism Research Database (NDAR),[2] and the Immunology Portal (ImmPort).[3] These datasets are generated by NIH-funded researchers and available for scientists around the world to use for new research. However, NIH had no coordinated plan for managing the public investment in these resources; assessing their accessibility, quality, and utility; or assuring the long-term sustainability of valued, strategic biomedical data research resources.

The Data and Informatics Working Group

In recognition of the need for a more comprehensive, NIH-wide plan, NIH director Francis Collins charged his Advisory Committee in 2011 to form a Data and Informatics Working Group (DIWG) to provide him with "expert advice on the management, integration, and analysis of large biomedical research datasets."[4] The DIWG's final report describes and contextualizes the significant transformation in the biomedical research enterprise in the last several years, driven in large part by new technologies that generate data at an unprecedented pace. As they note, "the 'omics' era is one in which a single experiment performed in a few hours generates terabytes (trillions of bytes) of data" and "translational and clinical research has experienced similar growth in data volume, in which gigabyte-scale digital images are common, and complex phenotypes derived from clinical data involve data extracted from millions of records with billions of observable attributes."[5] As a result of these changes to the scientific methods used in biomedical research, the DIWG suggests that "the bottleneck in scientific productivity [has shifted] from data production to data management, communication, and—most importantly—interpretation."[6]

Researchers can no longer rely on legacy tools for effective interpretation of these datasets; massive datasets require new types of interpretation methods, so the DIWG calls for "an environment that fosters the development, dissemination, and effective use of computational tools for the analysis of datasets whose size and complexity have grown by orders of magnitude in recent years."[7] In addition, modern science is often team driven, with collaborations among multiple researchers from different disciplines in disparate geographic locations becoming increasingly common, necessitating the creation of "an infrastructure and a set of policies and incentives to promote data sharing."[8]

Though many of the issues that the DIWG identified are common to most scientific disciplines, biomedical research faces its own set of unique challenges. As researchers gain a deeper understanding of the genetic and molecular factors that underlie and influence human health and disease, they will need to address how to integrate two very different types of data: basic science and clinical. Complicating this already challenging task are the many confidentiality issues that accompany clinical data associated with patients and containing personally identifiable information. As the DIWG notes, "fundamental differences between basic science and clinical investigation . . . create real challenges for the successful integration of molecular and clinical datasets."[9]

In order to address the challenges that they outlined, the DIWG made four recommendations relating to the research data generated by NIH-funded extramural researchers:

1. Promote data sharing through central and federated catalogs.
2. Support development, implementation, evaluation, maintenance, and dissemination of informatics methods and applications.
3. Build capacity by training the workforce in the relevant quantitative sciences, such as bioinformatics, biomathematics, biostatistics, and clinical informatics.
4. Provide a serious, substantial, and sustained funding commitment to enable these recommendations.[10]

The DIWG also made a fifth recommendation: that the NIH develop its own IT strategic plan that addresses these issues.[11] Specifically, they suggested that "some mechanism be designed and implemented that can provide sustained funding over multiple years in support of unified IT capacity, infrastructure, and human expertise in information sciences and technology."[12] This recommendation has helped inform actions that the NIH has since taken to establish a trans-NIH program of support for management of research data.

In closing, the committee noted that the challenges facing biomedical research were not only technological, but also cultural in nature, and emphasized the importance of "culture changes commensurate with recognition of the key role of informatics and computation for every IC's mission."[13] They also underlined the importance of these changes by encouraging a broad, NIH-wide focus, with "a distributed commitment to the use of advanced computation and informatics toward supporting the research portfolio of every IC."[14] Finally, the DIWG recognized the importance of funding to support new mandates that might arise from their recommendations, asserting that "funding the generation of data must absolutely require concomitant funding for its useful lifespan: the creation of methods and equipment to adequately represent, store, analyze, and disseminate these data."[15]

Implementing Change

Following acceptance of the DIWG's report, senior leaders and scientific staff from Institutes and Centers across NIH worked to create an implementation plan, under the interim leadership of Eric Green, director of the National Human Genome Research Institute. A search was launched to fill a new, permanent NIH leadership position, the associate director for data science (ADDS), and in March 2014, Philip Bourne was appointed as the NIH's first ADDS. In his first blog about the position, he summarized his long interest in digital science and outlined his vision for his new role.[16] He addressed the challenges inherent in preserving research data; not all data can or should be retained, but making decisions about retention requires an understanding not only of how data are used and managed today, but also how they might be used in the future. He also recognized that sustainability of data sharing is not a problem that can be dealt with by individual researchers, but must be a concern to institutions as well, suggesting that "mechanisms that reward institutions for their careful stewardship and open accessibility of biomedical data should be considered." In closing, he referenced an editorial he wrote in 2005 asking, "Is a biological database really different from a biological journal?" and noted that "in the world of digital scholarship the paper is a means to execute upon the underlying data and becomes a tool of interactive inquiry." These themes are probably familiar to health and science librarians, biomedical database curators, and other information professionals who work with biological and clinical data, as well as the published knowledge that pertains to them.

In addition to the work done within the ADDS office, additional support was needed from across the NIH. The emerging field of data science encompasses bioinformatics, computational biology, biomedical informatics, information science, and quantitative biology. Because the experts and funding streams for these various disciplines were scattered across all twenty-seven ICs, a new trans-NIH funding initiative, Big Data to Knowledge (BD2K), was formed to bring together stakeholders from across the NIH. BD2K addressed four programmatic goal areas, each with a dedicated committee of NIH staff recruited from different ICs. These programmatic areas included:

1. Facilitating Broad Use of Biomedical Big Data
2. Developing and Disseminating Analysis Methods and Software for Biomedical Big Data
3. Enhancing Training for Biomedical Big Data
4. Establishing Centers of Excellence for Biomedical Big Data

To support the funding initiatives that would evolve out of these goal areas, a seven-year funding plan was approved, through 2020, to be jointly funded by the NIH Common Fund and from funding contributed by each IC.

Roles for Librarians: BD2K and Beyond

Within BD2K's four goal areas, many activities of potential interest to librarians are planned, with some already underway. Much of the work of BD2K is conducted by institutions that have received funding through grants and contracts to accomplish specific outcomes. Librarians may be appropriate applicants for some of BD2K's funding opportunities, or they may be able to partner with BD2K grantees at their institutions. Many of the activities arising out of BD2K will have a significant impact on the research enterprise, thus affecting the communities with whom many biomedical librarians work.

In Goal 1, focusing on facilitating broad use of data, the creation of methods for citing datasets and assigning standard metadata to them is an important goal. A key award in this area supports development of BioCADDIE, a prototype data discovery index that will "play an important role in promoting data integration through the adoption of content standards and alignment to common data elements and high-level schema."[17] An additional award is planned for 2016 to support a national standards information resource for standards relevant to biomedicine. Such a resource would help researchers identify standards used in their particular research community, thus facilitating interoperability of data. Work in the area of citing data objects is also underway in conjunction with other national and international efforts.

The focus of Goal 2 includes not only tools to aid in sharing, analyzing, and managing biomedical research data[18] but also finding aids for software tools, similar to those being developed for finding data objects. Librarians who work closely with biomedical researchers may find many of these planned resources helpful in their work. For example, several awards support creating and validating data provenance information. Others support visualization of large or heterogeneous (or both) datasets.

Goal 3 is to enhance training across the biomedical sciences workforce and at all levels. The training activities developed in this area will address most individuals who work in the biomedical research enterprise, from graduate students interested in developing careers in data science, to faculty who explore their research data with data science tools, to researchers who design new data science methods, to technical staff who provide stewardship for the tools and resources needed for research data management. This latter group may include librarians, database managers, clinical informaticians, data curators, and others.

Finally, the BD2K Centers of Excellence (COEs) funded as part of Goal 4 can benefit health sciences libraries in their commitment to training. COEs develop and deliver webinars, short courses, and other activities that could be made available in local settings via remote access. Each Center has a website that provides information about current and upcoming offerings.[19]

Besides the training opportunities that will develop out of Goals 3 and 4, additional training grants offered through BD2K will help make training materials available, many of which could be of use to librarians for working with their research communities. As an aid to planning future funding and support initiatives, NIH sometimes issues a "request for information" or RFI inviting stakeholders and other interested parties to share insights, comment on proposed plans, or recommend directions. In February 2013, an RFI on training needs related to BD2K[20] generated over one hundred responses, including thoughts on which groups should be trained, when and how training should be delivered, and what topics should be included in the curriculum. Based on this public input, BD2K funding announcements for training were developed and issued in 2015. BD2K training initiatives provide widely accessible courses and open educational resources, institutional training for future data scientists, career development awards for scientists who wish to pursue careers in data science, and special educational events relating to data science.[21] As of February 2016, twenty-three awards had been made for developing instructional resources, six for university-based training for research careers in data science, and twenty-one for career transition into data science. Additional future awards in each category will expand the topics and access points for data science career training.

Roles for Librarians in Data Management

When the DIWG issued an RFI seeking information on the management, integration, and analysis of large biomedical datasets, in January 2012,[22] respondents offered nearly two hundred fifty suggestions on topics including the research information life cycle, standards development, secondary use of data, data accessibility, incentives for data sharing, and support needs.[23] One respondent addressed potential roles for librarians in expanding skills within the existing academic workforce:

> In partnership with computational bio-informaticists and statisticians, librarians undertaking additional training opportunities can address data stewardship principles and practices including: data archival methods; metadata creation and usage; and awareness of storage, statistical analysis, archives and other available resources as part of a data stewardship training curriculum.[24]

In today's health sciences and science libraries, it is common practice for library staff to offer courses in data management, use of information tools, and resources.[25] Given that the evolving digital research enterprise will require broad workforce training of scientists, students, and administrators on basics of research data management, librarians and other information specialists represent an installed base of talent that can be tapped to help all audiences attain the needed levels of skill and understanding in this important area.

The 1965 Medical Library Assistance Act gave the National Library of Medicine (NLM) authority to train librarians and other information specialists. In addition to its highly regarded Associate Fellowship Program for Librarians[26] and its Disaster Information Specialist Program,[27] NLM currently supports grant supplements to NIH-funded researchers who want to add an informationist (also called an in-context information specialist)[28] to the research team. An informationist works closely with the research team and can recommend and implement appropriate approaches for the acquisition, management, sharing, and use of research data.[29] Launched in 2012 with eight awards, NLM's informationist grant supplement program[30] has supported fifty librarian-informationists to date, providing valuable insights into the array of needs in research teams relating to data management, as well as the continuing education needs for librarians who work with them. Analysis of applications received in the first round of funding indicated a particular need for training and assistance in research data management and fostering team science.

Training for Librarians

The insights provided by these early awards led NLM representatives to draft a concept paper for presentation to the BD2K training team, proposing that BD2K expand its training portfolio to include the development of curriculum resources that librarians and other information specialists could use to update their own skills and to teach data management classes to the communities they serve.[31] As a result, an RFI about Online Resources for Teaching and Learning Biomedical Big Data Management and Data Science was issued in November 2014, aimed at identifying existing online learning resources in these areas.[32] Information was submitted about more than two hundred online and in-person courses, tutorials, guides and Massive Open Online Courses (MOOC).[33] MOOCs were the most common resource, and statistics and computer science the most common topics covered.

Based on the RFI responses and the concept paper, the BD2K training team recommended issuing two funding announcements relating to data management, aimed for use by librarians and information specialists. The first focused on developing MOOCs for training in the basics of data management for biomedical big data, with particular emphasis on working with a variety of different types of data, best practices for data management, and facilitating team science.[34] The second provided funding for the development of open educational resources for sharing, annotating, and curating biomedical big data.[35] These learning resources could be collected in a "community-owned virtual library" that could be easily reused, cited, and tracked. Five projects received funding as a result of these two opportunities, including a project that aims to develop a MOOC covering best practices in research data management[36] and another that will create a course designed to teach medical librarians how to understand and teach research data management.[37]

A defining concept of the BD2K initiative that ties everything together is the notion of the Commons. In October 2014, Bourne's blog addressed the Commons as a concept that is at the heart of NIH's long-term data management vision. "The Commons is a pilot experiment in the efficient storage, manipulation, analysis, and sharing of research output, from all parts of the research lifecycle."[38] Bourne characterized the Commons as a digital environment that makes access, manipulation, and sharing of biomedical research data efficient by storing datasets along with metadata about them, tools for analyzing and visualizing the data, and compute power (an approach that also supports replication of research findings). Research objects stored in the Commons would have unique identifiers that could also be used for finding them and for attribution when a dataset is used, giving credit to the team that created it.[39] Thus, the Commons has the basic features of a digital or virtual library.

More recent documents describe the Commons as a shared virtual space that takes advantage of cloud computing platforms and existing high-performance computing resources, one where digital objects (i.e., data, articles, workflows, methods, and the like) conform to the FAIR principles. That is, they are Findable, Accessible (and usable), Interoperable, and Reusable.[40] The idea is not to replace existing well-curated data repositories, but to expand and enhance access to research data and tools whose development is supported by NIH grants. One exciting outcome of this is the possibility of creating links among data, tools, workflows, and the articles that describe them or use them. This is a foundational concept of the digital ecosystem that will be enabled by the Commons. Another is that it will provide authors with the option to cite any type of digital object, not just articles, but all of the other objects accessible in the Commons. Each of the BD2K goal areas listed above is creating tools or resources that, collectively, will help bring the Commons to fruition. Thinking about the vision of the global digital research enterprise and the research data Commons, creating a ubiquitous, accessible research infrastructure at this scale will require commitment and expertise from many communities, working together to define and produce and update the resources that are developed.

In a recent report to the Advisory Committee to the NIH Director, the ACD Working Group on the Future of the National Library of Medicine recommended that "NLM should be the intellectual and programmatic epicenter for data science at NIH and stimulate its advancement throughout biomedical research and application."[41] Doing so would involve NLM becoming the programmatic and administrative home for the BD2K Initiative, and would mean that NLM would become the primary coordinator of all data science activities at the NIH. The report also suggested that NLM should facilitate the development of expertise and leadership in data science, within both the intramural and extramural communities. The report, with its emphasis on data science as part of NLM's strategic mission moving forward, can be seen as a planning roadmap for other health sciences libraries that are, and will continue to be, fundamental to making this vision a reality across the digital biomedical research enterprise. The librarians and information specialists who work in these organizations should be prepared to take new leadership roles in their home institutions and more broadly.

In addition to providing leadership to help their home institutions participate actively in the digital research ecosystem, health sciences librarians should consider their roles in other health initiatives mentioned in the ACD Report on the Future of NLM, such as the Precision Medicine Initiative (PMI). As described, PMI proposes to create a cohort of one million or more people whose health status and demographics matches that of the US population. The idea is that cohort members will contribute their own health data and be active participants in research that can lead to individualized therapies, approaches that take into account genomic, environmental, and social factors about an individual patient.[42] It is exciting to imagine the roles libraries and librarians might play as more and more individuals across the United States seek to find, use, and control information related to their own health.

Of course, research data management is only one of many important functions in health sciences libraries today. The ACD Report on the Future of NLM made a number of recommendations relating to the more traditional roles of libraries that are also worth broader consideration. The Report recognizes librarians' expertise in "assimilating and disseminating accessible and authoritative biomedical research findings and trusted health information to the public, healthcare professionals, and researchers worldwide" (Recommendation 1), as well as the library's responsibility to "maintain, preserve, and make accessible the nation's historical efforts in advancing biomedical research and medicine" (Recommendation 5).[43] Besides these more traditional roles for librarians, the report also suggests that librarians should take on new roles to support the evolving practice of biomedical research, including promoting openness in science through data sharing and transparency and reproducibility of research results (Recommendation 2).

Whether you are in a large academic health sciences library, a hospital library, a college library or other setting where research and learning take place, it is an exciting time to be a librarian. The scope of responsibilities for managing the data/information/knowledge spectrum is changing, the cast of stakeholders is changing, and the pace of change is breathtaking. Discussions are going on about retention and archiving policies for data, about standards and terminologies for describing digital objects, about access levels and rights—these and many related topics can and must benefit from the fundamental expertise librarians can bring to the discussion. There are many ways to contribute, from the backroom to the boardroom, but the important thing is to be in the room so your voice, and your ideas, can be heard.

Notes

1. National Center for Biotechnology Information, "dbGaP," http://www.ncbi.nlm.nih.gov/gap.
2. National Institutes of Health, "National Database for Autism Research," https://ndar.nih.gov/.
3. National Institutes of Health, "ImmPort: Bioinformatics for the Future of Immunology," https://immport.niaid.nih.gov/.
4. National Institutes of Health Data and Informatics Working Group (DIWG), "Draft Report to the Advisory Committee to the Director (ACD)," June 15, 2012. Section 1.1, p. 5. http://acd.od.nih.gov/Data%20and%20Informatics%20Working%20Group%20Report.pdf.
5. National Institutes of Health, ACD DIWG, p. 8.
6. National Institutes of Health, ACD DIWG, p. 8.
7. National Institutes of Health, ACD DIWG, p. 9.
8. National Institutes of Health, ACD DIWG, p. 9.
9. National Institutes of Health, ACD DIWG, p. 9.
10. National Institutes of Health, ACD DIWG, pp. 13–25.
11. National Institutes of Health, ACD DIWG, pp. 6–7.
12. National Institutes of Health, ACD DIWG, p. 25.
13. National Institutes of Health, ACD DIWG, p. 25.
14. National Institutes of Health, ACD DIWG, p. 25.
15. National Institutes of Health, ACD DIWG, p. 25.
16. Philip E. Bourne, "Taking on the Role of Associate Director for Data Science at the NIH—My Original Vision Statement," *PEBourne* (blog), December 21, 2013, https://pebourne.wordpress.com/2013/12/21/taking-on-the-role-of-associate-director-for-data-science-at-the-nih-my-original-vision-statement/.
17. BioCADDIE, which stands for Biomedical and HealthCare Data Discovery Index Ecosystem, is described at https://biocaddie.org/about.
18. See https://datascience.nih.gov/bd2k/funded-programs/software for examples of awards made in the area of targeted software.
19. https://datascience.nih.gov/bd2k/funded-programs/centers provides links to each Center. The foci of the centers differ, as do the types of activities supported.
20. National Institutes of Health, "Request for Information (RFI): Training Needs in Response to Big Data to Knowledge (BD2K) Initiative," NIH Guide for Grants and Contracts, February 20, 2013, https://grants.nih.gov/grants/guide/notice-files/NOT-HG-13-003.html.
21. Office of the NIH Associate Director of Data Science, "Training, Education, and Workforce Development," *Data Science at NIH*, February 18, 2016, https://datascience.nih.gov/bd2k/funded-programs/enhancing-training.
22. National Institutes of Health, "Request for Information (RFI): Input into the Deliberations of the Advisory Committee to the NIH Director Working Group on Data and Informatics," NIH Guide for Grants and Contracts, January 10, 2012, http://grants.nih.gov/grants/guide/notice-files/NOT-OD-12-032.html.

23. National Institutes of Health, ACD DIWG, pp. 28–76.
24. National Institutes of Health, ACD DIWG, p. 63.
25. Two examples among many: The Lamar Soutter Library at University of Massachusetts http://libraryguides.umassmed.edu/libclasses and the Eccles Health Sciences Library at University of Utah, http://campusguides.lib.utah.edu/further.
26. National Library of Medicine, "Associate Fellowship Program for Librarians," October 27, 2015, https://www.nlm.nih.gov/about/training/associate/index.html.
27. National Library of Medicine, "Disaster Information Specialist Program," September 26, 2015, https://www.sis.nlm.nih.gov/dimrc/disasterinfospecialist.html.
28. Valerie Florance, "Informationist Careers for Librarians—a Brief History of NLM's Involvement," *Journal of eScience Librarianship* 2, no. 1 (May 2013), http://escholarship.umassmed.edu/jeslib/vol2/iss1/2/.
29. The NIH Library has a vibrant consulting and teaching program that serves similar needs of intramural researchers and staff at the NIH. http://nihlibrary.nih.gov/Services/Pages/default.aspx.
30. National Library of Medicine, "Awards for NLM Administrative Supplements for Informationist Services in NIH-funded Research Projects," February 25, 2016, http://www.nlm.nih.gov/ep/InfoSplmnts.html.
31. Valerie Florance, "Roles for Libraries in BD2K, Concept Paper" (internal document, September 2, 2014).
32. National Institutes of Health, "Request for Information (RFI) on the NIH Big Data to Knowledge (BD2K) Initiative Resources for Teaching and Learning Biomedical Big Data Management and Data Science," November 4, 2014, http://grants.nih.gov/grants/guide/notice-files/NOT-LM-15-001.html.
33. Personal Communication, NLM Associate Fellow Ariel Deardorff, January 22, 2015.
34. National Institutes of Health, "NIH Big Data to Knowledge (BD2K) Initiative Research Education: Massive Open Online Course (MOOC) on Data Management for Biomedical Big Data (R25)," November 26, 2014, http://grants.nih.gov/grants/guide/rfa-files/RFA-LM-15-001.
35. National Institutes of Health, "NIH Big Data to Knowledge (BD2K) Initiative Research Education: Open Educational Resources for Sharing, Annotating and Curating Biomedical Big Data (R25)," November 26, 2014, http://grants.nih.gov/grants/guide/rfa-files/RFA-LM-15-002.html#sthash.Pgq5NSDp.dpuf.
36. Office of the NIH Associate Director of Data Science, "Massive Open Online Course (MOOC) on Data Management for Biomedical Big Data (R25)," *Data Science at NIH*, November 6, 2015, https://datascience.nih.gov/MOOC.
37. Office of the NIH Associate Director of Data Science, "Open Educational Resources for Sharing, Annotating and Curating Biomedical Big Data (R25)," *Data Science at NIH,* November 6, 2015, https://datascience.nih.gov/OER-Sharing.
38. Philip E. Bourne, "ADDS Current Vision Statement, October 2014," *PEBourne* (blog), October 31, 2014, https://pebourne.wordpress.com/2014/10/31/adds-current-vision-statement-october-2014/.
39. Office of the NIH Associate Director of Data Science, "The NIH Commons," *Data Science at the NIH*, December 30, 2015, https://datascience.nih.gov/commons.
40. FORCE11, "The FAIR Data Principles," http://www.force11.org/group/fairgroup/fairprinciples.
41. National Institutes of Health, Advisory Committee to the Director, National Library of Medicine Working Group (ACD NLMWG), Final Report, June 11, 2015. http://acd.od.nih.gov/meetings.htm.
42. National Institutes of Health, "Precision Medicine Initiative," http://www.nih.gov/precisionmedicine/index.htm.
43. National Institutes of Health, ACD NLMWG, pp. 1–2, http://acd.od.nih.gov/meetings.htm.

Bibliography

bioCADDIE. "Biomedical and HealthCare Data Discovery Index Ecosystem." 2016. https://biocaddie.org/about.

Bourne, Philip E. "ADDS Current Vision Statement, October 2014," *PEBourne* (blog), October 31, 2014. https://pebourne.wordpress.com/2014/10/31/adds-current-vision-statement-october-2014/.

———. "Taking on the Role of Associate Director for Data Science at the NIH—My Original Vision Statement." *PEBourne* (blog), December 21, 2013. https://pebourne.wordpress.com/2013/12/21/taking-on-the-role-of-associate-director-for-data-science-at-the-nih-my-original-vision-statement/.

Florance, V. "Roles for Libraries in BD2K, Concept Paper." Internal document, September 2, 2014.

National Center for Biotechnology Information. "dbGaP." http://www.ncbi.nlm.nih.gov/gap.

National Institutes of Health. "ImmPort: Bioinformatics for the Future of Immunology." https://immport.niaid.nih.gov/.

———. "National Database for Autism Research." https://ndar.nih.gov/.

———. "NIH Big Data to Knowledge (BD2K) Initiative Research Education: Massive Open Online Course (MOOC) on Data Management for Biomedical Big Data (R25)." November 26, 2014, http://grants.nih.gov/grants/guide/rfa-files/RFA-LM-15-001.

———. "NIH Big Data to Knowledge (BD2K) Initiative Research Education: Open Educational Resources for Sharing, Annotating and Curating Biomedical Big Data (R25)." November 26, 2014. http://grants.nih.gov/grants/guide/rfa-files/RFA-LM-15-002.html#sthash.Pgq5NSDp.dpuf.

———. "Precision Medicine Initiative." http://www.nih.gov/precisionmedicine/index.htm.

———. "Request for Information (RFI): Input into the Deliberations of the Advisory Committee to the NIH Director Working Group on Data and Informatics." NIH Guide for Grants and Contracts, January 10, 2012. http://grants.nih.gov/grants/guide/notice-files/NOT-OD-12-032.html.

———. "Request for Information (RFI) on the NIH Big Data to Knowledge (BD2K) Initiative Resources for Teaching and Learning Biomedical Big Data Management and Data Science." November 4, 2014. http://grants.nih.gov/grants/guide/notice-files/NOT-LM-15-001.html.

———. "Request for Information (RFI): Training Needs in Response to Big Data to Knowledge (BD2K) Initiative." NIH Guide for Grants and Contracts, February 20, 2013, https://grants.nih.gov/grants/guide/notice-files/NOT-HG-13-003.html.

National Institutes of Health Advisory Committee to the Director, National Library of Medicine Working Group (ACD NLMWG). "Final Report." June 11, 2015. http://acd.od.nih.gov/meetings.htm.

National Institutes of Health Data and Informatics Working Group (DIWG). "Draft Report to the Advisory Committee to the Director (ACD)." June 15, 2012, Section 1.1, p. 5. http://acd.od.nih.gov/Data%20and%20Informatics%20Working%20Group%20Report.pdf.

National Library of Medicine. "Associate Fellowship Program for Librarians." October 27, 2015. https://www.nlm.nih.gov/about/training/associate/index.html.

———. "Awards for NLM Administrative Supplements for Informationist Services in NIH-Funded Research Projects." February 25, 2016. http://www.nlm.nih.gov/ep/InfoSplmnts.html.

———. "Disaster Information Specialist Program." September 26, 2015. https://www.sis.nlm.nih.gov/dimrc/disasterinfospecialist.html.

Office of the NIH Associate Director of Data Science. "Massive Open Online Course (MOOC) on Data Management for Biomedical Big Data (R25)." *Data Science at NIH*, November 6, 2015. https://datascience.nih.gov/MOOC.

———. "The NIH Commons." *Data Science at the NIH*, December 30, 2015, https://datascience.nih.gov/commons.

———. "Open Educational Resources for Sharing, Annotating and Curating Biomedical Big Data (R25)." *Data Science at NIH*, November 6, 2015. https://datascience.nih.gov/OER-Sharing.

———. "Training, Education, and Workforce Development." *Data Science at the NIH*, February 18, 2016. https://datascience.nih.gov/bd2k/funded-programs/enhancing-training.

Chapter 2

What Could Possibly Go Wrong?

THE IMPACT OF POOR DATA MANAGEMENT

Chris Eaker, University of Tennessee Libraries

A Tibetan monk lost his life's work after posing for a photograph with London Mayor Boris Johnson.[1] A long-time Flickr user lost thousands of original digital photographs when the photo-sharing service erroneously deleted them.[2] The programmers of the movie *Toy Story 2* nearly lost the entire movie file when someone accidentally typed a wrong command.[3] A dataset containing mistakes from careless data entry forced a scientist to request retraction of seven articles.[4] What do these unfortunate situations all have in common? These are all situations in which poor data management practices caused problems that could have been avoided.

Why are data management skills so important? Should they matter more now than in the past? The answers to those questions may not always be apparent. Conceivably, some of the problems possible now were not possible when research data was primarily in paper form. On the one hand, the changes in the makeup of research and data from analog to digital have made collecting, processing, and analyzing data easier than ever.[5] On the other hand, the improvements offered by digital research bring ways to collect, process, and analyze data poorly, thereby creating more opportunities for problems.[6] If rates of article retractions are any indication, one study found that problems have increased tenfold since 1975.[7] Although about two-thirds (67.4 percent) of retractions in that study were caused by scientific misconduct, including fraud, duplicate publications, and plagiarism, the authors found retractions caused by error have also increased, including errors related to analysis and reproducibility.[8] Article retractions represent lost time, effort, and money in research projects, many of which were funded with public money through federal grants. Freedman, Cockburn, and Simcoe[9] estimate that the lack of reproducibility in scientific research costs $28 billion per year. The authors did not posit why these errors occurred or how they could have been avoided; it is possible rigorous data management practices may have mitigated some of the errors.

This chapter will highlight the importance of good data management practices by providing examples of problems a researcher may encounter when research data is poorly managed. It will provide examples of actual situations when bad data management led to serious problems with data loss, research integrity, and worse. It will also provide tips on how data management could have been done differently to encourage a more positive outcome.

Background

As research produces higher volumes of digital research data, effective management of these data is very important. Federal grant funding agencies require researchers to submit data management plans with grant proposals and share the results of their research, including the data, in part to increase the return on their investment. Stewardship of the data is the responsibility of the researcher.[10] However, data stewardship is typically not the first thing on researchers' minds. Busy researchers are often more focused on getting the research project finished, the data analyzed, and the articles published than they are on making sure the data are described and preserved for later reuse.[11]

Librarians have recognized the need for sound data management practices to support preservation and sharing of data. Within the last decade, in order to understand researchers' current data management practices and find opportunities to help, library and information science researchers have studied different groups of researchers' data management practices[12] and found that they often employ inconsistent practices.[13] In response to the need to improve data management practices among these researchers, librarians have developed training programs at different universities[14] to help improve these practices among faculty and students. These training programs are often framed around the data life cycle, such as the DataONE Data Life Cycle shown in figure 2.1, which puts the skills into the context of the research process.

Librarians are not the only ones who see the need for data management training; scientific researchers have published primers on data management for their fellow scientists in fields such as ecology[15] and earth sciences,[16] and even for the general public involved in citizen science initiatives.[17] Researchers are trained in the art of conducting research in their fields, but specific skills related to managing the data they collect are not always covered in their curricula.[18] The sheer proliferation of studies of researchers' data management skills and the number of training programs, books, and articles about data management best practices suggest a tacit admission that these skills need improvement.

Potential Problems from Poor Data Management

There are many opportunities for error to be introduced during a research project, even when data are managed well. However, when data are mismanaged, even inadvertently, the risks of errors are multiplied. The DataONE Data Life Cycle,[19] shown in figure 2.1, will be used as a model in this discussion of some of the things that can go wrong during a research project.

Of course, not every research project flows through every step of the life cycle, nor is each step of the life cycle passed through in the order shown in the model. For example, the analysis phase is often completed concurrent with or subsequent to the data collection and assurance phases, not after the preservation phase as the life cycle model shows. Nevertheless, the point of the life cycle model is to encourage a researcher to think about the issues involved in managing research data throughout a project. Each of these steps involves specific tasks associated with managing data, and when these tasks are not completed effectively, the potential for error arises. In this chapter, the following six phases will be discussed: planning, data collection, quality assurance, documentation, preservation, and analysis.

The Planning Stage

As the first step in the research data life cycle and the step upon which all the remaining steps are built, the planning stage is arguably the most important. With proper planning, research is more organized and leads to better-quality data. Researchers should allow ample time before they begin a project to write a data management plan that spells out who will be involved in various aspects of data collection, documentation, and analysis, and how the data will be preserved.

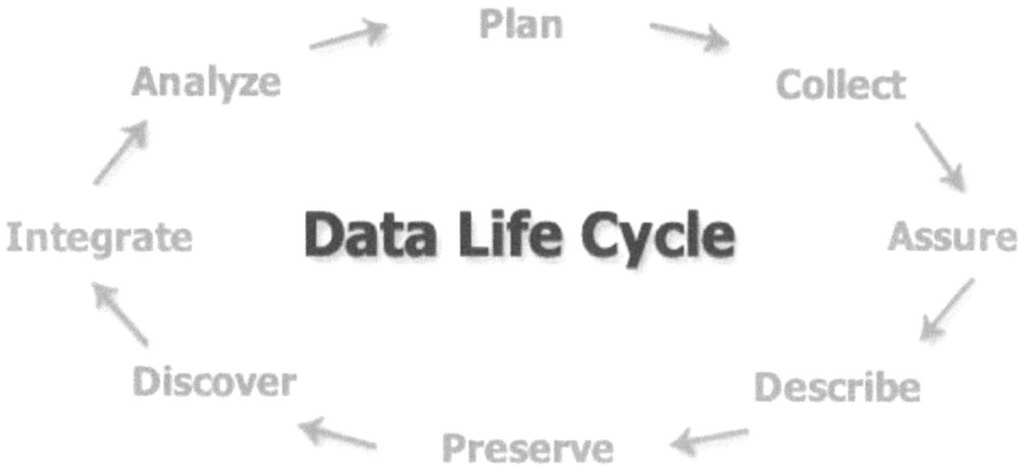

Figure 2.1. DataONE Data Life Cycle. DataONE Data Life Cycle (online at https://www.dataone.org/best-practices).

WHAT CAN GO WRONG?

Without a clear plan for how the research project will proceed, one might describe the situation as "flying by the seat of your pants." Researchers may never have a clear idea of how data should be collected, which can lead to data being collected inconsistently among project members. Different people may describe the variables and data files differently. People may save data in different places and in different formats, which makes it more difficult to locate data when needed. Roles among researchers may not be clearly defined; without clear roles, important tasks may be overlooked, as no one claims responsibility. This threat is higher in larger labs, as the possibility for human error is higher.[20] In a survey of graduate students, who are often tasked with data collection within laboratories and research groups,[21] Doucette and Fyfe found that almost 15 percent of their respondents had to collect data again that they knew had already been collected because the file was lost or corrupted. Worse, just over 17 percent indicated the data were permanently lost because they could not collect them again.[22] In each of these cases, lost data led to lost time and money. A thorough data management plan might have prevented these losses. Lastly, as many labs constantly deal with students graduating and new ones becoming involved in a project, without a clear transfer protocol, that changeover can be disorganized and may lead to missed tasks and lost data.

WHAT CAN BE DONE DIFFERENTLY?

Data management planning is an important step of the research process. It is the first step any researcher must complete in a research project. Most grant funding agencies, both public and private, now require that researchers complete a data management plan to accompany their grant proposals. However, many agencies require only brief or limited data management plans. Therefore, all researchers, even those not applying for grant funding, should consider completing a longer, more in-depth data management plan that covers detailed processes, steps, and roles. This planning step forces the researcher to think through the issues surrounding data, such as who will be involved in the project, what their roles will be, how often and where data will be backed up, how data will be cleaned and processed, how the data and processes will be described, and where that data will be shared upon completion of the project.

The Data Collection Stage

After the planning stage, during which processes and systems are established, data collection begins. The collected or generated data are the foundation upon which all future analysis and conclusions are built; therefore, it is important to collect the data consistently. As is the case with each consecutive step of the research data life cycle (figure 2.1), success during the data collection step depends on proper planning in the previous step.

WHAT CAN GO WRONG?

Without proper planning for data collection, a number of problems can occur. If the data collection steps and processes are not properly planned, the research project can ultimately end up with a dataset that does not serve the purpose for which it was intended. For example, if more than one person is involved in the data collection, but data collectors do not follow consistent data collection practices, they can end up with data with different units, collection processes, and variable names. One person may collect temperature using one device while another collects it using a different one. The difference in data collection device may not cause problems in later data analysis, especially if these differences are known and planned for. However, researchers should attempt to minimize these differences and collect data consistently among all members of the research team. If differences in data collection are not planned for, researchers may discover they have incompatible data sources. Problems of incompatibility are especially common when dealing with geospatial data of different coordinate projections.[23] If this incompatibility goes undetected, errors in analysis may occur.

In addition to consistency, data collection problems can be exacerbated by poor data entry techniques. Some popular data entry tools, such as Microsoft Excel and other spreadsheet software, make data entry easy. However, this ease of data entry can bring consequences, as these spreadsheet programs do not enforce any rules on data entry unless specifically told to do so. Without enforcement, people can input data into wrong fields, use incorrect formats, or leave data fields empty where there should be a value. It is important for researchers to be aware of the limitations of data entry in spreadsheet software so they can take precautions to eliminate opportunities for error.

WHAT CAN BE DONE DIFFERENTLY?

Data collection processes, procedures, and standards should be put in place early in the research process, preferably during the planning stage, so that all people involved collect data consistently. Examples of processes that should be established early on include consistent data collection procedures, an agreed-upon naming convention for all variables to be collected during the project, and a preferred unit convention and geodetic frame of reference. Researchers should document these standards in the data management plan, and periodically check that the research team is adhering to established procedures.

When using spreadsheets for data entry, three features in Excel improve the quality of data entry validity: dropdown lists, data validation, and data input forms. Dropdown lists of preset values make data entry easier by reducing the need to manually type repeated values and eliminate variation in the ways data collectors may record the same value. For example, if one of the pieces of information to be collected is the name of a particular species of plant and the set of species is already known and constant, the researcher can create a dropdown list of species' names to be selected from the list rather than typed repeatedly for each observation. Another helpful tool in data entry is data validation. Excel will allow the researcher to specify what type of information can go in a specific cell. For example, for a column of weights where the researcher wants two decimal places and knows the weights will always be within a certain range, the cells can be set to accept only numerical values with two decimal places within a certain numerical range. If a number that is input is out of that numerical range, Excel will display a warning. The last tool for more accurate data input is forms, which provide an easy way for data to be input into the spreadsheet. An example of an Excel input form is shown in figure 2.2.[24]

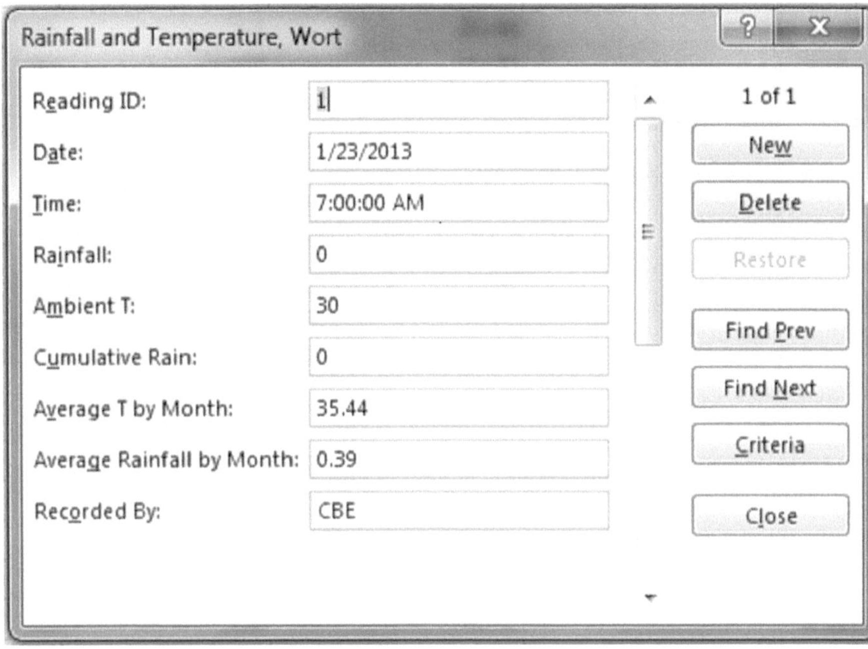

Figure 2.2. Example of an Excel input form.

The Quality Assurance Phase

Once data are collected and steps have been taken to reduce the opportunity for error during data input, the researcher still must undergo steps to assure the quality of the data. During data collection, two types of errors can occur: errors of omission and errors of commission.[25] Errors of omission occur when data or metadata are omitted from the dataset. These errors often occur inadvertently during data entry, such as when someone simply forgets to enter data for a specific observation. Errors of commission occur when incorrect data or metadata are entered. These errors also often occur inadvertently, such as when someone enters an incorrect value into a cell in the spreadsheet. In both cases, the researchers must take steps to eliminate these kinds of errors. These steps are discussed later in "What Can Be Done Differently?" It is important to note the goal of data quality assurance processes is not to eliminate legitimate outliers in the data, but to eliminate incorrect data. Legitimate outliers should be maintained and explained thoroughly in the documentation.

WHAT CAN GO WRONG?

Poor quality data can have serious effects on later analysis. Data containing errors of commission or omission have the potential of throwing off analytical calculations, which may then lead to incorrect conclusions. In addition to errors of commission or omission, careless handling of spreadsheet data can cause one column to be sorted out of order with the others, which is not always apparent at first glance.

Ultimately, poor quality datasets can have far-reaching implications and can lead to multiple article retractions. In one case, careless data entry caused retraction of seven articles.[26] In another case, a researcher who used a homemade computer model that erroneously reversed two columns of data had to request retraction of five articles.[27] Other researchers who had used the erroneous results from the original researcher then had to request retraction of several more articles. Additionally, other researchers who attempted to publish *correct* results in contradiction to the original researcher's *incorrect* results had difficulty getting their articles published.[28]

WHAT CAN BE DONE DIFFERENTLY?

There are several techniques to check the quality of data once they have been entered, two of which are discussed here. One way to reduce error during data input is for two people to input the same data into separate files. Once the data are entered twice, the researcher can compare the two files and identify and resolve any discrepancies.

Another powerful way to check data quickly is to use visualization techniques. For example, for geographic data, a simple visualization of all data points on a map will quickly identify any data that are geographically out of place. Then the researcher can flag those data and go back to check them for accuracy. Visualization can also be useful for identifying errors in data that can be plotted on a graph. If one data point shows up far away from the rest of the data points, it can be flagged for later verification.

The Documentation Phase

Although documentation is shown as one of many "steps" in the research life cycle in figure 2.1, in reality, it should be an ongoing process throughout the project. Data, people, instruments, processes, and more, should be described thoroughly using a standard metadata schema. Metadata is "structured information that describes the attributes of information resources[29] for the purposes of identification, discovery, selection, use, access, and management."[30] The data management plan must explain how this process will be completed and who is responsible for it.

WHAT CAN GO WRONG?

Many problems can occur when data are not documented and described properly. Reproducibility is an important cornerstone of scientific research, and without explicitly described methods and data, research projects are difficult to replicate. Without metadata, other researchers cannot know how the data were collected, processed, and analyzed, and therefore cannot replicate the study. This lack of reproducibility in scientific research has prompted the editors of the journal *Nature* to gather a list of articles about how to fix the problem[31] and strengthen their requirements for the methods sections for authors publishing in their journal.[32]

Data reuse also suffers when data and methods are not sufficiently described. Other researchers who were not involved in the data collection will lack important information necessary to reuse the data, such as the meaning of variable names, identification of instruments used to collect the data and their calibration, the spatial and temporal coverage of the data, and the accuracy of the dataset. Additionally, researchers wishing to reuse the data will not know the conditions under which the data were collected. These pieces of information are important when integrating data from several sources into one dataset for reuse.

Additionally, without documentation, it is even difficult for the researchers who conducted the research to reproduce their own efforts, should that become necessary, such as if data are lost. If analysis and processing steps were not adequately documented, re-creation of the lost dataset is much more difficult and time consuming.

Lastly, a researcher's recollection of the details of a research project are lost quickly after the end of the project. Michener, et al., demonstrate in figure 2.3 a phenomenon they call "Information Entropy." Soon after the article is published, researchers forget specific details about the conditions under which the data were collected and processed. As time goes on, they forget more general details about the data. Catastrophic losses of data can occur at any time when the media on which they are stored are lost. Later, as the researchers change positions or retire, their ability to remember details about the project drop substantially. Finally, if the researcher dies and there is no metadata for the project, the information dies along with the researcher.[33]

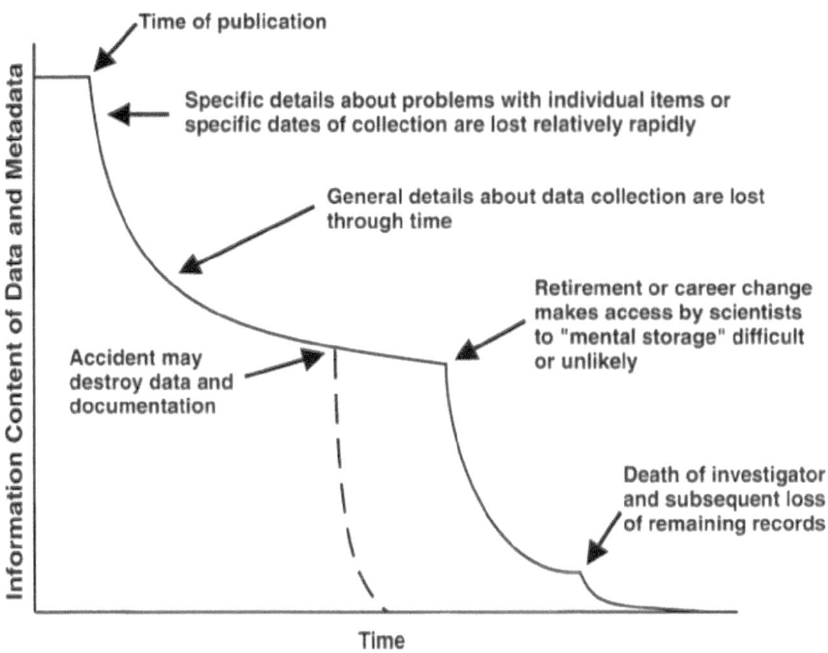

Figure 2.3. Information entropy. William K. Michener et al., "Nongeospatial Metadata for the Ecological Sciences," Ecological Applications 7, no. 1 (1997).

WHAT CAN BE DONE DIFFERENTLY?

Metadata standards are established to provide a standardized way for researchers within a field to describe their projects and datasets. Metadata standards also make datasets machine readable so they can be indexed and searched. Many disciplines have standardized metadata schemas. Examples of discipline-specific metadata schemas are Ecological Metadata Language for the ecological sciences,[34] Darwin Core for the biological sciences,[35] and ISO 19115 for the geographical sciences.[36] In cases where no standard format for metadata exists, researchers may describe their projects clearly and accurately using a simple Dublin Core metadata record. To provide more detailed information not contained in a metadata record, the researcher should include an accompanying "ReadMe" file.

Metadata records and other documentation, such as ReadMe files, contain different levels of granularity. Generally, the metadata should include information such as the overall purpose of the research, the people involved in the research, conditions on the use of the data, and structure of the data files, including how they are related to one another.[37] More detailed information may also be appropriate, including information on the research design, the data collection processes and methods, data processing processes and methods, and the spatial and temporal coverages of the dataset.[38]

Lastly, in the most granular, or detailed, view of the research project, information should be included about the variables within the dataset and how they relate to one another, the types of instruments used to collect each variable and the instruments' calibration, description of any codes used for missing values, explanation of any derived values, explanations of errors within the data files, and documentation of any outliers.[39]

The Preservation Phase

Preservation ensures that all the previous hard work is not lost and is thus perhaps even more important than data collection itself. Preservation includes both short-term backups of data files and long-term preservation of those files beyond the end of the project. During the planning stage, the researcher should devise a procedure for a regular backup schedule and location, as well as determine the most suitable format and location for long-term preservation.

WHAT CAN GO WRONG?

During the active research stage of a project, the researcher's primary concern is maintaining access to the data being collected. A study of 724 National Science Foundation grant awardees found that half of them had suffered a loss of data of some form or another ranging from human error to equipment error.[40] Therefore, redundancy of copies is crucial to maintaining access to important research data and supporting documents. Lack of a backup plan can result in the loss of data when hard drives fail or laptops are stolen; placing all of a project's data on one computer is risky. Lelung Rinpoche, the Tibetan monk mentioned in this chapter's introduction, exited the London Tube at his stop after snapping a photograph with London Mayor Boris Johnson. He accidentally left his laptop, and it was stolen. Rinpoche's computer contained "900 pages of rare Tibetan Buddhist scriptures he had travelled the world to find."[41] As they were his only copies of the material, his life's work was gone.

Many researchers are turning to cloud storage to maintain working copies of their current and past research data; however, cloud storage is not without faults. In 2014, Dedoose, a cloud storage system for academic research, suffered a major failure resulting in the loss of researchers' work over a three-week period prior to the crash.[42] These data were never recovered. Some researchers estimated the lost time to be about one hundred hours.[43] Unfortunately, this type of problem is not unique to this particular cloud storage service. Other cloud storage services also have had failures that caused users to lose valuable information. One Box.com user lost his files when the service gave access to his account to someone else and that new user deleted his files.[44] Likewise, Flickr erroneously deleted all (about four thousand) of one user's original digital photographs when the service mistook his account for one containing stolen photographs.[45]

While short-term storage of research data is of immediate importance to most researchers, long-term storage solutions are not always on their minds. Vines, et al. attempted to obtain datasets from 516 scholarly articles from 1991 to 2011. They found the older the publications were, the more likely that the data were not available. In fact, they found the data availability dropped 17 percent per year. They report one main reason the data were not available was because they were on inaccessible media.[46]

Digital files on electronic media are notorious for becoming inaccessible, both because of bit rot[47] and because the file formats and media themselves are highly susceptible to obsolescence.[48] Bit rot happens when physical storage media degrade, causing loss of access to the files stored on them. This degradation is a breakdown of the electrical, optical, or magnetic properties of the storage media, which causes them to lose their ability to hold the digital information. File format and media obsolescence is caused when software and hardware advancements cause older versions to no longer be accessible. Lotus 1-2-3, which was an extremely popular spreadsheet software throughout the 1980s and 1990s, is a perfect example of how file formats become obsolete. Researchers who have data in this file format from decades ago are no longer able to open them in modern spreadsheet packages. Moreover, those files may have been stored on floppy disks, which most modern computers lack the hardware to read.

WHAT CAN BE DONE DIFFERENTLY?

During the planning stage, the researcher should devise a plan for short-term and long-term preservation of the digital files from a research project. The first concern is to develop a regular backup schedule and a suitable location for the backups in order to maintain access to files throughout the research project and to ensure data are not lost. See table 2.1 for important questions to answer in developing a backup plan.[49] Ideally, three backup copies should be maintained to safeguard against the possibility

Table 2.1. Data Backup and Preservation Checklist

	Question	Possible Answers
1.	Where will you store your data?	PC or laptop Removable media External hard drives Network drives Remote storage (including Cloud)
2.	Where will you store backup copies?	PC or laptop Removable media External hard drives Network drives Remote storage (including Cloud)
3.	How will you create backup copies?	Automated system tools Manually
4.	What kind of backups will you run?	Full Incremental Differential
5.	How frequently will you run backups?	Daily Weekly Monthly
6.	Who will be responsible for running backups?	PI Data creators IT manager Post-doc or grad student Other ________________
7.	How will you organize backups?	Retain file naming conventions Label external media consistently
8.	What formats will files be stored in?	Non-proprietary Open documented Commonly used by research community As produced by instruments and software

of losing one copy. One copy can be local and internal, such as a hard drive on a laboratory or office computer, allowing easy access to the files most often used. A second copy can be local, but should be on an external device, such as an external hard drive. It is not recommended to save backup copies on devices such as CDs, DVDs, and USB drives, as they may suffer from bit rot over time. A third copy should be at an external, geographically separate location from the place the research is taking place. This location can be cloud storage or an off-site, physical server. If using cloud storage as an off-site backup copy, turn off automatic synchronization, as deletion or corruption of one copy will automatically duplicate that change in the other. Off-site backup is important to prevent loss due to fire or natural disasters.

Long-term preservation is the second important consideration. The main goal of preserving datasets for the long term is to facilitate reuse by other researchers. Researchers may be able to use data from another researcher to answer new research questions. When accompanied by adequate metadata and verified for accuracy, datasets have a higher potential to serve future research,[50] and as datasets are reused for additional research, their value increases.[51]

To facilitate long-term preservation and reuse, whenever possible, files should be saved in nonproprietary file formats. Proprietary file formats have the potential of becoming obsolete over time, as the software needed to read them may no longer be available, while nonproprietary, open-file formats are readable by many software packages. If the file format used to create the data must be preserved as is, the software required to open and use the data should be preserved along with the dataset. Additionally, a digital object identifier (DOI) should be assigned to the dataset for ease of discovery and citation.

The Analysis Phase

Once the data are collected and have been cleaned by eliminating errors of commission and correcting errors of omission, the dataset is ready for analysis. If the researcher has planned the project thoroughly, made efforts to reduce the possibility for error during data collection, and checked the data for accuracy during the quality assurance phase, the chance for error during the analysis phase is greatly reduced. However, there are still techniques the researcher can employ to reduce that chance even further.

WHAT CAN GO WRONG?

During the analysis phase, the researcher is processing and manipulating the dataset to find the information of interest to the research project. During this processing, the dataset may be transformed into a new form, such as converting a raw data file to a more usable spreadsheet format. This transformation is important for the analysis but can cause problems if not managed properly. A problem that can occur during dataset processing and analysis is that the dataset can be transformed to the wrong form, thereby requiring the researcher to revert to an earlier version. Geospatial data is especially susceptible to incorrect transformations when projecting a dataset of one coordinate projection to another. If earlier versions of data files were not backed up, reverting to an earlier version may be difficult or impossible.

WHAT CAN BE DONE DIFFERENTLY?

Borer, et al., recommend two best practices in maintaining proper versioning of datasets.[52] First, using a scripted software program, such as R, for processing will make a record of the steps necessary to recreate what has been done or make changes and reprocess the files. Second, the original, uncorrected file should always be saved, so that it will always be possible to go back to the beginning of the process and start over. Additionally, as files are processed and certain milestones are reached, those versions should be backed up in case it is necessary to revert to an earlier version. Milestones are points the researcher wants to preserve for easy retrieval. The first milestone that should be preserved is the original raw data generated by the research equipment. A subsequent important milestone may be set when the raw data is initially converted to a usable format, such as a spreadsheet. A final milestone may be set when the data is in its final format that supports a published journal article and that the researcher wants to share with other researchers.

Conclusion

The purpose of this chapter has been to highlight the importance of good data management practices from the viewpoint of what can go wrong if data are poorly managed. The examples in this chapter show a range of problems from minor to severe. Potential issues usually arise from neglectful or careless treatment of the datasets. While it is impossible to reduce the potential for error to zero, it is clear from these examples that managing data before, during, and after a research project will substantially reduce the chance for error. Estimates of the costs of irreproducible research range from $20 billion per year in one study of medical research[53] to $28 billion per year in one study of biological research.[54] Much of this research is irreproducible because of poor data management and lack of adequate metadata.

In addition to the financial costs, both researchers' and their institutions' reputations are on the line. Academic institutions both in the United States[55] and abroad[56] recognize how good data management practices ultimately help improve researchers' and institutions' reputations.

Pearls

- Plan as many details of your research as possible—from collection to processing to preservation—prior to beginning the project.
- Use data input tools such as data validation and input forms to reduce the chance for error during data collection.
- Stay current on documentation of processes and description of project details throughout the project; this work is more difficult to do at the end of a project.
- Always maintain three current backup copies of important work, such as the original unprocessed dataset and milestone versions of processed files.
- Give adequate attention to cleaning errors from the dataset prior to analysis, but maintain legitimate outliers.
- Understand the limitations of common statistical tests and provide as much supporting information as possible to support your claims.

Recommended Reading and Resources

Corti, Louise, Veerle Van den Eynden, Libby Bishop, and Matthew Woollard. *Managing and Sharing Research Data: A Guide to Good Practice*. London: Sage, 2014.

Pryor, Graham, ed. *Managing Research Data*. London: Facet Publishing, 2012.

Pryor, Graham, Sarah Jones, and Angus Whyte, eds. *Delivering Research Data Management Services: Fundamentals of Good Practice*. London: Facet Publishing, 2014.

Ray, Joyce, ed. *Research Data Management: Practical Strategies for Information Professionals*. West Lafayette, IN: Purdue University Press, 2014.

Notes

1. Ben Morgan and Rashid Razaq, "Tibetan Monk Loses His Life's Work in Tube Laptop Theft after Taking Selfie with Mayor Boris Johnson," *The London Evening Standard*, http://www.standard.co.uk/news/crime/tibetan-monk-loses-his-lifes-work-in-tube-laptop-theft-after-taking-selfie-with-mayor-boris-johnson-9285082.html.
2. Robin Wauters, "Flickr Accidentally Wipes Out Account: Five Years and 4,000 Photos Down the Drain," *Techcrunch*, http://techcrunch.com/2011/02/02/flickr-accidentally-wipes-out-account-five-years-and-4000-photos-down-the-drain/.
3. Stubby the Rocket, "How *Toy Story 2* Nearly Vanished," *Tor.com*, http://www.tor.com/2012/06/25/how-toy-story-2-nearly-vanished/.
4. Hans Rekers and Biran Affandi, "Letter to the Editor," *Contraception* 70, no. 5.
5. Joyce Ray, ed., *Research Data Management: Practical Strategies for Information Professionals* (West Lafayette, IN: Purdue University Press, 2014), 1.
6. Kara Woo, "Abandon All Hope, Ye Who Enter Dates in Excel," *Data Pub*, http://datapub.cdlib.org/2014/04/10/abandon-all-hope-ye-who-enter-dates-in-excel/; XLCalibre, "The Seven Deadly Sins of Data Entry (or How Not to Use Excel)," *DataScopic*, http://datascopic.net/xlcaliber-7deadlysins/.
7. Ferric C. Fang, R. Grant Steen, and Arturo Casadevall, "Misconduct Accounts for the Majority of Retracted Scientific Publications," *Proceedings of the National Academy of Sciences* 109, no. 42 (2012).
8. Arturo Casadevall, R Grant Steen, and Ferric C Fang, "Sources of Error in the Retracted Scientific Literature," *The FASEB Journal* 28, no. 9 (2014).
9. Leonard P. Freedman, Iain M. Cockburn, and Timothy S. Simcoe, "The Economics of Reproducibility in Preclinical Research," *PLoS Biol* 13, no. 6 (2015).
10. Louise Corti et al., *Managing and Sharing Research Data: A Guide to Good Practice* (London: Sage, 2014).
11. Christopher Eaker et al., "Data Sharing Practices of Agricultural Researchers: Implications for the Land-Grant University Mission" (paper presented at the Special Libraries Association Food and Agriculture Division Virtual Contributed Papers Session, May 13, 2015).
12. Katherine G. Akers and Jennifer Doty, "Disciplinary Differences in Faculty Research Data Management Practices and Perspectives," *International Journal of Digital Curation* 8, no. 2 (2013); John D'Ignazio and Jian Qin, "Faculty Data Management Practices: A Campus-Wide Census of Stem Departments" (2008) doi:citeulike-article-id:8241850; L. Doucette and B. Fyfe, "Drowning in Research Data: Addressing Data Management Literacy of Graduate Students," *ACRL 2013 Proceedings* (2013); Margaret Henty et al., *Investigating Data Management Practices in Australian Universities*" (Canberra: Australian Partnership for Sustainable Repositories, 2008); Merinda McLure et al., "Data Curation: A Study of Researcher Practices and Needs," *portal: Libraries and the Academy* 14, no. 2 (2014); Carol Tenopir et al., "Data Sharing by Scientists: Practices and Perceptions," *PLoS ONE* 6, no. 6 (2011).
13. C. Ward et al., "Making Sense: Talking Data Management with Researchers," *International Journal of Digital Curation* 6, no. 2 (2010).
14. Jessica Adamick, Rebecca Reznik-Zellen, and Matt Sheridan, "Data Management Training for Graduate Students at a Large Research University," *Journal of eScience Librarianship* 1, no. 1 (2012); Jake Carlson et al., "Developing an Approach for Data Management Education: A Report from the Data Information Literacy Project," *International Journal of Digital Curation* 8, no. 1 (2013); Christopher Eaker, "Educating Researchers for Effective Data Management," *Bulletin of the American Society for Information Science and Technology* 40, no. 3 (2014); "Planning Data Management Education Initiatives: Process, Feedback, and Future Directions," *Journal of eScience Librarianship*

3, no. 1 (2014); Lisa Johnston, Meghan Lafferty, and Beth Petsan, "Training Researchers on Data Management: A Scalable, Cross-Disciplinary Approach," *Journal of eScience Librarianship* 1, no. 2 (2012); Mary Piorun et al., "Teaching Research Data Management: An Undergraduate/Graduate Curriculum," *Journal of eScience Librarianship* 1, no. 1; Mark Scott et al., "Research Data Management Education for Future Curators," *International Journal of Digital Curation* 8, no. 1 (2013).

15. Elizabeth T. Borer et al., "Some Simple Guidelines for Effective Data Management," *Bulletin of the Ecological Society of America* 90, no. 2 (2009); Karina Kervin, William Michener; and Robert Cook, "Common Errors in Ecological Data Sharing," *Journal of eScience Librarianship* (2013).
16. C. Strasser et al., *Primer on Data Management: What You Always Wanted to Know, but Were Afraid to Ask* (Albuquerque, NM: DataONE, 2012).
17. Andrea Wiggins et al., *Data Management Guide for Public Participation in Scientific Research* (Albuquerque, NM: DataONE, 2013).
18. Lori Janke, Andrew Asher, and Spencer Keralis, "The Problem of Data," *Council on Library and Information Resources* CLIR Publication No. 154.
19. DataONE Data Life Cycle (online at https://www.dataone.org/best-practices).
20. Stacy Kowalczyk, "Before the Repository: Defining the Preservation Threats to Research Data in the Lab" (paper presented at the Joint Conference on Digital Libraries, Knoxville, TN, June 24, 2015 2015).
21. Jacob Carlson et al., "Determining Data Information Literacy Needs: A Study of Students and Research Faculty," *portal: Libraries and the Academy* 11, no. 2 (2011).
22. Doucette and Fyfe, "Drowning in Research."
23. Manfred Fischer, Henk Scholten, and David Unwin, *Spatial Analytical Perspectives on Gis* (London: Taylor & Francis, 1996).
24. Created by Christopher Eaker from a sample Microsoft Excel dataset.
25. DataONE, "Dataone Data Management Education Modules: Data Quality Control and Assurance," (2012), https://www.dataone.org/sites/all/documents/L05_DataQualityControlAssurance.pptx.
26. Rekers and Affandi, "Letter to the Editor."
27. Greg Miller, "A Scientist's Nightmare: Software Problem Leads to Five Retractions," *Science* 314, no. 1856 (2006).
28. Ibid.
29. Or in this case, a research project and its data.
30. Arlene G. Taylor and Daniel N. Joudrey, *The Organization of Information*, 3rd ed. (Westport, CT: Libraries Unlimited, 2009), 89.
31. "Challenges in Irreproducible Research," *Nature*, Special issue, http://www.nature.com/nature/focus/reproducibility/index.html.
32. "Availability of Data, Material and Methods," *Nature*, http://www.nature.com/authors/policies/availability.html.
33. William K. Michener et al., "Nongeospatial Metadata for the Ecological Sciences," *Ecological Applications* 7, no. 1 (1997).
34. The Knowledge Network for Biocomplexity, "Ecological Metadata Language," https://knb.ecoinformatics.org/#external//emlparser/docs/index.html.
35. Darwin Core Task Group, "Darwin Core," http://rs.tdwg.org/dwc/.
36. ISO/TC 211 Geographic Information/Geomatics Committee, "Iso 19115: Geographic Information—Metadata," International Standards Organization, http://www.iso.org/iso/home/store/catalogue_ics/catalogue_detail_ics.htm?csnumber=53798.
37. Corti et al., *Managing and Sharing Research Data*, 39.
38. Ibid.
39. Ibid., 41.

40. Stacy Kowalczyk, "Before the Repository: Defining the Preservation Threats to Research Data in the Lab" (paper presented at the Joint Conference on Digital Libraries, Knoxville, TN, June 24, 2015 2015).
41. Morgan and Razaq, "Tibetan Monk Loses His Life's Work."
42. Chris O'Brien, "Crash at Academic Cloud Service Dedoose May Wipe Out Weeks of Research," *Los Angeles Times*, May 12, 2014, http://www.latimes.com/business/technology/la-fi-tn-dedoose-crash-academic-cloud-20140512-story.html.
43. Steve Kolowich, "Hazards of the Cloud: Data-Storage Service's Crash Sets Back Researchers," *Chronicle of Higher Education*, May 12, 2014, http://chronicle.com/blogs/wiredcampus/hazards-of-the-cloud-data-storage-services-crash-sets-back-researchers/52571.
44. Dan Tynan, "How Box.Com Allowed a Complete Stranger to Delete All My Files," *IT World*, October 23, 2013, http://www.itworld.com/article/2833267/it-management/how-box-com-allowed-a-complete-stranger-to-delete-all-my-files.html.
45. Wauters, "Flickr Accidentally Wipes out Account: Five Years and 4,000 Photos Down the Drain."
46. Timothy H Vines et al., "The Availability of Research Data Declines Rapidly with Article Age," *Current Biology* 24, no. 1 (2014).
47. "Bit Rot," *Economist*, April 28, 2012, http://www.economist.com/node/21553445.
48. Adam Chandler, "A Warehouse Fire of Digital Memories," *Atlantic* (February 2015), http://www.theatlantic.com/technology/archive/2015/02/google-forgotten-century-digital-files-bit-rot/385500/; Jason Koebler, "Our Digital Memories Are Languishing on Obsolete Cd-Rs in Our Closets," *Motherboard*, January 2, 2015, http://motherboard.vice.com/read/our-digital-memories-are-languishing-on-obsolete-cd-rs-in-our-closets.
49. Modified from Lamar Soutter Library, University of Massachusetts Medical School, licensed under a Creative Commons Attribution-NonCommercial 3.0 Unported License (online at https://creativecommons.org/licenses/by-nc/3.0/deed.en_US).
50. Carole L Palmer, Nicholas M. Weber, and Melissa H. Cragin, "The Analytic Potential of Scientific Data: Understanding Re-Use Value," *Proceedings of the American Society for Information Science and Technology* 48, no. 1 (2011).
51. Paul F. Uhlir, "Information Gulags, Intellectual Straightjackets, and Memory Holes: Three Principles to Guide the Preservation of Scientific Data," *Data Science Journal* 9 (2010).
52. Borer et al., "Some Simple Guidelines for Effective Data Management."
53. Freedman, Cockburn, and Simcoe, "The Economics of Reproducibility in Preclinical Research."
54. Monya Baker, "Irreproducible Biology Research Costs Put at $28 Billion Per Year," *Nature*, June 9, 2015.
55. University of California Santa Barbara, "Data Curation and Management," http://www.library.ucsb.edu/scholarly-communication/data-curation-management.
56. LaTrobe University, "The Benefits of Data Management," http://www.latrobe.edu.au/research-infrastructure/eresearch/services/data-management/benefits; Royal Holloway University of London, "Research Data Management Policy," 2014; University of Leeds, "University of Leeds Research Data Management Policy," http://library.leeds.ac.uk/research-data-policies.

Bibliography

Adamick, Jessica, Rebecca Reznik-Zellen, and Matt Sheridan. "Data Management Training for Graduate Students at a Large Research University." *Journal of eScience Librarianship* 1, no. 1 (2012). doi:10.7191/jeslib.2012.1022.

Akers, Katherine G., and Jennifer Doty. "Disciplinary Differences in Faculty Research Data Management Practices and Perspectives." *International Journal of Digital Curation* 8, no. 2 (2013): 5–26. doi:10.2218/ijdc.v8i2.263.

Baker, Monya. "Irreproducible Biology Research Costs Put at $28 Billion Per Year." *Nature*, June 9, 2015. doi:10.1038/nature.2015.17711.

Borer, Elizabeth T., Eric W. Seabloom, Matthew B. Jones, and Mark Schildhauer. "Some Simple Guidelines for Effective Data Management." *Bulletin of the Ecological Society of America* 90, no. 2 (April 1, 2009): 205–14. doi:10.1890/0012-9623-90.2.205.

Carlson, Jacob, Michael Fosmire, C. C. Miller, and Megan Sapp Nelson. "Determining Data Information Literacy Needs: A Study of Students and Research Faculty." *portal: Libraries and the Academy* 11, no. 2 (2011): 629–57.

Carlson, Jake, Lisa Johnston, Brian Westra, and Mason Nichols. "Developing an Approach for Data Management Education: A Report from the Data Information Literacy Project." *International Journal of Digital Curation* 8, no. 1 (2013): 204–17. doi:10.2218/ijdc.v8i1.254.

Casadevall, Arturo, R. Grant Steen, and Ferric C Fang. "Sources of Error in the Retracted Scientific Literature." *FASEB Journal* 28, no. 9 (2014): 3847–55.

Chandler, Adam. "A Warehouse Fire of Digital Memories." *Atlantic*, February 13, 2015. http://www.theatlantic.com/technology/archive/2015/02/google-forgotten-century-digital-files-bit-rot/385500/.

Corti, Louise, Veerle Van den Eynden, Libby Bishop, and Matthew Woollard. *Managing and Sharing Research Data: A Guide to Good Practice*. London: Sage, 2014.

D'Ignazio, John, and Jian Qin. "Faculty Data Management Practices: A Campus-Wide Census of Stem Departments." *Proceedings of the American Society for Information Science and Technology*, annual meeting 2008. doi:citeulike-article-id:8241850.

DataONE. "Dataone Data Management Education Modules: Data Quality Control and Assurance." (2012). https://www.dataone.org/sites/all/documents/L05_DataQualityControlAssurance.pptx.

Doucette, L., and B. Fyfe. "Drowning in Research Data: Addressing Data Management Literacy of Graduate Students." *ACRL 2013 Proceedings* (2013).

Eaker, Christopher. "Educating Researchers for Effective Data Management." *Bulletin of the American Society for Information Science and Technology* 40, no. 3 (2014): 45–46. doi:10.1002/bult.2014.1720400314.

———. "Planning Data Management Education Initiatives: Process, Feedback, and Future Directions." *Journal of eScience Librarianship* 3, no. 1 (2014). doi:10.7191/jeslib.2014.1054.

Eaker, Christopher, Peter Fernandez, Shea Swauger, and Miriam Davis. "Data Sharing Practices of Agricultural Researchers: Implications for the Land-Grant University Mission." Paper presented at the Special Libraries Association Food and Agriculture Division Virtual Contributed Papers Session, May 13, 2015.

Economist. "Bit Rot." April 28, 2012. http://www.economist.com/node/21553445.

Fang, Ferric C., R. Grant Steen, and Arturo Casadevall. "Misconduct Accounts for the Majority of Retracted Scientific Publications." *Proceedings of the National Academy of Sciences* 109, no. 42 (2012): 17028-33. doi:10.1073/pnas.1212247109.

Fischer, Manfred, Henk Scholten, and David Unwin. *Spatial Analytical Perspectives on Gis*. London: Taylor & Francis, 1996.

Freedman, Leonard P., Iain M. Cockburn, and Timothy S. Simcoe. "The Economics of Reproducibility in Preclinical Research." *PLoS Biol* 13, no. 6 (2015): e1002165. doi:10.1371/journal.pbio.1002165.

Group, Darwin Core Task. "Darwin Core." http://rs.tdwg.org/dwc/.

Henty, Margaret, Belinda Weaver, Stephanie Bradbury, and Simon Porter. "*Investigating Data Management Practices in Australian Universities*." Canberra: Australian Partnership for Sustainable Repositories, 2008.

ISO/TC 211 Geographic Information/Geomatics Committee. "Iso 19115: Geographic Information—Metadata." International Standards Organization, http://www.iso.org/iso/home/store/catalogue_ics/catalogue_detail_ics.htm?csnumber=53798.

Janke, Lori, Andrew Asher, and Spencer Keralis. *The Problem of Data.* Council on Library and Information Resources CLIR Publication No. 154, August 2012. https://www.clir.org/pubs/reports/pub154/pub154.pdf.

Johnston, Lisa, Meghan Lafferty, and Beth Petsan. "Training Researchers on Data Management: A Scalable, Cross-Disciplinary Approach." *Journal of eScience Librarianship* 1, no. 2 (2012). doi:10.7191/jeslib.2012.1012.

Kervin, Karina, William Michener, and Robert Cook. "Common Errors in Ecological Data Sharing." *Journal of eScience Librarianship* (2013). doi:10.7191/jeslib.2013.1024.

Knowledge Network for Biocomplexity, The. "Ecological Metadata Language." https://knb.ecoinformatics.org/#external//emlparser/docs/index.html.

Koebler, Jason. "Our Digital Memories Are Languishing on Obsolete Cd-Rs in Our Closets." *Motherboard,* January 2, 2015. http://motherboard.vice.com/read/our-digital-memories-are-languishing-on-obsolete-cd-rs-in-our-closets.

Kolowich, Steve. "Hazards of the Cloud: Data-Storage Service's Crash Sets Back Researchers." *Chronicle of Higher Education,* May 12, 2014. http://chronicle.com/blogs/wiredcampus/hazards-of-the-cloud-data-storage-services-crash-sets-back-researchers/52571.

Kowalczyk, Stacy. "Before the Repository: Defining the Preservation Threats to Research Data in the Lab." Paper presented at the Joint Conference on Digital Libraries, Knoxville, TN, June 24, 2015 2015. doi:10.1145/2756406.2756909.

LaTrobe University. "The Benefits of Data Management." http://www.latrobe.edu.au/research-infrastructure/eresearch/services/data-management/benefits.

McLure, Merinda, Allison V. Level, Catherine L. Cranston, Beth Oehlerts, and Mike Culbertson. "Data Curation: A Study of Researcher Practices and Needs." *portal: Libraries and the Academy* 14, no. 2 (2014): 139–64. doi:10.1353/pla.2014.0009.

Michener, William K., James W. Brunt, John J. Helly, Thomas B. Kirchner, and Susan G. Stafford. "Nongeospatial Metadata for the Ecological Sciences." *Ecological Applications* 7, no. 1 (1997): 330–42. doi:10.2307/2269427.

Miller, Greg. "A Scientist's Nightmare: Software Problem Leads to Five Retractions." *Science* 314, no. 1856 (2006). doi:10.1126/science.314.5807.1856.

Morgan, Ben, and Rashid Razaq. "Tibetan Monk Loses His Life's Work in Tube Laptop Theft after Taking Selfie with Mayor Boris Johnson." *The London Evening Standard,* April 25, 2014. http://www.standard.co.uk/news/crime/tibetan-monk-loses-his-lifes-work-in-tube-laptop-theft-after-taking-selfie-with-mayor-boris-johnson-9285082.html.

Nature. "Availability of Data, Material and Methods." Special issue, http://www.nature.com/authors/policies/availability.html.

———. "Challenges in Irreproducible Research." Special issue, http://www.nature.com/nature/focus/reproducibility/index.html.

O'Brien, Chris. "Crash at Academic Cloud Service Dedoose May Wipe Out Weeks of Research." *Los Angeles Times,* May 12, 2014. http://www.latimes.com/business/technology/la-fi-tn-dedoose-crash-academic-cloud-20140512-story.html.

Palmer, Carole L, Nicholas M Weber, and Melissa H Cragin. "The Analytic Potential of Scientific Data: Understanding Re-Use Value." *Proceedings of the American Society for Information Science and Technology* 48, no. 1 (2011): 1–10. doi:10.1002/meet.2011.14504801174.

Piorun, Mary, Donna Kafel, Tracey Leger-Hornby, Siamak Najafi, Elaine Martin, Paul Colombo, and Nancy LaPelle. "Teaching Research Data Management: An Undergraduate/Graduate Curriculum." *Journal of eScience Librarianship* 1, no. 3 (2012). doi:10.7191/jeslib.2012.1003.

Ray, Joyce, ed. *Research Data Management: Practical Strategies for Information Professionals.* West Lafayette, IN: Purdue University Press, 2014.

Rekers, Hans, and Biran Affandi. "Letter to the Editor." *Contraception* 70, no. 5 (October 26, 2004): 433. doi:10.1016/j.contraception.2004.07.004.
Royal Holloway University of London. "Research Data Management Policy." 2014.
Scott, Mark, Richard Boardman, Philippa Reed, and Simon Cox. "Research Data Management Education for Future Curators." *International Journal of Digital Curation* 8, no. 1 (2013): 288–94. doi:10.2218/ijdc.v8i1.261.
Strasser, C., R. B. Cook, W. K. Michener, and A. Budden. *Primer on Data Management: What You Always Wanted to Know, but Were Afraid to Ask*. Albuquerque, NM: DataONE, 2012.
Stubby the Rocket. "How Toy Story 2 Nearly Vanished." *Tor.com*, June 25, 2012. http://www.tor.com/2012/06/25/how-toy-story-2-nearly-vanished/.
Taylor, Arlene G., and Daniel N. Joudrey. *The Organization of Information*. 3rd ed. Westport, CT: Libraries Unlimited, 2009.
Tenopir, Carol, Suzie Allard, Kimberly Douglass, Arsev Umur Aydinoglu, Lei Wu, Eleanor Read, Maribeth Manoff, and Mike Frame. "Data Sharing by Scientists: Practices and Perceptions." *PLoS ONE* 6, no. 6 (2011): e21101. doi:10.1371/journal.pone.0021101.
Tynan, Dan. "How Box.Com Allowed a Complete Stranger to Delete All My Files." *IT World*, October 23, 2013. http://www.itworld.com/article/2833267/it-management/how-box-com-allowed-a-complete-stranger-to-delete-all-my-files.html.
Uhlir, Paul F. "Information Gulags, Intellectual Straightjackets, and Memory Holes: Three Principles to Guide the Preservation of Scientific Data." *Data Science Journal* 9 (2010): ES1-ES5. doi:10.2481/dsj.Essay-001-Uhlir.
University of California Santa Barbara. "Data Curation and Management." http://www.library.ucsb.edu/scholarly-communication/data-curation-management.
University of Leeds. "University of Leeds Research Data Management Policy." http://library.leeds.ac.uk/research-data-policies.
Vines, Timothy H., Arianne Y. K. Albert, Rose L. Andrew, Florence Débarre, Dan G. Bock, Michelle T. Franklin, Kimberly J. Gilbert, et al. "The Availability of Research Data Declines Rapidly with Article Age." *Current Biology* 24, no. 1 (1/6/ 2014): 94–97. doi:10.1016/j.cub.2013.11.014.
Ward, C., L. Freiman, S. Jones, L. Molloy, and K. Snow. "Making Sense: Talking Data Management with Researchers." *International Journal of Digital Curation* 6, no. 2 (2010).
Wauters, Robin. "Flickr Accidentally Wipes Out Account: Five Years and 4,000 Photos Down the Drain." *Techcrunch*, February 2, 2011. http://techcrunch.com/2011/02/02/flickr-accidentally-wipes-out-account-five-years-and-4000-photos-down-the-drain/.
Wiggins, Andrea, Rick Bonney, Eric Graham, Sandra Henderson, Steve Kelling, Gretchen LeBuhn, Richard Littauer, et al. *Data Management Guide for Public Participation in Scientific Research*. Albuquerque, NM: DataONE, 2013.
Woo, Kara. "Abandon All Hope, Ye Who Enter Dates in Excel." *Data Pub*, April 10, 2014. http://datapub.cdlib.org/2014/04/10/abandon-all-hope-ye-who-enter-dates-in-excel/.
XLCalibre. "The Seven Deadly Sins of Data Entry (or How Not to Use Excel)." *DataScopic*, n.d., http://datascopic.net/xlcaliber-7deadlysins/.

Chapter 3

Research Data as Record

Bethany Myers, Louise M. Darling Biomedical Library, University of California, Los Angeles

Research libraries and librarians are well positioned to offer a variety of data management support services,[1] and demand for these services is expected to increase.[2] Library services in support of research data fall under the umbrella term of "digital curation." Digital curation encompasses all data management activities, including planning, preservation for future discovery and reuse, and active management of data.[3] Many different types of professionals have roles in digital curation, including librarians.[4] Librarians are being "upskilled" and "reskilled" in order to apply their knowledge of bibliographic techniques, information literacy instruction, reference assistance, and other library services to research data.[5]

As librarians examine the knowledge and skills that will be needed for their expanding future role as curators of scientific data, they would do well to look to the hard-won insight provided by other information management traditions. Archivists in particular have much to offer, since "it has been archivists, not librarians, who historically have served as 'keepers of the record,' seeking to balance the stewardship and protection of collections with the pragmatics of managing an ever-growing corpus of paper and electronic information."[6] Over the past three centuries, the archival profession has developed and refined theories and techniques for the management of administrative and personal records. These archival methods for appraisal and selection, authentication, arrangement and description, and preservation are also applicable to the practical management of scientific research data.[7] In fact, as Nielsen and Hjørland point out in their analysis of institutional roles in data curation, "archives already occupy a functional niche that research libraries are now trying to access."[8] This chapter will define some fundamental principles of the archives field and offer suggestions on applying archival methods to research data management.

Archives

Archives are the noncurrent records of human activity that have been set aside for permanent preservation. The word "archives" (or archive) can also refer to a building, organization, program, or department that is responsible for housing these records. Archives are documents that record transactions made by the creating body, whether organizational (such as those produced by a business, government, or other group) or personal (such as those produced by families and individuals).[9] Archives are differentiated from active, or current, records by their deliberately continued existence, as opposed to their destruction. They are also distinguished by their availability. While active records are normally accessed only by the creating body, and only to support its primary functional purpose, archives may be used by historical researchers, genealogists, journalists, writers, lawyers, and any others who seek information about the former activities of the creating body.

There are two major types of archives in the American archival tradition: manuscript archives and public archives. Manuscript archives often consist of premodern or pre-twentieth-century documents; or more recent, non-administrative materials that reflect the life, work, and interests of the creator or collector. The uniqueness of these collections may demand close, item-level attention on the part of the archivist. In contrast, public archives typically consist of voluminous official records, which must be managed on a much larger scale.[10]

The rise of electronic recordkeeping has disrupted the traditional, static, hierarchical conception of print archives. The mass and ubiquity of digital information has provoked new discussion among archival theorists on the definition of a record.[11]

What Is a Record?

Despite (or perhaps because of) the record's centrality to the concept of archives, precisely defining a record has been an intellectual challenge within archival science.[12] Communicating the archival concept of a record to other information professions has also presented a problem for archivists.[13] Nevertheless, some generally accepted properties of records can be discussed.

Records consist of content, form or structure, and context.[14] They have two types of values: primary and secondary. The primary value of records is to facilitate their capacity to facilitate their creator's functional objectives. This purpose is achieved during the record's active life. The secondary value, unique to archival records, is the "enduring value"[15] the records provide to researchers. Records with secondary value are identified through their evidential nature; that is, their existence serves as documentation of a particular activity (i.e., documentation of their primary value). In defining the notion of evidential value, the archivist and archival theorist T. R. Schellenberg emphasized the importance of the organic nature of records:

> Records that are the product of organic activity have a value that derives from the way they were produced. Since they were created in consequence of the actions to which they relate, they often contain an unconscious and therefore impartial record of the action. Thus the evidence they contain of the actions they record has a peculiar value. It is the *quality* of this evidence that is our concern here. Records, however, also have a value for the evidence they contain of the actions that resulted in their production. It is the *content* of the evidence that is our concern here.[16]

The first aspect of evidential value derives from the records' having been produced as a by-product of an activity, and thus bearing witness to the occurrence of that activity. The second aspect derives from the records' content regarding the function, structure, workflow, and other administrative properties of the creating body.

In addition, records may contain informational value. Informational value comes from the content of the record apart from its creating body's activities or function, that is, the information it contains regarding "persons, things, or phenomena."[17] Discovering informational value is often the objective of researchers. In some cases, such as statistical data or artificially assembled groups of documents brought together by a collector, records may be of mostly informational value, with little evidence of the action of collecting. Informational value and evidential value are not mutually exclusive, and many records support a wide variety of research interests.[18]

Do research data meet this definition for records? This too is an ongoing discussion with much confusion around archival professional jargon.[19] Some archivists consider research data to be records of informational value.[20] Others disagree, noting that data represent pure information, and lack evidential value.[21] A difference in terminology between archivists and scientists has been observed—while archivists use the term "electronic record" to describe an object slated for digital preservation, scientists refer to their content as "data."[22] Other authors have confirmed that some scientists consider their data synonymous with the archival record,[23] while others consider the research publication as the true record, with their data consisting of the daily documentation of the research process.[24] To further complicate the issue, there is also contention on the definition of the word *data*![25]

Vague terminology continues to hinder discussions on data management,[26] hampering communication between disciplines, and impeding progress in the field. As Lauriault et al. point out,

> One of the most serious problems in this respect is that for most scientists the term "record" means data, databases, and related information. . . . For many archivists, these are not considered records. . . . This is not simply a matter of semantics. It is a fundamental difference in perspective between creators and preservers, compounded by the emergence in all disciplines of ephemeral interactive information, which exists only in cyberspace. If this problem is not resolved, the increasing volume of interactive, social, and personalized information in the Web 2.0 environment, which does not meet the archival definition of record, may never find its way into archives. This is already happening, and as the interactive, experimental, and dynamic information environment becomes the dominant source of information on many aspects of life in the twenty-first century, we are in danger of losing our cultural heritage. . . .
>
> . . . The nature of the "record" is changing dramatically and traditional archival science will have to adapt to these changes in both theoretical and practical terms if they are to preserve this new information environment in the archives of the twenty-first century.[27]

This chapter assumes a definition of data likely to be pertinent to health information professionals: data are "information used in scientific, engineering, and medical research as inputs to generate research conclusions."[28]

Archivists

Archivists are the practitioners responsible for establishing physical and intellectual control over records of enduring value. Though archival education often overlaps with the related fields of records management and library science, and archivists often integrate aspects of records management and librarianship into their daily work, the archivist's core professional role is distinct from either. Unlike traditional records managers, who primarily control active records that are still being used for their original administrative purpose, archivists manage only those records that have been selected for permanent retention. Unlike traditional librarians, who primarily control published, discrete bibliographic volumes and electronic products, archivists manage largely unpublished materials, and take a very different approach to the organization of their collections.[29]

Archivists have a wide range of responsibilities, but typically are responsible for the appraisal and selection, acquisition, arrangement and description, and preservation of archival materials. Appraisal is a judgment of the value of records, while selection involves determining which records should be preserved. The archivist must have a knowledge of the creating body's functional context to make these decisions. Acquisition refers to the physical or electronic transfer of custody from the records' current location to the archive, a process often referred to as accessioning. Arrangement, description, and preservation are techniques for the archivist to gain physical and intellectual control over the records: these three tasks are known as processing. The end product of processing is usually a finding aid, a document for researchers that describes the hierarchical organization of the records. The top level of hierarchy is usually known as the record group (or sometimes the fonds), which may represent the entire creating organization. The record group is divided into subgroups (e.g., one subgroup for each department), which are then divided into series (e.g., one for each departmental activity: reports, correspondence, etc.), subseries, and finally files.[30] The archivist also physically re-houses printed materials into preservation-quality folders and boxes. On the finding aid, the type and location of each file is noted (e.g., "Box 4, folder 12"). A finding aid usually also includes a narrative description of the creating body's significance, and may include a summary of the records' informational and evidential value. The final finding aid is made available for researchers to help them identify which boxes and files they are interested in requesting. Archivists may also be responsible for public service, such as answering reference inquiries and promoting access to their collections.

Archival Science

The Society of American Archivists defines archival science from the perspective of the working archivist, as the "systematic body of theory that supports the practice of appraising, acquiring, authenticating, preserving, and providing access to recorded materials."[31] Duranti and MacNeil focus instead on archival science as a theoretical field of study apart from any practical implementation: "a body of concepts and methods directed toward the study of records in terms of their documentary and functional relationships and the ways in which they are controlled and communicated."[32] Gilliland-Swetland unifies these perspectives: "Archival theory, methodology, and practice together constitute archival science . . . the disciplinary and professional aspects of archival science together compose the archival paradigm—a set of assumptions, principles, and practices that are common to the archival community and are a model for its activities and outlook."[33] Archival science forms the foundation of archival work.

Archival Theory Background

The "twin pillars of classical archival theory," provenance and original order, were widely disseminated throughout the international archives community in the nineteenth and early twentieth centuries.[34] The principle of provenance, or "respect des fonds," requires that records remain grouped according to their originating body. Archival materials from the same source must be retained together, with their relationship to the creating body preserved intact. Provenance provides administrative, legal, and historical context to the creation of all materials,[35] and archival records depend on this context for their evidential value.[36] Without the principles of provenance to guide archival arrangement, the materials' original source could be obfuscated, destroying the "chain of custody" that is crucial to understanding the meaning of the records. Closely related to provenance is the concept of original order, meaning that, as far as possible, records should be maintained in the order imposed upon them by their creator. This articulation of archival principles represented a significant break from archivists' previous practice of dividing and classifying archival material based on subject (a tactic borrowed from the library bibliographic tradition).[37]

The twentieth century created an enormous amount of bureaucratic administrative records. New archival techniques had to be developed for the management of so many records. Since most records could no longer be saved, they needed to be appraised to inform the selection decision. One approach, advocated by T. R. Schellenberg, was to encourage archivists to participate earlier in the records life cycle. This active participation allowed them to identify which records had enduring value, and provided time for preservation planning before they entered the custody of the archives.[38]

However, despite archival efforts, the tremendous volume of records led to an inevitable backlog of unprocessed, inaccessible archival material. Archivists continued to wrestle with the problem of too many records and not enough management capacity. In their influential 2005 paper "More Product, Less Process," Greene and Meissner noted that archivists' focus on detailed physical processing and lower-level description had been ineffective in reducing the ever-growing backlog of unprocessed collections. Instead, they suggested that archivists focus on series or higher-level description, and (when appropriate) reduce expensive item-level conservation: the transfer of documents from regular folders to acid-free folders, the removal of staples and paperclips, and the photocopying of news clippings, among other common tasks. The MPLP philosophy is that archives are better off providing high-level descriptive access to minimally conserved holdings than they are spending their dwindling financial and human resources on overly detailed description and item-level conservation.[39] Like archivists in an overwhelming deluge of records, digital curators face a data deluge on an unprecedented scale. The lessons of "more product, less process" are to automate accession with a minimum of human processing—facilitated by archival input into systems design—and to make accessibility a top priority.

Archival Theory into Data Management Practice

William J. Maher, former president of the Society of American Archivists, contrasted the essential values of librarianship and archival work: "Librarianship is an information profession wherein data are valued as independent entities, separate from the context that created them. By contrast, archivists must focus on unique documents created often as the accident rather than object of an action. We are not information professionals like librarians—we are evidence professionals."[40] The archival focus on evidential documents brings a provenance-centered perspective to the current discussion around data curation.

As a type of recorded evidential document, research data "should be included in the sphere of interest of research libraries. . . . The discussion of data selection and management is thus in principle just part of the general discussion of document collection, indexing and preservation in libraries and other kinds of 'memory institutions.'"[41] Document management has long been modeled as a records life cycle. In the first phase of the life cycle, the records are used by their creating body to facilitate its organizational function—their primary use. Often, records managers are in charge of the active records during this phase. Over time, the records are needed less often for their primary purposes, and are either destroyed or taken into the custody of the archives, where they are arranged, described, preserved, and made available for secondary use by researchers.[42] Research data management has also been modeled as a life cycle, a series of stages that cover data creation, appraisal and selection, ingestion, preservation, storage, access, use, and reuse, providing a foundation for continuing research.[43]

Later archival theorists developed new records models that blur the distinction between active and inactive records, placing archivists within a "bigger picture" of responsibilities. These approaches increased the archivists' involvement in record creation and active management,[44] including designing systems that support archival standards of recordkeeping.[45] This creates a much more active, rather than passive, role for archivists.[46] In accordance with this charge to participate more actively earlier in the life cycle, archivists have begun to work directly with scientists to make sure that their data are preserved with its full context, or provenance.[47]

Provenance has emerged as a critical aspect of data preservation. The computer science field has developed applications to ensure provenance information can be captured and transmitted along with the data. Their concern is the preservation, in metadata, of the data lineage—its origin and intermediate transformations—for the purpose of verifying the data's trustworthiness. In contrast, the archival perspective on provenance is concerned not only with trustworthiness, but also with the social and environmental origins of the records that provide interpretive context.[48] Scientific research is a highly collaborative, distributed environment, with data collection and creation occurring in different places and teams.[49] These environmental factors are included in a more archival-centric explanation of provenance: "Data provenance is meaningfully communicated to users not solely through metadata but through the *arrangement* of a set of records, in this case datasets and associated manuscripts. The importance of connecting the multiple records generated in the course of an activity is well known to archivists."[50]

The following sections discuss archival responsibilities and data curation in five areas: appraisal and selection, authentication of material, arrangement and description, preservation, and access.

Appraisal and Selection

Appraisal is the process of determining the evidential and informational values of the records. Selection is a disposition decision—whether to destroy or preserve inactive records.[51] Appraisal and selection are foundational tasks for digital curation as well as print archives. Like the paper records of the twentieth century, data are everywhere, and appraisal and selection becomes ever more difficult as more data are generated. There is a tradeoff between the costs of creating new data from new research, and the costs of preserving previous data from previous research.[52] Since not all data can be curated, decisions must be made about which data to preserve. The criteria for appraisal and selection should depend on the specific research community.[53]

Appraisal, like all other archival tasks, relies on an understanding of the whole fonds, its context and documentation. For digital records, appraisal also relies on descriptive information, since the archivists need to "identify records in the often undifferentiated mass of digital information."[54] Once the archivist has appraised the record group, a selection decision must be made. The Dutch SURFshare project summarized three "groups of reasons" for preserving research data: reuse of the data (secondary use); verification of the data (to repeat published research findings); and heritage (either scientific heritage or general cultural heritage). Reuse and verification potential can be estimated by assessing the informational value of the data, the uniqueness of the data, and the legal or contractual value of the data. They also acknowledged several "necessary preconditions" for selection decisions: preservation format, metadata management, legal and ethical limitations, infrastructure and expertise, and financial resources. These preconditions do not automatically prescribe a certain decision, but they should be assessed along with the data's potential value.[55]

Authentication

Authentication refers to records being what they claim to be—not counterfeit, corrupted, or otherwise altered from the genuine state. Scientists may prefer different terminology to describe this concept, such as data lineage, data provenance, or data integrity.[56] Digital records and digital data are more susceptible to corruption than paper records. The goal of digital preservation is to preserve the content of the record (rather than the form), necessitating periodic migrations to new technology. Information is vulnerable to changes at each of these migration points.[57] These changes may compromise the authenticity of a record. Changes may also be inflicted deliberately, by researchers fabricating or manipulating their findings.[58]

From the user perspective, Fear and Donaldson have researched the attitude of proteomics researchers in their approach to provenance information. The scientists using the database performed their own assessments of accuracy by looking at the instrument used to generate the sample, the sample itself, and processing methods. These scientists had personal familiarity with the techniques used to generate the data, and so were able to, for instance, gauge the accuracy based on the brand of instrument used. Other considerations for the researchers were the provision of contact information for the scientists who uploaded the data, and whether the data had supported a previously published manuscript. Some users also needed to directly interact (i.e., download and process on their own) with the data in order to convince themselves of the data's credibility.[59]

It must be mentioned that archival theory does not provide a reference for appraising the accuracy or quality of scientific data. In archival theory, accuracy is secondary to authenticity: a record that makes the same error consistently will be accepted as authentic, despite its inaccuracy. However, for scientists, data accuracy or quality is of prime importance, and each scientific discipline has different standards for determining quality.[60] This poses a challenge to archivists, who despite a model for assessing authenticity may have difficulty assessing quality without deep disciplinary knowledge. Data quality must be verified by the data creators, the scientists, and preserved in metadata.[61]

Arrangement and Description

As discussed, archivists abandoned the idea of arrangement by subject, and focused on provenance-based arrangement. Record groups consist of a single creating body's records, with no intermixed content from other creators (with the exception of archival materials received as artificially created collections). The archivist maintains the original order of the records, and arranges them into hierarchical strata. This arrangement is an important part of provenance, since it reflects the creating body's activities and demonstrates the evidential value of the records.

To capture the original order arrangement of research records, data archivists are experimenting with "sheer" data curation, an approach that seamlessly works technical solutions for workflow and metadata capture into the daily research process, with little to no effort on the part of the researchers. This invisible capture of data along with detailed provenance information allows for semantic reconstruction of the meaning of the files based on their context—the date, time, action, surrounding files, and more. This sheer curation requires a high level of knowledge of researchers' work.[62]

Like unprocessed collections, raw data are difficult for users to access. The archival collection must be described to make the collection findable and usable. As with appraisal and selection, archivists must have a familiarity with the whole fonds before a collection can be processed. Likewise, digital curators need a holistic understanding of the work and workflow of scientists to be able to manage the data.[63] Descriptive information for electronic materials is stored as *metadata*, or data about data, which documents its "content, structure, processing, access conditions, and source."[64] A finding aid, which may be paper or electronic, is one example of metadata.[65] Many metadata standards exist, depending on what type of material needs to be described. Descriptive metadata provides critical provenance information for the discoverability and reuse of data.[66]

Description is often thought of as synonymous with this descriptive metadata, but as we have seen, archival provenance is concerned with much more than simply descriptive metadata. For scientists, the fonds of research may include more than the datasets, particularly the published papers arising from the research,[67] which some scientists consider to be the true record of the research.[68] It is important to maintain (via the arrangement of the data and its associated records), and describe (via detailed metadata) these relationships.

Preservation

Preservation is "communication with the future,"[69] and as such, it has always been a core responsibility of archivists. The preservation of print materials is largely environmental in nature. Considerations of light, temperature, humidity, acidity, pests, and other potentially destructive factors influence print preservation decisions. In contrast, the preservation of digital data faces serious challenges related to "technological dependency." Since digital data cannot be accessed as readily as paper, the archivist and the digital preservation system must ensure operability of the data over many changes to the original technology.[70] This requirement for ongoing data transformation means that provenance is an important part of preservation. Changes to the data, including migrations to new technologies, must be documented not only for authenticity purposes but also for future accessibility. The researchers themselves must participate in this documentation during the course of their daily work.[71]

The DigitalPreservationEurope project provided an overview of core issues that bring digital preservation alongside analogue preservation. The nine themes of this project were: restoration (how do we assess digital loss, and what processes can be used to restore the object?); conservation (how do we prevent digital loss?); collection and repository management (how should digital collections be built and maintained?); preservation as risk management (how do we assess the risk to the digital objects?); preserving the interoperability and functionality of digital objects (how do we validate different digital objects' properties?); collection cohesion and interoperability (how do we integrate disparate collections into seamless and usable systems?); automation in preservation (how do we automate as much of the preservation process as possible?); preserving the context (how do we preserve or retrieve provenance information?); and storage technology and methods (where do we keep the digital objects?).[72]

Much has been written about these and other issues surrounding the long-term digital preservation of data, but they all rely on the quality and trustworthiness of digital repositories. In his review of digital data curation literature, Poole described current repository trustworthiness criteria and noted that "just as archives have built up currency as trustworthy, so should repositories curating data."[73] One common standard for repositories is the Reference Model for an Open Archival Information System, generally referred to as the OAIS Reference Model. The OAIS Reference Model is widely applied in digital archives research and development.[74] It specifies the core concepts of digital preservation and provides two types of models that define the entities involved and the data flow process. The functional model essentially describes what an Open Archival Information System must *do*, while the information model describes what an OAIS must *have* in its collections.[75] The information model requires the OAIS to store the digital object as well as the supporting information "that should be associated with the digital object in order to preserve and provide meaningful access to it over time."[76] This provenance information, familiar to archival preservation practices, is essential for long-term access to the data.[77] Lee and Tibbo summarized this digital sea change in archives:

> A common theme of both the OAIS Reference Model and the archival literature on electronic records is the importance of attending not only to individual information objects, but also to the wider, socio-technical systems in which the objects are embedded. Within an archival context, this has meant a shift from focusing primarily on aggregations of records to placing much more emphasis on characteristics of, and requirements for, entire recordkeeping systems; this is an important move, because care for digital records usually requires successful interactions with a much wider and more diverse set of system components—people, hardware, and software—than care for analogue records.[78]

Building on the foundation of OAIS, the Trusted Digital Repository Checklist provides a specific list of requirements that trusted repositories must meet for certification.[79]

Access

Application of best practices in appraisal and selection, authentication, arrangement and description, and preservation ultimately facilitates accessibility. Archival institutions recognize that they exist to be used, as do scientific data repositories.[80] Secondary use of research data is of increasing importance to many fields of research.[81] Data sharing offers multiple benefits. Society at large benefits from data sharing, since open access to data promotes further research. As the National Board of Science stated, "[digital data] democratizes research by providing the opportunity for all who have access to these data collections to make a contribution."[82] Archives are also often seen as contributors to the public good, particularly in democratic societies, where they offer governmental accountability.[83] Other beneficiaries of data sharing are the data themselves, since reuse increases both the data's validity and likelihood of preservation,[84] as well as their value.[85]

Archival processing and storage incur labor and facility costs. Collection use justifies these costs, but dormant, inaccessible, unprocessed collections incur costs without the benefits to society, the research field, and the archival institutions. Likewise, data curation also incurs costs, but the costs of unshared data may be even higher: repetitive research, delayed innovation, and other limitations on progress.[86] While there are many incentives for open data sharing, there are also many reasons why data may need to be restricted. Archivists have experience redacting or restricting files for a variety of reasons, including intellectual property, national security, and personal privacy.[87] Data may need to be de-identified before sharing, or only made available to IRB-approved, authorized researchers.

Once again, provenance emerges as an important enabler of access.[88] Provenance's significance for retrieval purposes reiterates and extends its descriptive value—"provenance information should be thought of as a means for providing access points to records" that specify the *relationships* between creating activities and organizations.[89] As we have seen, these relationships can be preserved through detailed documentation and automated systems, such as sheer curation applications.[90]

Conclusion

The concept of an archive only makes sense in the plural. One archival document does not an archive make—the significance of any one record comes from the fonds as a whole. The context of all the surrounding records is imperative to understanding archives.[91] Research data also only exist in plural form. One datum does not a dataset make, and data's interpretation and application also come from the context of their creation. Like data curation, archival work is inherently aggregate—"[archivists] have developed descriptive tools designed to work with aggregates. We believe that aggregation is both an essential reflection of the organic nature of recordkeeping, and a recognition that context matters in fully understanding individual items."[92] The archival theories of provenance and original order, along with other archival science concepts, are directly applicable to the fonds of research inquiry.

In discussing the development of the DigCCurr (Digital Curation Curriculum) at the University of North Carolina, Chapel Hill, Lee and Tibbo acknowledged the multidisciplinary role of the digital curator: "Both the ability to understand information technology colleagues, and to explain the importance of archival concepts to those individuals stand as some of the most important—and often challenging—aspects of the digital curation professional's job. Educational grounding and practical experience in applying traditional archival concepts are fundamental elements of this equation."[93] They go on to assert that "archivists have long-standing experience with managing materials as aggregates, conveying contextual information, documenting provenance, engaging with creators, and attending to projected secondary use needs. These are all considerations that have become widely recognized in the interdisciplinary space of digital curation."[94]

In 1958, T. R. Schellenberg presciently told the Society of American Archivists, in essence, that the medium is the message; that the archival field will be shaped by the characteristics of the materials in its custody.[95] These theories and practices, shaped by the materials of the past, now support the future—and continue to be shaped by new information forms. The essential principles of the archival perspective—an understanding of the sanctity of evidence; *respect des fonds* (provenance and original order); the records life cycle model; and the organic nature of records—continue to influence and support digital curation.[96]

Pearls

- It is critical for curators to become involved in the data life cycle as early as possible. Contribution to the planning stage will directly affect the long-term preservation of the material: "The effect of decisions made at each stage of the lifecycle is cumulative."[97]
- Provenance information is key to the understanding and future reuse of data. Provenance includes not only basic descriptive metadata, but also information that preserves original order and original relationships between documents and entities.

- Data curators need an understanding of the research domain in order to apply effective appraisal and selection criteria. It is important to consider researcher input for the development of these criteria.
- Researchers have their own values and norms regarding data collection, documentation, sharing, and reuse. Data curators will need to collaborate with researchers to promote new practices.[98] When researchers look for data for reuse, they may dismiss uninformative metadata and apply their own personal authenticity evaluation.
- Repositories must establish and maintain their trustworthiness. Digital curators must adhere to a repository's standards, and users seeking to deposit data should look for trusted repositories that exhibit recognized core principles.
- To users, digital services may be more ambiguous than traditional archival services. It is very important for every service provider to be aware of other institutional resources, since many units may provide different services that span different phases of the data life cycle.[99]

Recommended Readings and Resources

Akmon, Dharma, Ann Zimmerman, Morgan Daniels, and Margaret Hedstrom. "The Application of Archival Concepts to a Data-Intensive Environment: Working with Scientists to Understand Data Management and Preservation Needs." Archival Science 11, nos. 3–4 (October 11, 2011): 329–48. doi:10.1007/s10502-011-9151-4.

BioSharing Standards Registry. https://www.biosharing.org/standards/

CRL, Digital Preservation Metrics. http://www.crl.edu/archiving-preservation/digital-archives/metrics

Decision Tree for Selection of Digital Materials for Long-Term Retention. http://www.dpconline.org/advice/preservationhandbook/decision-tree

Digital Curation Centre (UK)—Introduction to Digital Curation: http://www.dcc.ac.uk/resources/briefing-papers/introduction-curation

Gilliland-Swetland, Anne J. *Enduring Paradigm, New Opportunities: The Value of the Archival Perspective in the Digital Environment*. Washington, DC: Council on Library and Information Resources, 2000.

Lauriault, Tracey P., Barbara L. Craig, D. R. Fraser Taylor, and Peter L. Pulsifer. "Today's Data Are Part of Tomorrow's Research: Archival Issues in the Sciences." *Archivaria* 64 (Fall 2007): 123–79.

Lee, Christopher A., and Helen Tibbo. "Where's the Archivist in Digital Curation? Exploring the Possibilities through a Matrix of Knowledge and Skills." *Archivaria* 72 (Fall 2011). http://www.synergiescanada.org/journals/bcn/archivaria/454/13362.

Library of Congress—National Digital Information Infastructure and Preservation Program. http://www.digitalpreservation.gov/

Morris, Sammie. "Applying Archival Science to Digital Curation: Advocacy for the Archivist's Role in Implementing and Managing Trusted Digital Repositories." *Libraries Faculty and Staff Presentations*, Paper 93, January 1, 2015. http://docs.lib.purdue.edu/lib_fspres/93.

Purdue Data Curation Profiles Toolkit. http://datacurationprofiles.org/

Tjalsma, H. D. *Selection of Research Data. Guidelines for Appraising and Selecting Research Data. A Report by DANS and 3TU.Datacentrum*. The Hague, Netherlands: DANS, 2011. http://www.dans.knaw.nl/nl/over/organisatie-beleid/publicaties/DANSselectionofresearchdata.pdf.

W3C Provenance Incubator Group report. http://www.w3.org/2005/Incubator/prov/XGR-prov-20101214/

Notes

1. Andrew Cox, Eddy Verbaan, and Barbara Sen, "Upskilling Liaison Librarians for Research Data Management," *Ariadne* 70 (November 2012), http://www.ariadne.ac.uk/issue70/cox-et-al.

2. Carol Tenopir, Ben Birch, and Suzie Allard, "Academic Libraries and Research Data Services: Current Practices and Plans for the Future. An ACRL White Paper." (The Center for Information and Communication Studies, 2012), 29, http://www.ala.org/acrl/sites/ala.org.acrl/files/content/publications/whitepapers/Tenopir_Birch_Allard.pdf.
3. Daisy Abbot, "What Is Digital Curation?," *DCC Briefing Papers: Introduction to Curation*, 2008, http://www.dcc.ac.uk/resources/briefing-papers/introduction-curation; Daniel Noonan and Tamar Chute, "Data Curation and the University Archives," *American Archivist* 77, no. 1 (April 1, 2014): 201–40, doi:10.17723/aarc.77.1.m49r46526847g587.
4. Abbot, "What Is Digital Curation?"; Alex H. Poole, "How Has Your Science Data Grown? Digital Curation and the Human Factor: A Critical Literature Review," *Archival Science* 15, no. 2 (November 23, 2014): 101–39, doi:10.1007/s10502-014-9236-y; Christopher A. Lee and Helen Tibbo, "Where's the Archivist in Digital Curation? Exploring the Possibilities through a Matrix of Knowledge and Skills," *Archivaria* 72 (Fall 2011), http://www.synergiescanada.org/journals/bcn/archivaria/454/13362.
5. Mary Auckland, "Re-Skilling for Research" (Research Libraries UK, 2012), http://www.rluk.ac.uk/wp-content/uploads/2014/02/RLUK-Re-skilling.pdf; Cox, Verbaan, and Sen, "Upskilling Liaison Librarians for Research Data Management"; Andrew M. Cox and Stephen Pinfield, "Research Data Management and Libraries: Current Activities and Future Priorities," *Journal of Librarianship and Information Science* 46 (2014): 299; Michael J. Giarlo, "Academic Libraries as Data Quality Hubs," *Journal of Librarianship and Scholarly Communication* 1, no. 3 (2013); P. Bryan Heidorn, "The Emerging Role of Libraries in Data Curation and E-Science," *Journal of Library Administration* 51, no. 7–8 (October 1, 2011): 662–72, doi:10.1080/01930826.2011.601269.
6. Marisa L. Ramírez, "Whose Role Is It Anyway? A Library Practitioner's Appraisal of the Digital Data Deluge," *Bulletin of the American Society for Information Science and Technology* 37, no. 5 (2011), http://digitalcommons.calpoly.edu/cgi/viewcontent.cgi?article=1080&context=lib_fac.
7. Anne J. Gilliland-Swetland, *Enduring Paradigm, New Opportunities: The Value of the Archival Perspective in the Digital Environment* (Washington, DC: Council on Library and Information Resources, 2000), http://www.clir.org/pubs/reports/pub89/pub89.pdf; S. Ross, "Digital Preservation, Archival Science and Methodological Foundations for Digital Libraries" (Keynote Address, ECDL2007, Budapest, 2007), http://eprints.erpanet.org/131/01/Keynote_ECDL2007_SROSS.pdf.
8. Hans Jørn Nielsen and Birger Hjørland, "Curating Research Data: The Potential Roles of Libraries and Information Professionals," *Journal of Documentation* 70, no. 2 (March 4, 2014): 221–40, doi:10.1108/JD-03-2013-0034.
9. Richard Pearce-Moses, "A Glossary of Archival and Records Terminology: Archives," *Society of American Archivists*, 2005, http://www2.archivists.org/glossary/terms/a/archives.
10. Luke J. Gilliland-Swetland, "The Provenance of a Profession: The Permanence of the Public Archives and Historical Manuscripts Traditions in American Archival History," *American Archivist* 54, no. 2 (April 1, 1991): 160–75.
11. Randall C. Jimerson and Linda J. Henry, eds., "Schellenberg in Cyberspace," in *American Archival Studies: Readings in Theory and Practice* (Chicago: Society of American Archivists, 2002), 569–88; Frank Upward et al., "Recordkeeping Informatics: Re-figuring a Discipline in Crisis with a Single Minded Approach," *Records Management Journal* 23, no. 1 (March 22, 2013): 37–50, doi:10.1108/09565691311325013; Tracey P. Lauriault et al., "Today's Data Are Part of Tomorrow's Research: Archival Issues in the Sciences," *Archivaria* 64 (Fall 2007): 123–79.
12. Richard J. Cox, *Managing Records as Evidence and Information* (Westport, CT: Quorum Books, 2001), 1; Lauriault et al., "Today's Data Are Part of Tomorrow's Research."
13. K. Abukhanfusa, ed., *The Concept of Record: Report from the Second Stockholm Conference on Archival Science and the Concept of Record, 30–31 May 1996*, Skrifter Utgivna Av Riksarkivet 4 (Stockholm: Riksarkivet, 1998), 47.

14. Cox, *Managing Records as Evidence and Information*, 46.
15. Gilliland-Swetland, *Enduring Paradigm, New Opportunities*, 2.
16. T. R. Schellenberg, "Archival Principles of Arrangement," in *A Modern Archives Reader: Basic Readings on Archival Theory and Practice*, ed. Maygene F. Daniels and Timothy Walch (Washington, DC: National Archives and Records Service, U.S. General Services Administration, 1984), 149–61.
17. T. R. Schellenberg, "The Appraisal of Modern Public Records: Introduction," *Bulletins of the National Archives*, no. 8 (October 1956), http://www.archives.gov/research/alic/reference/archives-resources/appraisal-intro.html.
18. Ibid.
19. Abukhanfusa, *The Concept of Record*, 147–48.
20. T. R. Schellenberg, "The Appraisal of Modern Public Records: Informational Value," *Bulletins of the National Archives*, no. 8 (October 1956), http://www.archives.gov/research/alic/reference/archives-resources/appraisal-informational-values.html.
21. Abukhanfusa, *The Concept of Record*, 19–20.
22. J. Esanu et al., "Selection, Appraisal, and Retention of Digital Scientific Data: Highlights of an ERPANET/CODATA Workshop," *Data Science Journal* 3 (December 30, 2004): 226–32.
23. Lauriault et al., "Today's Data Are Part of Tomorrow's Research."
24. Kalpana Shankar, "Order from Chaos: The Poetics and Pragmatics of Scientific Recordkeeping," *Journal of the American Society for Information Science and Technology* 58, no. 10 (August 1, 2007): 1457–66, doi:10.1002/asi.20625.
25. Nielsen and Hjørland, "Curating Research Data"; Committee on Science, Engineering, and Public Policy and Committee on Ensuring the Utility and Integrity of Research Data in a Digital Age, *Ensuring the Integrity, Accessibility, and Stewardship of Research Data in the Digital Age* (Washington, DC: National Academy of Sciences, 2009), 22, http://www.nap.edu/catalog/12615/ensuring-the-integrity-accessibility-and-stewardship-of-research-data-in-the-digital-age.
26. Nicholas M. Weber, Carole L. Palmer, and Tiffany C. Chao, "Current Trends and Future Directions in Data Curation Research and Education," *Journal of Web Librarianship* 6, no. 4 (October 1, 2012): 305–20, doi:10.1080/19322909.2012.730358.
27. Lauriault et al., "Today's Data Are Part of Tomorrow's Research," 160.
28. Committee on Science, Engineering, and Public Policy and Committee on Ensuring the Utility and Integrity of Research Data in a Digital Age, *Ensuring the Integrity*, 22.
29. Society of American Archivists, "So You Want to Be an Archivist: An Overview of the Archives Profession," *Society of American Archivists*, accessed May 29, 2015, http://www2.archivists.org/profession.
30. Schellenberg, "Archival Principles of Arrangement."
31. Richard Pearce-Moses, "A Glossary of Archival and Records Terminology: Archival Science," *Society of American Archivists*, 2005, http://www2.archivists.org/glossary/terms/a/archival-science.
32. Luciana Duranti and Heather McNeil, "The Protection of the Integrity of Electronic Records: An Overview of the UBC-MAS Research Project," *Archivaria* 42 (1995): 47.
33. Gilliland-Swetland, *Enduring Paradigm, New Opportunities*, 7.
34. Samuel Muller, Johan Adriaan Feith, and R. Fruin, *Manual for the Arrangement and Description of Archives*, Archival Classics Series (Chicago: Society of American Archivists, 2003); Terry Cook, "What Is Past Is Prologue: A History of Archival Ideas Since 1898, and the Future Paradigm Shift," *Archivaria* 43 (Spring 1997), http://journals.sfu.ca/archivar/index.php/archivaria/article/viewFile/12175/13184.
35. Gilliland-Swetland, "The Provenance of a Profession."
36. Schellenberg, "Archival Principles of Arrangement."
37. Ibid.
38. Gilliland-Swetland, *Enduring Paradigm, New Opportunities*, 9.

39. Mark Greene and Dennis Meissner, "More Product, Less Process: Revamping Traditional Archival Processing," *The American Archivist* 68, no. 2 (2005): 208-63.
40. William J. Maher, "Archives, Archivists, and Society," *American Archivist*, Presidential Address, 61 (Fall 1998): 262-63.
41. Nielsen and Hjørland, "Curating Research Data," 236-37.
42. Gilliland-Swetland, *Enduring Paradigm, New Opportunities*, 14-15; The U.S. National Archives and Records Administration, "What's a Record?," accessed June 14, 2015, http://www.archives.gov/about/info/whats-a-record.html.
43. Sarah Higgins, "The DCC Curation Lifecycle Model," *International Journal of Digital Curation* 3, no. 1 (February 12, 2008): 134-40, doi:10.2218/ijdc.v3i1.48.
44. Lee and Tibbo, "Where's the Archivist in Digital Curation?," 160-61.
45. Cox, *Managing Records as Evidence and Information*, 27, 109.
46. Lee and Tibbo, "Where's the Archivist in Digital Curation?," 161.
47. Dharma Akmon et al., "The Application of Archival Concepts to a Data-Intensive Environment: Working with Scientists to Understand Data Management and Preservation Needs," *Archival Science* 11, nos. 3-4 (October 11, 2011): 329-48, doi:10.1007/s10502-011-9151-4.
48. Kathleen Fear and Devan Ray Donaldson, "Provenance and Credibility in Scientific Data Repositories," *Archival Science* 12, no. 3 (April 15, 2012): 319-39, doi:10.1007/s10502-012-9172-7.
49. Brian Matthews et al., "Towards the Preservation of the Scientific Memory," *International Journal of Digital Curation* 10, no. 1 (2015): 196-209, doi:10.2218/ijdc.v10i1.361.
50. Fear and Donaldson, "Provenance and Credibility in Scientific Data Repositories" (emphasis added), 333.
51. H. D. Tjalsma, *Selection of Research Data, Guidelines for Appraising and Selecting Research Data: A Report by DANS and 3TU.Datacentrum* (The Hague: Netherlands: DANS, 2011), 10, http://www.dans.knaw.nl/nl/over/organisatie-beleid/publicaties/DANSselectionofresearchdata.pdf.
52. Committee on Science, Engineering, and Public Policy and Committee on Ensuring the Utility and Integrity of Research Data in a Digital Age, *Ensuring the Integrity*, 98.
53. Poole, "How Has Your Science Data Grown?"; Tjalsma, *Selection of Research Data*, 18.
54. Gilliland-Swetland, *Enduring Paradigm, New Opportunities*, 9.
55. Tjalsma, *Selection of Research Data*.
56. Lauriault et al., "Today's Data Are Part of Tomorrow's Research."
57. Gilliland-Swetland, *Enduring Paradigm, New Opportunities*.
58. Committee on Science, Engineering, and Public Policy and Committee on Ensuring the Utility and Integrity of Research Data in a Digital Age, *Ensuring the Integrity*, 34.
59. Fear and Donaldson, "Provenance and Credibility in Scientific Data Repositories."
60. Committee on Science, Engineering, and Public Policy and Committee on Ensuring the Utility and Integrity of Research Data in a Digital Age, *Ensuring the Integrity*, 42.
61. Lauriault et al., "Today's Data Are Part of Tomorrow's Research"; Ross, "Digital Preservation, Archival Science and Methodological Foundations for Digital Libraries."
62. Mark Hedges et al., "Sheer Curation of Experiments: Data, Process, Provenance," *Journal of Digital Information* 13, no. 1 (March 8, 2012), https://journals.tdl.org/jodi/index.php/jodi/article/view/5883.
63. Nielsen and Hjørland, "Curating Research Data."
64. Committee on Science, Engineering, and Public Policy and Committee on Ensuring the Utility and Integrity of Research Data in a Digital Age, *Ensuring the Integrity*, 106.
65. Kristi Kiesling, "Metadata, Metadata, Everywhere—but Where Is the Hook?," *OCLC Systems & Services: International Digital Library Perspectives* 17, no. 2 (June 1, 2001): 84-88, doi:10.1108/10650750110395007.

66. David J. Bearman and Richard H. Lytle, "The Power of the Principle of Provenance," *Archivaria* 21 (Winter 1985–1986), http://journals.sfu.ca/archivar/index.php/archivaria/article/viewFile/11231/12170.
67. Fear and Donaldson, "Provenance and Credibility in Scientific Data Repositories."
68. Shankar, "Order from Chaos."
69. Reagan Moore, "Towards a Theory of Digital Preservation," *International Journal of Digital Curation* 3, no. 1 (February 12, 2008): 64, doi:10.2218/ijdc.v3i1.42.
70. Lee and Tibbo, "Where's the Archivist in Digital Curation?," 127.
71. Esanu et al., "Selection, Appraisal, and Retention of Digital Scientific Data."
72. Ross, "Digital Preservation, Archival Science and Methodological Foundations for Digital Libraries."
73. Poole, "How Has Your Science Data Grown?," 20.
74. Christopher A. Lee, "Open Archival Information System (OAIS) Reference Model," 2010, http://www.statearchivists.org/seri/STEP/IntroInstitute/OAIS_Reference_Model%20-%20Cal%20Lee.pdf.
75. Lee and Tibbo, "Where's the Archivist in Digital Curation?," 132–36.
76. Lee, "Open Archival Information System (OAIS) Reference Model," 4026.
77. Sammie Morris, "Applying Archival Science to Digital Curation: Advocacy for the Archivist's Role in Implementing and Managing Trusted Digital Repositories," January 1, 2015, *Libraries Faculty and Staff Presentations*, Paper 93, http://docs.lib.purdue.edu/lib_fspres/93.
78. Lee and Tibbo, "Where's the Archivist in Digital Curation?," 138.
79. CCSDS Secretariat, *Recommended Practice for Requirements for Bodies Providing Audit and Certification of Candidate Trustworthy Digital Repositories*, Recommended Practice, Issue 2 (Washington, DC: CCSDS, March 2014), http://public.ccsds.org/publications/archive/652x1m2.pdf; Center for Research Libraries: Global Resources Networks, "Digital Preservation Metrics," accessed June 19, 2015, http://www.crl.edu/archiving-preservation/digital-archives/metrics.
80. Poole, "How Has Your Science Data Grown?"
81. Committee on Science, Engineering, and Public Policy and Committee on Ensuring the Utility and Integrity of Research Data in a Digital Age, *Ensuring the Integrity*, 95.
82. National Science Board, *Long-Lived Data Collections* (Arlington, VA: National Science Foundation, 2005), 14, http://www.nsf.gov/nsb/documents/2005/LLDDC_report.pdf.
83. Richard J. Cox and David A. Wallace, *Archives and the Public Good: Accountability and Records in Modern Society* (Westport, CT: Quorum Books, 2002).
84. Committee on Science, Engineering, and Public Policy and Committee on Ensuring the Utility and Integrity of Research Data in a Digital Age, *Ensuring the Integrity*, 63.
85. Paul F. Uhlir, "Information Gulags, Intellectual Straightjackets, and Memory Holes: Three Principles to Guide the Preservation of Scientific Data," *Data Science Journal* 9 (2010): ES1–5, doi:10.2481/dsj.Essay-001-Uhlir.
86. Committee on Science, Engineering, and Public Policy and Committee on Ensuring the Utility and Integrity of Research Data in a Digital Age, *Ensuring the Integrity*, 70; Uhlir, "Information Gulags."
87. Richard Pearce-Moses, "Caught in the Middle: Access to State Government Records in the United States" (paper presented at Access to Archives: The Japanese and American Practices, conference Tokyo, May 7-11, 2007); Cox, *Managing Records as Evidence and Information*, 156–71.
88. Angelika Menne-Haritz, "Access—The Reformulation of an Archival Paradigm," *Archival Science* 1, no. 1 (March 1, 2001): 74, doi:10.1007/BF02435639.
89. Bearman and Lytle, "The Power of the Principle of Provenance."
90. Hedges et al., "Sheer Curation of Experiments."
91. Maygene F. Daniels, Timothy Walch, and Mary Jo Pugh, eds., "The Illusion of Omniscience: Subject Access and the Reference Archivist," in *A Modern Archives Reader: Basic Readings on Archival Theory and Practice* (Washington, DC: National Archives and Records Service, U.S. General Services Administration, 1984), 264-77.

92. Mark A. Greene, "The Power of Archives: Archivists' Values and Value in the Post-Modern Age," *American Archivist* 72, no. 1 (2009), http://www.archivists.org/governance/presidential/GreeneAddressAug08.pdf, 4.
93. Lee and Tibbo, "Where's the Archivist in Digital Curation?," 160.
94. Ibid., 163.
95. Gilliland-Swetland, *Enduring Paradigm, New Opportunities*, 2.
96. Ibid., 9.
97. Poole, "How Has Your Science Data Grown?," 16; Jullian C. Wallis et al., "Moving Archival Practices Upstream: An Exploration of the Life Cycle of Ecological Sensing Data in Collaborative Field Research," *International Journal of Digital Curation* 3, no. 1 (February 12, 2008): 114–26, doi:10.2218/ijdc.v3i1.46.
98. Esanu et al., "Selection, Appraisal, and Retention of Digital Scientific Data."
99. Christie Peters and Anita Riley Dryden, "Assessing the Academic Library's Role in Campus-Wide Research Data Management: A First Step at the University of Houston," *Science & Technology Libraries* 30, no. 4 (September 1, 2011): 387–403, doi:10.1080/0194262X.2011.626340.

Bibliography

Abbot, Daisy. "What Is Digital Curation?" *DCC Briefing Papers: Introduction to Curation.* 2008. http://www.dcc.ac.uk/resources/briefing-papers/introduction-curation.

Abukhanfusa, K. *The Concept of Record: Report from the Second Stockholm Conference on Archival Science and the Concept of Record, 30–31 May 1996*. Skrifter Utgivna Av Riksarkivet 4. Stockholm: Riksarkivet, 1998.

Akmon, Dharma, Ann Zimmerman, Morgan Daniels, and Margaret Hedstrom. "The Application of Archival Concepts to a Data-Intensive Environment: Working with Scientists to Understand Data Management and Preservation Needs." *Archival Science* 11, nos. 3–4 (October 11, 2011): 329–48. doi:10.1007/s10502-011-9151-4.

Auckland, Mary. "Re-Skilling for Research." Research Libraries UK, 2012. http://www.rluk.ac.uk/wp-content/uploads/2014/02/RLUK-Re-skilling.pdf.

Bearman, David J., and Richard H. Lytle. "The Power of the Principle of Provenance." *Archivaria* 21 (Winter 1985–1986). http://journals.sfu.ca/archivar/index.php/archivaria/article/viewFile/11231/12170.

CCSDS Secretariat. *Recommended Practice for Requirements for Bodies Providing Audit and Certification of Candidate Trustworthy Digital Repositories*. Recommended Practice, Issue 2. Washington, DC: CCSDS, March 2014. http://public.ccsds.org/publications/archive/652x1m2.pdf.

Center for Research Libraries, Global Resources Networks. "Digital Preservation Metrics." Accessed June 19, 2015. http://www.crl.edu/archiving-preservation/digital-archives/metrics.

Committee on Science, Engineering, and Public Policy, and Committee on Ensuring the Utility and Integrity of Research Data in a Digital Age. *Ensuring the Integrity, Accessibility, and Stewardship of Research Data in the Digital Age*. Washington, DC: National Academy of Sciences, 2009. http://www.nap.edu/catalog/12615/ensuring-the-integrity-accessibility-and-stewardship-of-research-data-in-the-digital-age.

Cook, Terry. "What Is Past Is Prologue: A History of Archival Ideas Since 1898, and the Future Paradigm Shift." *Archivaria* 43 (Spring 1997). http://journals.sfu.ca/archivar/index.php/archivaria/article/viewFile/12175/13184.

Cox, Andrew M., and Stephen Pinfield. "Research Data Management and Libraries: Current Activities and Future Priorities." *Journal of Librarianship and Information Science* 46 (2014): 299.

Cox, Andrew, Eddy Verbaan, and Barbara Sen. "Upskilling Liaison Librarians for Research Data Management." *Ariadne* 70 (November 2012). http://www.ariadne.ac.uk/issue70/cox-et-al.

Cox, Richard J. *Managing Records as Evidence and Information*. Westport, CT: Quorum Books, 2001.

Cox, Richard J., and David A. Wallace. *Archives and the Public Good: Accountability and Records in Modern Society*. Westport, CT: Quorum Books, 2002.

Daniels, Maygene F., Timothy Walch, and Mary Jo Pugh, eds. "The Illusion of Omniscience: Subject Access and the Reference Archivist." In *A Modern Archives Reader: Basic Readings on Archival Theory and Practice*, 264–77. Washington, D.C: National Archives and Records Service, U.S. General Services Administration, 1984.

Duranti, Luciana, and Heather McNeil. "The Protection of the Integrity of Electronic Records: An Overview of the UBC-MAS Research Project." *Archivaria* 42 (1995): 46–67.

Esanu, J., J. Davidson, S. Ross, and W. Anderson. "Selection, Appraisal, and Retention of Digital Scientific Data: Highlights of an ERPANET/CODATA Workshop." *Data Science Journal* 3 (December 30, 2004): 226–32.

Fear, Kathleen, and Devan Ray Donaldson. "Provenance and Credibility in Scientific Data Repositories." *Archival Science* 12, no. 3 (April 15, 2012): 319–39. doi:10.1007/s10502-012-9172-7.

Giarlo, Michael J. "Academic Libraries as Data Quality Hubs." *Journal of Librarianship and Scholarly Communication* 1, no. 3 (2013).

Gilliland-Swetland, Anne J. *Enduring Paradigm, New Opportunities: The Value of the Archival Perspective in the Digital Environment*. Washington, DC: Council on Library and Information Resources, 2000. http://www.clir.org/pubs/reports/pub89/pub89.pdf.

Gilliland-Swetland, Luke J. "The Provenance of a Profession: The Permanence of the Public Archives and Historical Manuscripts Traditions in American Archival History." *American Archivist* 54, no. 2 (April 1, 1991): 160–75.

Greene, Mark A. "The Power of Archives: Archivists' Values and Value in the Post-Modern Age." *American Archivist* 72, no. 1 (2009). http://www.archivists.org/governance/presidential/GreeneAddressAug08.pdf.

Greene, Mark, and Dennis Meissner. "More Product, Less Process: Revamping Traditional Archival Processing." *American Archivist* 68, no. 2 (2005): 208–63.

Hedges, Mark, Tobias Blanke, Stella Fabiane, Gareth Knight, and Eric Liao. "Sheer Curation of Experiments: Data, Process, Provenance." *Journal of Digital Information* 13, no. 1 (March 8, 2012). https://journals.tdl.org/jodi/index.php/jodi/article/view/5883.

Heidorn, P. Bryan. "The Emerging Role of Libraries in Data Curation and E-Science." *Journal of Library Administration* 51, nos. 7–8 (October 1, 2011): 662–72. doi:10.1080/01930826.2011.601269.

Higgins, Sarah. "The DCC Curation Lifecycle Model." *International Journal of Digital Curation* 3, no. 1 (February 12, 2008): 134–40. doi:10.2218/ijdc.v3i1.48.

Jimerson, Randall C., and Linda J. Henry, eds. "Schellenberg in Cyberspace." In *American Archival Studies: Readings in Theory and Practice*, 569–88. Chicago: Society of American Archivists, 2002.

Kiesling, Kristi. "Metadata, Metadata, Everywhere—but Where Is the Hook?" *OCLC Systems & Services: International Digital Library Perspectives* 17, no. 2 (June 1, 2001): 84–88. doi:10.1108/10650750110395007.

Lauriault, Tracey P., Barbara L. Craig, D. R. Fraser Taylor, and Peter L. Pulsifer. "Today's Data Are Part of Tomorrow's Research: Archival Issues in the Sciences." *Archivaria* 64 (Fall 2007): 123–79.

Lee, Christopher A. "Open Archival Information System (OAIS) Reference Model," 2010. http://www.statearchivists.org/seri/STEP/IntroInstitute/OAIS_Reference_Model%20-%20Cal%20Lee.pdf.

Lee, Christopher A., and Helen Tibbo. "Where's the Archivist in Digital Curation? Exploring the Possibilities through a Matrix of Knowledge and Skills." *Archivaria* 72 (Fall 2011). http://www.synergiescanada.org/journals/bcn/archivaria/454/13362.

Maher, William J. "Archives, Archivists, and Society." *American Archivist*, Presidential Address, 61 (Fall 1998): 252–65.

Matthews, Brian, Shirley Crompton, Catherine Jones, and Simon Lambert. "Towards the Preservation of the Scientific Memory." *International Journal of Digital Curation* 10, no. 1 (2015): 196–209. doi:10.2218/ijdc.v10i1.361.

Menne-Haritz, Angelika. "Access—the Reformulation of an Archival Paradigm." *Archival Science* 1, no. 1 (March 1, 2001): 57–82. doi:10.1007/BF02435639.

Moore, Reagan. "Towards a Theory of Digital Preservation." *International Journal of Digital Curation* 3, no. 1 (February 12, 2008): 63–75. doi:10.2218/ijdc.v3i1.42.

Morris, Sammie. "Applying Archival Science to Digital Curation: Advocacy for the Archivist's Role in Implementing and Managing Trusted Digital Repositories." *Libraries Faculty and Staff Presentations*, Paper 93, January 1, 2015. http://docs.lib.purdue.edu/lib_fspres/93.

Muller, Samuel, Johan Adriaan Feith, and R. Fruin. *Manual for the Arrangement and Description of Archives*. Archival Classics Series. Chicago: Society of American Archivists, 2003.

National Science Board. *Long-Lived Data Collections*. Arlington, VA: National Science Foundation, 2005. http://www.nsf.gov/nsb/documents/2005/LLDDC_report.pdf.

Nielsen, Hans Jørn, and Birger Hjørland. "Curating Research Data: The Potential Roles of Libraries and Information Professionals." *Journal of Documentation* 70, no. 2 (March 4, 2014): 221–40. doi:10.1108/JD-03-2013-0034.

Noonan, Daniel, and Tamar Chute. "Data Curation and the University Archives." *American Archivist* 77, no. 1 (April 1, 2014): 201–40. doi:10.17723/aarc.77.1.m49r46526847g587.

Pearce-Moses, Richard. "A Glossary of Archival and Records Terminology: Archival Science." *Society of American Archivists*, 2005. http://www2.archivists.org/glossary/terms/a/archival-science.

———. "A Glossary of Archival and Records Terminology: Archives." *Society of American Archivists*, 2005. http://www2.archivists.org/glossary/terms/a/archives.

———. "Caught in the Middle: Access to State Government Records in the United States." Paper presented at Access to Archives: The Japanese and American Practices, conference Tokyo, May 7–11, 2007.

Peters, Christie, and Anita Riley Dryden. "Assessing the Academic Library's Role in Campus-Wide Research Data Management: A First Step at the University of Houston." *Science & Technology Libraries* 30, no. 4 (September 1, 2011): 387–403. doi:10.1080/0194262X.2011.626340.

Poole, Alex H. "How Has Your Science Data Grown? Digital Curation and the Human Factor: A Critical Literature Review." *Archival Science* 15, no. 2 (November 23, 2014): 101–39. doi:10.1007/s10502-014-9236-y.

Ramírez, Marisa L. "Whose Role Is It Anyway? A Library Practitioner's Appraisal of the Digital Data Deluge." *Bulletin of the American Society for Information Science and Technology* 37, no. 5 (2011). http://digitalcommons.calpoly.edu/cgi/viewcontent.cgi?article=1080&context=lib_fac.

Ross, S. "Digital Preservation, Archival Science and Methodological Foundations for Digital Libraries." Keynote Address presented at the ECDL2007, Budapest, 2007. http://eprints.erpanet.org/131/01/Keynote_ECDL2007_SROSS.pdf.

Schellenberg, T. R. "Archival Principles of Arrangement." In *A Modern Archives Reader: Basic Readings on Archival Theory and Practice*, edited by Maygene F. Daniels and Timothy Walch, 149–61. Washington, DC: National Archives and Records Service, U.S. General Services Administration, 1984.

———. "The Appraisal of Modern Public Records: Informational Value." *Bulletins of the National Archives*, no. 8 (October 1956). http://www.archives.gov/research/alic/reference/archives-resources/appraisal-informational-values.html.

———. "The Appraisal of Modern Public Records: Introduction." *Bulletins of the National Archives*, no. 8 (October 1956). http://www.archives.gov/research/alic/reference/archives-resources/appraisal-intro.html.

Shankar, Kalpana. "Order from Chaos: The Poetics and Pragmatics of Scientific Recordkeeping." *Journal of the American Society for Information Science and Technology* 58, no. 10 (August 1, 2007): 1457–66. doi:10.1002/asi.20625.

Society of American Archivists. "So You Want to Be an Archivist: An Overview of the Archives Profession." *Society of American Archivists*. Accessed May 29, 2015. http://www2.archivists.org/profession.

Tenopir, Carol, Ben Birch, and Suzie Allard. "Academic Libraries and Research Data Services: Current Practices and Plans for the Future. An ACRL White Paper." The Center for Information and Communication Studies, 2012. http://www.ala.org/acrl/sites/ala.org.acrl/files/content/publications/whitepapers/Tenopir_Birch_Allard.pdf.

Tjalsma, H. D. *Selection of Research Data, Guidelines for Appraising and Selecting Research Data: A Report by DANS and 3TU.Datacentrum*. The Hague: Netherlands: DANS, 2011. http://www.dans.knaw.nl/nl/over/organisatie-beleid/publicaties/DANSselectionofresearchdata.pdf.

Uhlir, Paul F. "Information Gulags, Intellectual Straightjackets, and Memory Holes: Three Principles to Guide the Preservation of Scientific Data." *Data Science Journal* 9 (2010): ES1–5. doi:10.2481/dsj.Essay-001-Uhlir.

Upward, Frank, Barbara Reed, Gillian Oliver, and Joanne Evans. "Recordkeeping Informatics: Re-figuring a Discipline in Crisis with a Single Minded Approach." *Records Management Journal* 23, no. 1 (March 22, 2013): 37–50. doi:10.1108/09565691311325013.

U.S. National Archives and Records Administration. "What's a Record?" Accessed June 14, 2015. http://www.archives.gov/about/info/whats-a-record.html.

Wallis, Jullian C., Christine L. Borgman, Matthew S. Mayernik, and Alberto Pepe. "Moving Archival Practices Upstream: An Exploration of the Life Cycle of Ecological Sensing Data in Collaborative Field Research." *International Journal of Digital Curation* 3, no. 1 (February 12, 2008): 114–26. doi:10.2218/ijdc.v3i1.46.

Weber, Nicholas M., Carole L. Palmer, and Tiffany C. Chao. "Current Trends and Future Directions in Data Curation Research and Education." *Journal of Web Librarianship* 6, no. 4 (October 1, 2012): 305–20. doi:10.1080/19322909.2012.730358.

Chapter 4

Raising Researchers' Awareness of Biomedical Data Journals to Promote Data Sharing

Katherine G. Akers, Shiffman Medical Library, Wayne State University

Despite expectations from funding agencies and journals that researchers provide access to the data underlying their findings to enable reproducibility and reuse,[1] researchers often do not share their data beyond a small circle of collaborators. For instance, when Savage and Vickers requested data from ten authors of articles published in *PLoS Medicine* or *PLoS Clinical Trials*, which explicitly state that authors should make their data available to other researchers for academic purposes, they were successful in receiving only one dataset.[2] Similarly, Alsheikh-Ali et al. found that 59 percent of authors did not fully comply with various journal policies on the public deposition of microarray, nucleic acid, protein, or macromolecular data.[3] These examples provide evidence that the practice of sharing data with the greater scientific community is not yet common among biomedical and health sciences researchers.

As champions of access to information, academic librarians are stepping up to promote data sharing, in part by reaching out to and educating researchers about the benefits of and avenues for data sharing.[4] To communicate effectively with researchers about why and how to share their research data, it is important to understand the barriers that prevent data sharing from becoming common practice. Surveys and interviews have identified several reasons why scientists may be wary of or disinterested in sharing their data, including concerns about the privacy of human subjects, fears that data might be misinterpreted or used without proper acknowledgment, and a desire to publish as many papers as possible before relinquishing the data.[5] However, across surveys, the most consistently reported reason why researchers do not share their data is that it takes too much time.[6] This unwillingness of researchers to spend time cleaning, organizing, and documenting their data in preparation for public release may result from the lack of strong mandates from funders, institutions, and journals[7] and the lack of scholarly reward for data sharing.[8]

Currently, the prestige and promotion of academic researchers hinges on their ability to publish journal articles and secure grant funding, whereas acts of data sharing are neither reflected on CVs nor valued by hiring or tenure and promotion committees. However, by co-opting the traditional system of scholarly publication, the emergence of journals that publish data papers ("data journals") may provide a mechanism by which researchers can earn scholarly credit for sharing their data.[9] Rather than reporting research findings based on the critical analysis of data, data papers draw attention to and describe the context, content, and quality of research datasets, thereby increasing the likelihood of their reuse by other researchers. Data papers are published in scholarly journals and are typically subject to peer review, allowing them to be listed on CVs just like traditional research articles. Therefore, the opportunity to publish a data paper could motivate researchers to share their data and provide an incentive for spending time and effort toward readying datasets for use by a wider audience.[10]

The number of journals that publish data papers has rapidly increased over the last fifteen years.[11] Of the approximately two hundred data journals now in existence, the majority of data journals are either aimed at biological, medical, or health care fields or are general-science journals that also serve the biomedical community (see table 4.1). These data journals include both those that publish data papers as one possible article type ("mixed" data journals) and those that only publish data papers ("pure" data journals). Despite the growing number of data journal publishers and titles, however, most researchers and librarians are not aware of this emerging avenue for data dissemination. This chapter will highlight features of biomedical, health sciences, and general science data journals; identify the types of researchers that might be most interested in publishing data papers; and suggest how librarians could promote data sharing by raising awareness of data journals among researchers.

Table 4.1. Data Journals Serving the Biomedical and Health Sciences Communities

Publisher	Journal Title
BioMed Central	*Biology of Sex Differences*
BioMed Central	*BMC Anesthesiology*
BioMed Central	*BMC Biochemistry*
BioMed Central	*BMC Bioinformatics*
BioMed Central	*BMC Biology*
BioMed Central	*BMC Biophysics*
BioMed Central	*BMC Biotechnology*
BioMed Central	*BMC Cancer*
BioMed Central	*BMC Cardiovascular Disorders*
BioMed Central	*BMC Cell Biology*
BioMed Central	*BMC Clinical Pathology*
BioMed Central	*BMC Complementary & Alternative Medicine*
BioMed Central	*BMC Dermatology*
BioMed Central	*BMC Developmental Biology*
BioMed Central	*BMC Ear, Nose and Throat Disorders*
BioMed Central	*BMC Emergency Medicine*
BioMed Central	*BMC Endocrine Disorders*
BioMed Central	*BMC Family Practice*
BioMed Central	*BMC Gastroenterology*
BioMed Central	*BMC Genetics*
BioMed Central	*BMC Genomics*
BioMed Central	*BMC Geriatrics*
BioMed Central	*BMC Health Services Research*

(continued)

Publisher	Journal Title
BioMed Central	*BMC Hematology*
BioMed Central	*BMC Immunology*
BioMed Central	*BMC Infectious Diseases*
BioMed Central	*BMC International Health and Human Rights*
BioMed Central	*BMC Medical Education*
BioMed Central	*BMC Medical Ethics*
BioMed Central	*BMC Medical Genetics*
BioMed Central	*BMC Medical Genomics*
BioMed Central	*BMC Medical Imaging*
BioMed Central	*BMC Medical Informatics & Decision Making*
BioMed Central	*BMC Medical Research Methodology*
BioMed Central	*BMC Medicine*
BioMed Central	*BMC Microbiology*
BioMed Central	*BMC Molecular Biology*
BioMed Central	*BMC Musculoskeletal Disorders*
BioMed Central	*BMC Nephrology*
BioMed Central	*BMC Neurology*
BioMed Central	*BMC Neuroscience*
BioMed Central	*BMC Nursing*
BioMed Central	*BMC Obesity*
BioMed Central	*BMC Ophthalmology*
BioMed Central	*BMC Oral Health*
BioMed Central	*BMC Palliative Care*
BioMed Central	*BMC Pediatrics*
BioMed Central	*BMC Pharmacology & Toxicology*
BioMed Central	*BMC Physiology*
BioMed Central	*BMC Pregnancy & Childbirth*
BioMed Central	*BMC Psychiatry*
BioMed Central	*BMC Public Health*
BioMed Central	*BMC Pulmonary Medicine*
BioMed Central	*BMC Research Notes*
BioMed Central	*BMC Sports Science, Medicine and Rehabilitation*
BioMed Central	*BMC Structural Biology*
BioMed Central	*BMC Surgery*
BioMed Central	*BMC Systems Biology*
BioMed Central	*BMC Urology*

(continued)

Publisher	**Journal Title**
BioMed Central	*BMC Women's Health*
BioMed Central	*Cell & Bioscience*
BioMed Central	*Chiropractic & Manual Therapies*
BioMed Central	*Genome Medicine*
BioMed Central	*GigaScience*
BioMed Central	*Human Genomics*
BioMed Central	*Journal of Occupational Medicine and Toxicology*
BioMed Central	*Standards in Genomic Sciences*
BioMed Central	*Substance Abuse Treatment, Prevention, and Policy*
BioMed Central	*Theoretical Biology and Medical Modelling*
Elsevier	*Data in Brief*
Elsevier	*Genomics Data*
Faculty of 1000	*F1000Research*
Frontiers	*Frontiers in Aging Neuroscience*
Frontiers	*Frontiers in Behavioral Neuroscience*
Frontiers	*Frontiers in Bioengineering and Biotechnology*
Frontiers	*Frontiers in Cell and Developmental Biology*
Frontiers	*Frontiers in Cellular and Infection Microbiology*
Frontiers	*Frontiers in Cellular Neuroscience*
Frontiers	*Frontiers in Computational Neuroscience*
Frontiers	*Frontiers in Endocrinology*
Frontiers	*Frontiers in Evolutionary Neuroscience*
Frontiers	*Frontiers in Genetics*
Frontiers	*Frontiers in Human Neuroscience*
Frontiers	*Frontiers in Immunology*
Frontiers	*Frontiers in Integrative Neuroscience*
Frontiers	*Frontiers in Microbiology*
Frontiers	*Frontiers in Molecular Biosciences*
Frontiers	*Frontiers in Molecular Neuroscience*
Frontiers	*Frontiers in Neural Circuits*
Frontiers	*Frontiers in Neuroanatomy*
Frontiers	*Frontiers in Neuroenergetics*
Frontiers	*Frontiers in Neuroengineering*
Frontiers	*Frontiers in Neuroinformatics*
Frontiers	*Frontiers in Neurology*
Frontiers	*Frontiers in Neurorobotics*

(continued)

Publisher	Journal Title
Frontiers	*Frontiers in Neuroscience*
Frontiers	*Frontiers in Oncology*
Frontiers	*Frontiers in Pediatrics*
Frontiers	*Frontiers in Pharmacology*
Frontiers	*Frontiers in Physiology*
Frontiers	*Frontiers in Psychiatry*
Frontiers	*Frontiers in Public Health*
Frontiers	*Frontiers in Surgery*
Frontiers	*Frontiers in Synaptic Neuroscience*
Frontiers	*Frontiers in Systems Neuroscience*
Hindawi Publishing Corporation	*Dataset Papers in Science*
MDPI	*Data*
Nature Publishing Group	*Scientific Data*
Procon	*Biomedical Data Journal*
Public Library of Science	*PLoS ONE*
Springer	*Neuroinformatics*
SpringerOpen	*Applied Informatics*
SpringerOpen	*Health and Justice*
SpringerOpen	*In Silico Pharmacology*
SpringerOpen	*SpringerPlus*
Ubiquity Press	*Open Health Data*

Features of Data Journals

Names for Data Papers

Although the term "data paper" will be used throughout this chapter for simplicity, data papers actually go by a variety of names depending on the journal in which they are published. *Open Health Data* and *Biomedical Data Journal* use the term "data paper;" *Dataset Papers in Science* and *Data* use the term "dataset paper;" *Scientific Data* uses the term "data descriptor;" *F1000Research* and BioMed Central's *GigaScience* use the term "data note;" Elsevier's *Data in Brief* and *Genomics Data* use the term "data in brief article;" *Neuroinformatics* uses the term "data original article;" and Frontiers journals use the term "data report." SpringerOpen journals and other BioMed Central journals publish "database articles," and SpringerOpen's *SpringerPlus* publishes both "data notes" and "database articles." Finally, *PLoS ONE* publishes articles with the primary purpose of describing databases, but these are classified as a type of regular "research article." Despite having different names, the purpose of these articles is the same—to describe available research datasets or databases that may be of use to other researchers.

Open Access

Consistent with their intent to encourage public access to research datasets, nearly all data journals are open access. The one exception is *Neuroinformatics*, which provides authors with an open-access option for a fee. Most of the data journals serving the biomedical and health sciences communities are listed in the Directory for Open Access Journals (DOAJ) except for Elsevier's *Data in Brief* and *Genomics Data*, BioMed Central's *Genomic Medicine*, MDPI's *Data*, and SpringerOpen's *Applied Informatics* and *Health and Justice*. The *Biomedical Data Journal* is currently in the process of being indexed by DOAJ.

Because most data journals are open access, authors typically must pay an article processing charge (APC) to publish a data paper, the cost of which varies depending on the journal. Some new data journals temporarily offered free or reduced APCs to encourage submission. Specifically, the APC for *Biomedical Data Journal* was waived through 2015, Elsevier's *Data in Brief* and *Genomics Data* offered a 50 percent discount on their $500 APC until the end of 2015, and the APC for *Data* is waived through 2015 and 2016. *Data in Brief* offers the additional opportunity to publish ten data papers at the same time for the price of one. The APC for *Open Health Data* is £100, but this fee can be waived if the authors have no available funding. The APC is $250 for Frontiers journals, $500 for *Dataset Papers in Science*, $1,350 for *Scientific Data* and *PLoS ONE*, and $1,085–$1,290 for SpringerOpen journals. BioMed Central APCs range from $1,015–$2,770, although there is no charge for publishing in *Chiropractic and Manual Therapies* because professional chiropractic societies cover the cost of article processing. The APC for papers published in *F1000Research* depends on word count—$150 for up to 1,000 words, $500 for 1,000–2,500 words, and $1,000 for over 2,500 words. *F1000Research* also offers discounts for authors who perform various activities such as serving as a peer reviewer for *F1000Research* or submitting a poster to *F1000Posters*. Finally, the open access option for *Neuroinformatics* costs $3,000.

The explosion in the number of open-access journals in recent years has unfortunately fueled the launch of open access journals that exist merely to extract APCs from authors without providing any value added in return. These suspected "predatory" journals are tracked by Jeffrey Beall, a librarian from the University of Colorado Denver. Of the data journal publishers discussed in this chapter, only MDPI, which publishes the journal *Data*, makes it onto Beall's list. MDPI is suspected of being predatory due to its practice of using respected researchers as figureheads on editorial boards and its history of accepting questionable articles, among other reasons.[12]

Indexing in Article Databases and Impact Factors

Most data journals serving the biomedical and health sciences communities are indexed in PubMed, Scopus, or Web of Science, indicating that their contents are readily discoverable by other researchers. Some exceptions include *Biomedical Data Journal, Dataset Papers in Science, Data, Open Health Data*, and *Applied Informatics*, which are not indexed by any of these databases, although *Biomedical Data Journal* is currently undergoing indexing by PubMed. Also, many of these data journals have received impact factors as calculated by Thomson Reuters' Journal Citation Index. Specifically, the 2014 impact factor of BioMed Central data journals ranges from 0.95 to 7.98, the impact factor of *Neuroinformatics* is 2.85, the impact factor of *PLoS ONE* is 3.23, and the impact factor of Frontiers data journals ranges from 2.20 to 4.29. Data journals with no 2014 impact factors include *Data in Brief, Genomics Data, F1000Research, Data, Dataset Papers in Science, Scientific Data, Biomedical Data Journal, Open Health Data*, and SpringerOpen journals. However, because several of these journals did not launch until midway through 2012 or thereafter, this lack of an impact factor is often due to the absence of a full three years of citation data and does not necessarily reflect low journal quality.

Data Paper Structure

Because the purpose of data papers is to call attention to and describe research datasets rather than to form arguments or draw conclusions from the data, data papers do not usually adopt the traditional article structure of Abstract, Introduction, Methods, Results, and Discussion. Rather, they often consist of sections describing the motivation for collecting the data, the methods used to generate and/

or process the data, a description of the content of the dataset, suggestions for how the data could be reused, and information on where and how data can be accessed. For example, *Dataset Papers in Science* instructs authors to arrange their data paper according to the following structure: Abstract, Introduction (i.e., motivations for conducting the study and any necessary background information), Methodology, Dataset Description (i.e., a detailed description of each table, image, or gene sequence in the dataset; a label for and description of each column header in a tabular dataset; and as much additional metadata as possible), Concluding Remarks, and Dataset Availability (i.e., web address of database and/or accession number of a dataset in a data repository). As another example, Frontiers journals do not require authors to use particular sections for their data paper, but indicate that the manuscript must include a description of how the data were acquired, the data collection period, an overview of the data files and their formats, a description of the methods used to collect the data, and information on how readers should interpret or could reuse the data.

As the structure of data papers differs from that of traditional research articles, some data journals provide templates that can assist authors in writing data papers. For instance, *Scientific Data* encourages authors to use a Word document template consisting of an Abstract, Background and Summary (i.e., overview of the study design and data generated, any background information needed to place the study into the context of previous research, motivation for collecting the data, and potential reuse value of the data), Methods (i.e., detailed methods for producing the data), Data Records (i.e., information on the repository in which the data are housed and an overview of the individual data files and formats), Technical Validation (i.e., any experimental, observational, or statistical techniques for confirming the reliability of the data), and an optional Usage Notes section (i.e., brief tips to assist other researchers in reusing the data and/or instructions on how to access data containing sensitive information). Similar templates are provided by *Open Health Data*, *Biomedical Data Journal*, and Elsevier's *Data in Brief* and *Genomics Data*.

Access to Data

An important distinction among data journals is how they instruct authors to provide access to the data described in the data papers, either allowing authors to host the data themselves, requesting that the data be submitted along with the data paper as supplemental files, or requiring the deposit of data in a publicly accessible data repository.

Journals that publish "database papers" describing freestanding databases allow authors to host the databases themselves. That is, *PLoS ONE* and journals published by BioMed Central and SpringerOpen rely on authors to host the described database on a personal or institutional server and to provide a web address for the database within the body of the paper. As a backup, BioMed Central and SpringerOpen journals use the WebCite service to archive the web pages. However, not surprisingly, this strategy often fails,[13] and readers are confronted with dead links and no ability to access the databases that were intended for public use.

Providing greater assurance that the underlying data will remain accessible in the future, some journals require that data files be deposited in a trustworthy, publicly accessible repository at the time of data paper submission or acceptance. These journals can be considered "overlay journals" in that their content overlays material (i.e., data) stored in other locations.[14] For instance, *Scientific Data* provides authors with a list of over seventy recommended data repositories that meet certain requirements for data access, preservation, and stability. Authors are encouraged to use discipline-specific data repositories when available and instructed to use a general repository such as Figshare or Dryad if no appropriate discipline-specific repository exists. In the latter case, *Scientific Data* offers an integrated submission option whereby authors can deposit their dataset into Figshare or Dryad as a step in the data paper submission process, and the journal covers the repository fees for data submission (up to 5 GB in Figshare or 10 GB in Dryad). Similarly, *F1000Research* requires authors to deposit their dataset in a stable, recognized, and open repository and provides a list of journal-approved repositories that allow access to the dataset, ensure its stability and persistence, and enable dataset searching and retrieval. If no appropriate discipline-specific data repository exists, authors of *F1000Research* data papers are instructed to submit their data files directly to the journal, which mediates their deposit into a general repository and crosslinks the data paper and the data files so that the data can be previewed within the article. *Open Health Data* also requires authors to deposit their data in one of several recommended disciplinary, general, or institutional repositories. *Genomics Data* and Frontiers journals state that the data described by a data paper must be deposited in a public repository, but do not recommend particular repositories.

Some data journals provide their own dedicated repositories for hosting the data described in data papers. *Open Health Data* and *Data in Brief* are associated with their own Dataverses, which are web applications developed by Harvard University's Institute for Quantitative Social Science for the sharing and preservation of research data.[15] *Gigascience* also provides its own open data repository called GigaDB, although authors are instructed to submit their data to other repositories when appropriate (e.g., if required or expected by funding agencies or particular scientific communities). Furthermore, data papers published by *Biomedical Data Journal* and the underlying data files are both hosted by the OpenScienceLink platform, which is the outcome of a European Union–funded project that aims to utilize new technologies and procedures to support the more effective, timely, and comprehensive open access to scientific information.[16]

Other journals provide authors with multiple options for providing access to the data described in data papers. Authors of data papers published in *Data in Brief* can submit their data to the journal as supplementary material, deposit their data in the Data in Brief Dataverse, or link to their data in an external public database or repository. *Dataset Papers in Science* and *Data* instruct authors to submit the dataset to the journal as supplementary material and/or to provide information in the data paper on the location of data if deposited in a publicly available repository. For *BMC Research Notes* and several other BMC-series journals, BioMed Central provides authors with 100 MB of free data storage in LabArchives, which is an electronic laboratory notebook system that allows researchers to publicly share data files.[17] Alternatively, these journals will also accept data files as supplementary material or allow authors to deposit data in an external repository with a link to the dataset in the body of data papers. In addition, *Neuroinformatics* requires an "Information Sharing Statement" that explains where and how the data can be accessed (i.e., through a public data repository or database) and accepts data as supplementary material.

Data Containing Sensitive Information

A significant barrier to data sharing among biomedical researchers is their concern about releasing private patient information.[18] However, the sharing of data from human participants is also viewed as important for maximizing the utility of research datasets and enhancing the efficiency of biomedical research and its impact on health-related treatments, technologies, and policies.[19] As the aim of data journals is to describe research datasets that are potentially useful to the broader scientific community, most data journals require that the data are made accessible without restrictions. Only a few data journals speak directly to the issue of protecting data that contain personal information. For instance, the OpenScienceLink platform that hosts the *Biomedical Data Journal* takes the position that personal data should be made fully anonymous, as the destruction of links between datasets and the individuals on which they are based makes datasets exempt from data protection regulations.[20] *GigaScience* recommends the deposit of data into its open GigaDB repository but also allows the deposit of data containing sensitive clinical information into external repositories that provide restricted access. Also, although *Scientific Data* recommends that authors provide open access to their data, they also recognize that sometimes clinical research data cannot be made fully anonymous and therefore cannot be made open access. Therefore, a working group is focusing on establishing a practical approach to allowing detailed descriptions of clinical research datasets to be published without making the full data publicly available.[21]

Code Availability

Beyond the sharing of data, the sharing of computer code and research software is also considered important for promoting the reuse of tools that may be helpful to other researchers and for ensuring the replicability of research results.[22] Many data journals direct authors to provide access to any software or code necessary for viewing, interpreting, or analyzing the data described in data papers. For example, *Open Health Data* states that any specific script or software needed to manipulate the data should be archived and made accessible through a repository, and *Genomics Data* requires that any related software or code be submitted alongside data papers. For studies using custom code to generate or process datasets, *Scientific Data*, *GigaScience*, *F1000Research*, and *BMC Research Notes* expect authors to include a code availability statement explaining how the code can be accessed and requirements for its execution. Also, *Data in Brief* and *Genomics Data* require authors to submit any code used in the analysis of data to the journal as supplementary material or to a data repository.

Some data journals also publish stand-alone software papers that describe pieces of research software that may be of broader use to the scientific community. For these types of articles, BioMed Central and SpringerOpen journals state that authors must make the tools freely available to any researcher who wishes to use them for noncommercial purposes without enforcing restrictions such as a material transfer agreement. These journals advise authors of open-source projects to host their project with an open-source repository (e.g., SourceForge) and strongly recommend that authors include a backup copy of the source code as a supplementary file along with the software paper to guarantee its availability in the future. The body of the software paper includes sections describing the specific issue that the software was intended to address, the overall architecture of the software implementation, how its functionality and performance compare with that of previously created software, and the benefits of using the software and any planned future development. *F1000Research* and *GigaScience* also require that the source code for new software described by software papers is made openly and persistently available and encourages authors to upload code to a code repository with version control (e.g., GitHub, BitBucket, or SourceForge). Furthermore, *GigaScience* has its own GitHub page for storing the software described in software papers. Software articles describing publicly accessible research software are also published by *Neuroinformatics* and *PLoS ONE*.

Peer Review

Despite its shortcomings, most researchers consider peer review essential to scholarly communication, providing a "stamp of approval" and improving the quality of publications.[23] Therefore, an important feature of data journals is that nearly all of them employ peer review. Most commonly, both the data paper and the underlying dataset are reviewed to ensure their completeness and technical rigor. However, as the concept and practice of data peer review are still evolving, different data journals take varying approaches to peer review.[24]

For many data journals, the review of data papers differs from that of a traditional research article. The purpose of peer review at *GigaScience* is to assure that the rationale and methods for collecting the data are well described, that the data are of high quality and conform to minimum standards in the field, and that the data can be easily accessed. In addition to external peer reviewers, *GigaScience* data papers are also assessed by an in-house data reviewer who evaluates technical aspects of the data, its documentation, and its availability. Peer review at *Open Health Data* is meant to ensure that the paper adequately describes that data and that the data are openly archived in accordance with best practices. The data paper must sufficiently report how the dataset was created, correctly describe the contents of the dataset, provide concrete suggestions for how the dataset could be reused, and explain any policies for accessing datasets containing sensitive information, if applicable. Also, the underlying dataset must be deposited in a repository that is suitable for the subject matter and that has a satisfactory sustainability model, be accessible without restrictions when appropriate, include nonproprietary file formats when possible, and be thoroughly documented (with understandable column headers, accompanying "readme" files, etc.) so that the data can be understood by others. Likewise, peer review at *Scientific Data* serves to verify that the procedures used to generate the dataset are technically sound, that the dataset has reuse value, and that the description of the dataset is complete. Most data papers in *Scientific Data* are reviewed by at least one expert in the research methods described in the data paper and one expert in data standards. All three of these journals state that data papers should not be evaluated based on the perceived importance or novelty of the findings associated with the data; rather, the purpose of peer review is to confirm the reliability of the techniques used to generate and/or process the data and that enough information is provided to allow other researchers to interpret and reuse the data.

Similarly, peer reviewers of data papers published in Elsevier's *Data in Brief* and *Genomics Data* are asked to judge whether the data are in a standard format, whether the data are well-documented, whether the methods for generating the data are sound, and whether the authors adequately explain how the data might be useful to the scientific community. However, whereas stand-alone data papers submitted to *Data in Brief* are sent to external peer reviewers, data papers submitted as an accompaniment to a research article submitted to another Elsevier journal are reviewed only by the *Data in Brief* editor, who uses the same review criteria described above, assuming that the underlying dataset will be subject to peer review by the other Elsevier journal. Likewise, data papers submitted to *Genomics Data* are reviewed by members of the editorial board but not external peer reviewers.

Biomedical Data Journal, Dataset Papers in Science, Data, F1000Research, PLoS ONE, Frontiers journals, SpringerOpen journals, and most BioMed Central journals provide no explicit information on the peer review process for data papers and how it might differ from that for traditional research articles. However, as *F1000Research, PLoS ONE,* and Frontiers journals employ "non-selective review," a review process that assesses articles based on their scientific quality rather than their perceived importance, novelty, or potential impact, it can be assumed that the peer review of data papers also adheres to this practice.[25]

Redundant Publication

Redundant publication (also known as duplicative publication) is a type of scientific misconduct that can occur when the same results are presented in more than one publication.[26] Therefore, it is important to consider whether a data paper describing a dataset might be redundant with a traditional research article analyzing the same dataset and how this might be viewed by publishers. Several data journals and their publishers have explicitly addressed this issue. *Scientific Data* states that data papers are designed to complement research articles, and Nature-titled journals would not consider a data paper to be a prior publication that would impede subsequent publication of a research article that reports new scientific findings from the same dataset. Frontiers journals also consider data papers complementary to research articles and will link research articles to related data papers. Likewise, Elsevier encourages authors to submit a data paper to *Data in Brief* alongside an associated research article submitted to another Elsevier journal. Furthermore, staff at *F1000Research* confirmed that several major journal publishers (e.g., BioMed Central, BMJ, Lancet, PLoS, Sage) and prominent journals (e.g., *Science, Proceedings of the National Academy of Sciences, New England Journal of Medicine, Journal of Neuroscience*) would not consider a data paper as a prior publication that would prevent the publication of a research article based on the same dataset, although *Annals of Oncology* and journals published by Cell Press would potentially view data papers as prior publications.

Recommended Users

Because data papers add to one's publication record and provide scholarly credit for data sharing, they hold great potential for adoption by researchers who otherwise might not have strong motivation to provide public access to their data. Although any biomedical or health sciences researcher might be interested in publishing data papers, this opportunity might be especially appealing to certain populations of researchers. For example, graduate students and postdoctoral fellows may be particularly good authors of data papers, as these researchers are generally the ones who collect, process, and analyze research data on a daily basis and therefore may be best prepared for describing the data acquisition process and documenting data files so that they are understandable by others. In addition to graduate students and postdoctoral fellows who may be preparing to face a competitive academic job market, assistant professors who face the prospect of receiving tenure may also be interested in expanding their CVs by publishing data papers. Also, as clinical faculty are often expected to engage in scholarship in addition to their patient care and medical education demands,[27] these faculty might be interested in the possibility of doubling their publication output from a single research project—by publishing a traditional research article drawing conclusions from a dataset and then publishing a data paper describing that same dataset for potential use by other researchers. Furthermore, the publication of data papers may be well-suited to researchers who generate "small data" as opposed to "big data."[28] That is, data papers can highlight and describe datasets produced by small-scale studies conducted by individual or small teams of researchers who lack a robust infrastructure supporting data preservation and dissemination (e.g., a single knock-out mouse experiment vs. large-scale astronomy or high-energy physics research projects). Despite its name, "small data" collectively makes up the bulk of research data generated by the scientific community.[29]

Roles for Librarians

Raising Researchers' Awareness of Data Journals

Despite potentially high interest in data journals from researchers, most researchers are unaware of this emerging publication venue. For example, 67 percent of researchers in the atmospheric sciences stated that they would deposit their data in a data repository if they could obtain scholarly credit through a data journal.[30] However, a recent survey of scientists across disciplines revealed that only 16 percent could name a specific data journal.[31] Therefore, librarians could play an important role in raising researchers' awareness of data journals as an avenue of data dissemination.

Health sciences and medical librarians could rely on already established routes of communication to introduce data journals to researchers, such as departmental newsletters, presentations at faculty meetings, and informal conversations with individual faculty members and research trainees. As most data journals are open access and require open access to the data described in data papers, information about data journals could be incorporated into various Open Access Week activities, such as those described by Johnson.[32] Furthermore, attempts to raise awareness of data journals could easily be integrated into the research data services already provided by many academic libraries. For example, librarians could tell researchers about data journals during consultations on data management or sharing plans for grant applications, during "data interviews" to understand researchers' data management needs, and during the ingest of research datasets into institutional data repositories.[33] Furthermore, librarians could bring attention to data papers as a way to disseminate research data during data management training aimed at graduate students, such as that developed by librarians at Massachusetts Medical School and Worcester Polytechnic Institute.[34]

To capture the interest of researchers, librarians may wish to convey the following key points about data journals.

- *Data papers are easy to write.* Data papers are generally brief, and many data journals provide article templates that are simple to complete.
- *Data papers are peer reviewed.* Because data papers are typically peer reviewed, they can be listed on CVs just like traditional research articles. Thus, publishing a data paper can transform the act of data sharing into scholarship.
- *Data papers can facilitate data discovery.* Data journals are often indexed in major article databases, such as PubMed, Web of Science, and Scopus, meaning that data papers and their associated datasets can be found by other researchers.
- *Data papers can be cited.* Data papers can be cited just like traditional journal articles, enabling authors to track the reuse of their data and allowing data paper citations to contribute to one's h-index.
- *Data papers can enhance research productivity.* Many journals do not view data papers as a redundant publication, meaning that researchers can publish both a research article and a data paper from the same dataset.

Assisting with Data Preparation

One of the major barriers to widespread data sharing is that preparing datasets for public release is time-consuming.[35] Pressed for time, many researchers clean, organize, and document their data only to an extent that permits their own analysis. In practice, therefore, many research datasets are "messy," containing errors or missing values, possessing inconsistent file names and contents, and lacking sufficient documentation to allow others to understand or reuse the data. Furthermore, medical research datasets may contain personal identifiers that would need to be removed before the data could be shared outside of the original research team. Health sciences and medical librarians could assist in the creation of data papers by helping researchers prepare their datasets for a wider audience, including scouring the data for missing values or obvious mistakes, renaming files, ensuring that spreadsheet columns have understandable headers, preparing codebooks or "readme" files, and applying metadata standards as required by particular data repositories. For clinical data, librarians could help anonymize datasets by looking for and removing direct and indirect patient identifiers following guidelines proposed by journal editors and statisticians.[36] After having become intimately familiar with the dataset, librarians could also help write relevant portions of the data paper, such as those describing the content and organization of the dataset. By playing a key role in dataset preparation and writing of the data paper, librarians could even be credited as a coauthor on the data paper. Thus, by taking the burden of data preparation off the shoulders of researchers, librarians could play a valuable role in facilitating the dissemination of research data.

Subsidizing Costs of Data Paper Publication and Data Deposit

Another way that health sciences or medical librarians could promote the publication of data papers and the sharing of research data is to take advantage of institutional memberships to subsidize authors' costs of publishing data papers and submitting associated datasets to data repositories. For example, BioMed Central and SpringerOpen offer several tiers of institutional memberships, allowing the institution to cover APCs in full, to split the cost of APCs with authors, or to provide authors with a 15 percent discount on APCs. Hindawi, Frontiers, and PLoS also offer institutional memberships that allow institutions to pay reduced-rate APCs on behalf of affiliated authors. Likewise, some data repositories offer institutional memberships so that institutions can help pay for the costs of data deposit. In particular, the general data repository Dryad allows institutions to purchase reduced-rate vouchers ($65 per data package) that cover researchers' costs of data submission,[37] which is a service that is currently provided by the University of Rochester River Campus Libraries.[38] Similar to the open-access funds established by many academic libraries,[39] becoming an institutional member of data journal publishers and data repositories could be a strategy for helping researchers publish in data journals and thus encouraging open access to data.

Conclusion

Besides providing scholarly credit for data sharing, data papers have several other benefits. Previously described as a "somewhat unfamiliar bundle of scholarly output with a familiar façade,"[40] the concept of data papers will be familiar to researchers due to their similarity to traditional journal articles. As the purpose of data papers is to thoroughly describe datasets, they force researchers to sufficiently document their data so that they can be understood by others. Also, by often encouraging or requiring the deposit of data into data repositories, data journals increase the likelihood of persistent data access. Although data papers also have some drawbacks, such as their reliance on the notoriously slow peer review process and their inability to scale to the accelerating pace at which research data is generated,[41] the publication of data papers may serve as a good stop-gap for incentivizing and mainstreaming the practice of data sharing among researchers. After learning about the data journals serving the biomedical and health sciences communities, academic and medical librarians can promote data sharing by raising researchers' awareness of data journals, helping researchers ready their data for public release, and subsidizing the costs of data paper publication.

Pearls

- Data papers are a type of journal article that call attention to and describe publicly available research datasets that may be useful to the broader scientific community.
- Currently, there are approximately one hundred twenty data journals serving the biomedical and health sciences communities.
- Data papers are generally peer reviewed and can be listed on CVs just like traditional research articles, thus providing an incentive for researchers to share their data.
- Many publishers of data journals encourage or require authors to submit the data described by data papers into an open and trustworthy data repository.
- Librarians can promote data sharing by raising researchers' awareness of data journals, assisting in preparing data for public release, and subsidizing the cost of data paper publication fees.

Recommended Reading and Resources

- *Biomedical Data Journal*, http://www.biomed-data.eu/. The purpose of Procon's *Biomedical Data Journal* is to provide access to biomedical datasets that can be used for the computational modeling of biological processes and diseases. Both the peer-reviewed data papers and the associated data sets are hosted by European Union-funded OpenScienceLink platform (http://openscience link.eu/).
- *Data in Brief*, http://www.journals.elsevier.com/data-in-brief/. Elsevier's *Data in Brief* publishes peer-reviewed or editorially reviewed data in brief articles that describe research data to facilitate research reproducibility. The associated dataset can be deposited in the dedicated Data in Brief Dataverse repository (https://dataverse.harvard.edu/dataverse/dib). Data in Brief articles are also published in Elseiver's *Genomics Data* (http://www.journals.elsevier.com/genomics-data/).
- *Gigascience*, http://www.gigasciencejournal.com/. GigaScience, published by BioMed Central, seeks to "revolutionize data dissemination, organization, understanding, and use." It is a peer-reviewed journal that publishes research articles and data notes describing "big data" studies and datasets in the life and biomedical sciences. The associated data and analysis tools are placed in

a dedicated GigaScience database (GigaDB, http://gigadb.org/), providing a direct link between manuscripts and their supporting data.

- *Open Health Data,* http://openhealthdata.metajnl.com/. Ubiquity Press's *Open Health Data* publishes peer-reviewed data papers describing health datasets with high potential for reuse. The associated datasets can be deposited in the dedicated Open Health Data Dataverse repository (https://dataverse.harvard.edu/dataverse/openhealthdata). In addition to research data, *Open Health Data* encourages the submission of gray literature, including research study protocols, data mangement plans, and consent forms.
- *Scientific Data*, http://www.nature.com/sdata/. Launched by the prestigious Nature Publishing Group, *Scientific Data* is a peer-reviewed journal that publishes data descriptors describing research datasets that are potentially valuable to the scientific community. Covering all fields of natural science, *Scientific Data* aims to "address the increasing need to make research data more available, citable, discoverable, interpretable, resuable, and reproducible".

Notes

1. J Kaye, C Heeney, N Hawkins, J de Vries, and P Boddington. 2009. "Data sharing in genomics—reshaping scientific practice." *Nature Reviews Genetics* 10; PN Schofield, T Bubela, T Weaver, L Portilla, SD Brown, JM Hancock, D Einhorn, G Tocchini-Valentini, M Hrabe de Angelis, N Rosenthal, and CASIMIR Rome Meeting participants. 2009. "Post-publication sharing of data and tools." *Nature* 461; HA Piwowar and WW Chapman. 2008. A review of journal policies for sharing research data. In *Open Scholarship: Authority, community, and sustainability in the age of Web 2.0. Proceedings of the 12th International Conference on Electronic Publishing (ELPUB), June 25-27 2008, Toronto, Canada.* http://elpub.scix.net/data/works/att/001_elpub2008.content.pdf.
2. CJ Savage and AJ Vickers. 2009. "Empirical study of data sharing by authors publishing in PLoS journals." *PLoS ONE* 4:e7078.
3. AA Alsheikh-Ali, W Qureshi, MH Al-Mallah, and JPA Ioannidis. 2011. "Public availability of published research data in high-impact journals." *PLoS ONE* 6:e24357.
4. KG Akers and JA Green. 2014. "Towards a symbiotic relationship between academic libraries and disciplinary data repositories: A Dryad and University of Michigan case study." *International Journal of Digital Curation* 9:119–131; D Fearon, B Gunia, S Lake, BE Pralle, and AL Sallans. 2013. Research Data Management Services (SPEC Kit No. 334).
5. C Tenopir, S Allard, K Douglass, AU Aydinoglu, L Wu, E Read, M Manoff, and M Frame. 2011. "Data sharing by scientists: Practices and perceptions." *PLos ONE* 6:e21101; V Rathi, K Dzara, CP Gross, I Hrynaszkiewicz, S Joffe, HM Krumholz, KM Strait, and JS Ross. 2012. "Sharing of clinical trial data among trialists: A cross sectional survey." *The BMJ* 345:e7570; Y Kim, and JM Stanton. 2012. "Institutional and individual influences on scientists' data sharing practices." *Journal of Computational Science Education* 3:47–56; Akers, KG, and J Doty. 2013. "Disciplinary differences in faculty research data management practices and perspectives." *International Journal of Digital Curation* 8(2):5–26.
6. JE Kratz and C Strasser. 2015. "Researcher perspectives on publication and peer review of data." *PLoS ONE* 10:e0117619.
7. I Hrynaszkiewicz and D.G. Altman. 2009. "Towards agreement on best practice for publishing raw clinical trial data." *Trials* 10:17; TH Vines, RL Andrew, DG Bock, MT Franklin, KJ Gilbert, NC Kane, J-S Moore, BT Moyers, S Renaut, DJ Rennison, T Veen, and S Yeaman. 2013. "Mandated data archiving greatly improves access to research data." *The FASEB Journal* 27:1304-1308; AJ Vickers. 2006. "Whose data set is it anyway? Sharing raw data from randomized trials." *Trials* 7:15.
8. V Chavan and L Penev. 2011. "The data paper: A mechanism to incentivize data publishing in biodiversity science." *BMC Bioinformatics* 12(Suppl 15):S2; K Gorgolewski, DS Marguiles, and MP

Milham. 2013. "Making data sharing count: a publication-based solution." *Frontiers in Neuroscience* 7:1–7; B Fecher, S Friesike, and M Hebing. 2015. "What drives academic data sharing?" *PLoS ONE* 10:e0118053.
9. V Chavan and L Penev. 2011. "The data paper: A mechanism to incentivize data publishing in biodiversity science." *BMC Bioinformatics* 12(Suppl 15):S2; J Rees. 2010. Recommendations for independent scholarly publication of data sets; K Gorgolewski, DS Marguiles, and MP Milham. 2013. "Making data sharing count: a publication-based solution." *Frontiers in Neuroscience* 7:1–7; JL Breeze, J-B Poline, and DN Kennedy. 2012. "Data sharing and publishing in the field of neuroimaging." *GigaScience* 1:9; I Mourouzis and C Pantos. 2015. "The Biomedical Data Journal in the new era of open access to scientific information." *Biomedical Data Journal* 1:5–11.
10. JE Kratz and C Strasser. 2015. "Researcher perspectives on publication and peer review of data." *PLoS ONE* 10:e0117619.
11. L Candela, D Castelli, P Manghi, and A Tani. 2015. "Data journals: A survey." *Journal of the Association for Information Science and Technology* Published online ahead of print.
12. J Beall. 2014. "Chinese publisher MDPI added to list of questionable publishers." http://scholarlyoa.com/2014/02/18/chinese-publishner-mdpi-added-to-list-of-questionable-publishers.
13. Dellavalle, RP, EJ Hester, LF Heilig, AL Drake, JF Kunztman, M Graber, and LM Schilling. 2003. "Going, going, gone: Lost internet references." *Science* 302:787-788.
14. B Lawrence, C Jones, B Matthews, S Pepler, and S Callaghan. 2011. "Citation and peer review of data: Moving towards formal data publication." *International Journal of Digital Curation* 6(2):5–37; S Callaghan, F Hewer, S Pepler, P Hardaker, and A Gadian. 2009. "Overlay journals and data publishing in the meterological sciences." *Ariadne* 60.
15. M Crosas. 2011. "The Dataverse network: An open-source application for sharing, discovering and preserving data." *D-Lib Magazine* 17:1–2.
16. D Eisinger, G Tsatsaronis, A Petrova, E Karanastasis, V Andronikou, and E Chondrogiannis. 2015. "OSL Platform: A link to open-access scientific information and structured data." *Biomedical Data Journal* 1:52–54.
17. I Hrynaszkiewicz, ML Norton, AJ Vickers, and DG Altman. 2010. "Preparing raw clinical data for publication: Guidance for journal editors, authors, and peer reviewers." *BMJ* 340:c181.
18. KG Akers and J Doty. 2013. "Disciplinary differences in faculty research data management practices and perspectives." *International Journal of Digital Curation* 8(2):5–26.
19. S Brown Trinidad, SM Fullerton, JM Bares, GP Jarvik, EB Larson, and W Burke. 2010. "Genomic research and wide data sharing: Views of prospective participants." *Genetics in Medicine* 12:486–495; T Lang. 2011. "Advancing global health research through digital technology and sharing data." *Science* 331:714–717; HM Krumholz. 2012. "Open science and data sharing in clinical research: Basing informed decisions on the totality of the evidence." *Circulation: Cardiovascular Quality and Outcomes* 5:141–142.
20. S Hugelier. 2015. "Publishing open-access biomedical data: legal challenges." *Biomedical Data Journal* 1:43–51.
21. Hrynaszkiewicz, I. 2014. "Trialling a pragmatic approach to clinical data disclosure." http://blogs.nature.com/scientificdata/2014/11/27/trialling-a-pragmatic-approach-to-clinical-data-disclosure/.
22. A Prlic and JB Procter. 2012. "Ten simple rules for the open development of scientific software." *PLoS Computational Biology* 8:e1002802; Nature Editorial. 2014. "Code share." *Nature* 514:536.
23. A Mulligan, L Hall, and E Raphael. 2013. "Peer review in a changing world: An international study measuring the attitudes of researchers." *Journal of the American Society for Information Science and Technology* 84:132-161; D Nicholas, A Watkinson, HR Jamali, E Herman, C Tenopir, R Volentine, S Allard, and K Levine. 2015. "Peer review: Still king in the digital age." *Learned Publishing* 28:15–21.
24. B Lawrence, C Jones, B Matthews, S Pepler, and S Callaghan. 2011. "Citation and peer review of data: Moving towards formal data publication." *International Journal of Digital Curation* 6(2):5–37;

J Kratz and C Strasser. 2014. "Data publication consensus and controversies [v3; ref status: indexed, http://f1000r.es/4ja]." *F1000Research* 3:94.
25. R Walker and P Rocha da Silva. 2015. "Emerging trends in peer review—a survey." *Frontiers in Neuroscience* 9:169.
26. V Yank and D Barnes. 2003. "Consensus and contention regarding redundant publications in clinical research: Cross-sectional survey of editors and authors." *Journal of Medical Ethics* 29:109-114.
27. RA Young, MJ Dehaven, C Passmore, and JG Baumer. 2006. "Research participation, protected time, and research output by family physicians in family medicine residencies." *Family Medicine* 38:341–348; DM Rubio, BA Primack, GE Switzer, C Bryce, DL Seltzer, and WN Kapoor. 2011. "A comprehensive career-success model for physician-scientists." *Academic Medicine* 86:1571–1576.
28. AR Ferguson, JL Nielson, MH Cragin, AE Bandrowski, and ME Martone. 2014. "Big data from small data: Data-sharing in the 'long tail' of neuroscience." *Nature Neuroscience* 17:1442–1448; V Chavan and L Penev. 2011. "The data paper: A mechanism to incentivize data publishing in biodiversity science." *BMC Bioinformatics* 12(Suppl 15):S2.
29. PB Heidorn. 2008. "Shedding light on the dark data in the long tail of science." *Library Trends* 57:280–299.
30. S Callaghan, F Hewer, S Pepler, P Hardaker, and A Gadian. 2009. "Overlay journals and data publishing in the meterological sciences." *Ariadne* 60.
31. JE Kratz and C Strasser. 2015. "Researcher perspectives on publication and peer review of data." *PLoS ONE* 10:e0117619.
32. PC Johnson. 2014. "International Open Access Week at small to medium U.S. academic libraries: The first five years." *Journal of Academic Librarianship* 40:626–631.
33. J Carlson. 2012. "Demystifying the data interview." *Reference Services Review* 40:7–23.
34. E Martin, T Leger-Hornby, and D Kafel. 2012. "Frameworks for a data management curriculum: Course plans for data management instruction to undergraduate and graduate students in science, health sciences, and engineering programs." http://library.umassmed.edu/data_management_frameworks.pdf
35. JE Kratz and C Strasser. 2015. "Researcher perspectives on publication and peer review of data." *PLoS ONE* 10:e0117619.
36. I Hrynaszkiewicz, ML Norton, AJ Vickers, and DG Altman. 2010. "Preparing raw clinical data for publication: Guidance for journal editors, authors, and peer reviewers." *BMJ* 340:c181.
37. KG Akers and JA Green. 2014. "Towards a symbiotic relationship between academic libraries and disciplinary data repositories: A Dryad and University of Michigan case study." *International Journal of Digital Curation* 9:119–131.
38. University of Rochester River Campus Libraries. 2014. "River Campus Libraries partner with Dryad repository to offer vouchers." http://www.library.rochester.edu/news/dryad.
39. CD Eckman and BT Weil. 2010. "Institutional open access funds: Now is the time." *PLoS Biology* 8:e1000375.
40. J Kunze, T Cruse, R Hu, S Abrams, K Hastings, C Mitchell, and L Schiff. 2011. Practices, trends, and recommendations in technical appendix usage for selected data-intensive disciplines. http://escholarship.org/uc/item/9jw4964t.
41. MA Parsons and PA Fox. 2013. "Is data publication the right metaphor?" *Data Science Journal* 12:WDS32-WDS46.

Bibliography

Akers, KG, and J Doty. 2013. "Disciplinary differences in faculty research data management practices and perspectives." *International Journal of Digital Curation* 8(2):5–26.

Akers, KG, and JA Green. 2014. "Towards a symbiotic relationship between academic libraries and disciplinary data repositories: A Dryad and University of Michigan case study." *International Journal of Digital Curation* 9:119–131.

Akers, KG, FC Sferdean, NH Nicholls, and JA Green. 2014. "Building support for research data management: biographies of eight research universities." *International Journal of Digital Curation* 9:171–191.

Alsheikh-Ali, AA, W Qureshi, MH Al-Mallah, and JPA Ioannidis. 2011. "Public availability of published research data in high-impact journals." *PLoS ONE* 6:e24357.

Beall, J. 2014. "Chinese publisher MDPI added to list of questionable publishers." http://scholarlyoa.com/2014/02/18/chinese-publishner-mdpi-added-to-list-of-questionable-publishers.

Breeze, JL, J-B Poline, and DN Kennedy. 2012. "Data sharing and publishing in the field of neuroimaging." *GigaScience* 1:9.

Brown Trinidad, S, SM Fullerton, JM Bares, GP Jarvik, EB Larson, and W Burke. 2010. "Genomic research and wide data sharing: Views of prospective participants." *Genetics in Medicine* 12:486–495.

Callaghan, S, F Hewer, S Pepler, P Hardaker, and A Gadian. 2009. "Overlay journals and data publishing in the meterological sciences." *Ariadne* 60.

Candela, L, D Castelli, P Manghi, and A Tani. 2015. "Data journals: A survey." *Journal of the Association for Information Science and Technology* Published online ahead of print.

Carlson, J. 2012. "Demystifying the data interview." *Reference Services Review* 40:7–23.

Chavan, V, and L Penev. 2011. "The data paper: A mechanism to incentivize data publishing in biodiversity science." *BMC Bioinformatics* 12(Suppl 15):S2.

Crosas, M. 2011. "The Dataverse network: An open-source application for sharing, discovering and preserving data." *D-Lib Magazine* 17:1–2.

Dellavalle, RP, EJ Hester, LF Heilig, AL Drake, JF Kunztman, M Graber, and LM Schilling. 2003. "Going, going, gone: Lost internet references." *Science* 302:787–788.

Eckman, CD, and BT Weil. 2010. "Institutional open access funds: Now is the time." *PLoS Biology* 8:e1000375.

Eisinger, D, G Tsatsaronis, A Petrova, E Karanastasis, V Andronikou, and E Chondrogiannis. 2015. "OSL Platform: A link to open-access scientific information and structured data." *Biomedical Data Journal* 1:52–54.

Fearon, D, B Gunia, S Lake, BE Pralle, and AL Sallans. 2013. Research Data Management Services (SPEC Kit No. 334).

Fecher, B, S Friesike, and M Hebing. 2015. "What drives academic data sharing?" *PLoS ONE* 10:e0118053.

Ferguson, AR, JL Nielson, MH Cragin, AE Bandrowski, and ME Martone. 2014. "Big data from small data: Data-sharing in the 'long tail' of neuroscience." *Nature Neuroscience* 17:1442–1448.

Gorgolewski, K, DS Marguiles, and MP Milham. 2013. "Making data sharing count: a publication-based solution." *Frontiers in Neuroscience* 7:1–7.

Heidorn, PB. 2008. "Shedding light on the dark data in the long tail of science." *Library Trends* 57:280–299.

Hrynaszkiewicz, I. 2014. "Trialling a pragmatic approach to clinical data disclosure." http://blogs.nature.com/scientificdata/2014/11/27/trialling-a-pragmatic-approach-to-clinical-data-disclosure/.

Hrynaszkiewicz, I. 2012. "LabArchives and BioMed Central: A new platform for publishing scientific data." http://blogs.biomedcentral.com/bmcblog/2012/04/04/labarchives-and-biomed-central-a-new-platform-for-publishing-scientific-data/.

Hrynaszkiewicz, I, and D.G. Altman. 2009. "Towards agreement on best practice for publishing raw clinical trial data." *Trials* 10:17.

Hrynaszkiewicz, I, ML Norton, AJ Vickers, and DG Altman. 2010. "Preparing raw clinical data for publication: Guidance for journal editors, authors, and peer reviewers." *BMJ* 340:c181.

Hugelier, S. 2015. "Publishing open-access biomedical data: legal challenges." *Biomedical Data Journal* 1:43–51.

Johnson, PC. 2014. "International Open Access Week at small to medium U.S. academic libraries: The first five years." *Journal of Academic Librarianship* 40:626–631.

Kaye, J, C Heeney, N Hawkins, J de Vries, and P Boddington. 2009. "Data sharing in genomics—reshaping scientific practice." *Nature Reviews Genetics* 10:331–335.

Kim, Y, and JM Stanton. 2012. "Institutional and individual influences on scientists' data sharing practices." *Journal of Computational Science Education* 3:47–56.

Kratz, J, and C Strasser. 2014. "Data publication consensus and controversies [v3; ref status: indexed, http://f1000r.es/4ja]." *F1000Research* 3:94.

Kratz, JE, and C Strasser. 2015. "Researcher perspectives on publication and peer review of data." *PLoS ONE* 10:e0117619.

Krumholz, HM. 2012. "Open science and data sharing in clinical research: Basing informed decisions on the totality of the evidence." *Circulation: Cardiovascular Quality and Outcomes* 5:141–142.

Kunze, J, T Cruse, R Hu, S Abrams, K Hastings, C Mitchell, and L Schiff. 2011. Practices, trends, and recommendations in technical appendix usage for selected data-intensive disciplines. http://escholarship.org/uc/item/9jw4964t.

Lang, T. 2011. "Advancing global health research through digital technology and sharing data." *Science* 331:714–717.

Lawrence, B, C Jones, B Matthews, S Pepler, and S Callaghan. 2011. "Citation and peer review of data: Moving towards formal data publication." *International Journal of Digital Curation* 6(2):5–37.

Martin, E, T Leger-Hornby, and D Kafel. 2012. "Frameworks for a data management curriculum: Course plans for data management instruction to undergraduate and graduate students in science, health sciences, and engineering programs." http://library.umassmed.edu/data_management_frameworks.pdf

Mourouzis, I, and C Pantos. 2015. "The Biomedical Data Journal in the new era of open access to scientific information." *Biomedical Data Journal* 1:5–11.

Mulligan, A, L Hall, and E Raphael. 2013. "Peer review in a changing world: An international study measuring the attitudes of researchers." *Journal of the American Society for Information Science and Technology* 84:132–161.

Nature Editorial. 2014. "Code share." *Nature* 514:536.

Nicholas, D, A Watkinson, HR Jamali, E Herman, C Tenopir, R Volentine, S Allard, and K Levine. 2015. "Peer review: Still king in the digital age." *Learned Publishing* 28:15–21.

Parsons, MA, and PA Fox. 2013. "Is data publication the right metaphor?" *Data Science Journal* 12:WDS32-WDS46.

Piwowar, HA, and WW Chapman. 2008. A review of journal policies for sharing research data. In *Open Scholarship: Authority, community, and sustainability in the age of Web 2.0. Proceedings of the 12th International Conference on Electronic Publishing (ELPUB), June 25–27 2008, Toronto, Canada*. http://elpub.scix.net/data/works/att/001_elpub2008.content.pdf.

Prlic, A, and JB Procter. 2012. "Ten simple rules for the open development of scientific software." *PLoS Computational Biology* 8:e1002802.

Rathi, V, K Dzara, CP Gross, I Hrynaszkiewicz, S Joffe, HM Krumholz, KM Strait, and JS Ross. 2012. "Sharing of clinical trial data among trialists: A cross sectional survey." *The BMJ* 345:e7570.

Rees, J. 2010. Recommendations for independent scholarly publication of data sets.

Rubio, DM, BA Primack, GE Switzer, C Bryce, DL Seltzer, and WN Kapoor. 2011. "A comprehensive career-success model for physician-scientists." *Academic Medicine* 86:1571–1576.

Savage, CJ, and AJ Vickers. 2009. "Empirical study of data sharing by authors publishing in PLoS journals." *PLoS ONE* 4:e7078.

Schofield, PN, T Bubela, T Weaver, L Portilla, SD Brown, JM Hancock, D Einhorn, G Tocchini-Valentini, M Hrabe de Angelis, N Rosenthal, and CASIMIR Rome Meeting participants. 2009. "Post-publication sharing of data and tools." *Nature* 461:171–173.

Tenopir, C, S Allard, K Douglass, AU Aydinoglu, L Wu, E Read, M Manoff, and M Frame. 2011. "Data sharing by scientists: Practices and perceptions." *PLos ONE* 6:e21101.

University of Rochester River Campus Libraries. 2014. "River Campus Libraries partner with Dryad repository to offer vouchers." http://www.library.rochester.edu/news/dryad.

Vickers, AJ. 2006. "Whose data set is it anyway? Sharing raw data from randomized trials." *Trials* 7:15.

Vines, TH, RL Andrew, DG Bock, MT Franklin, KJ Gilbert, NC Kane, J-S Moore, BT Moyers, S Renaut, DJ Rennison, T Veen, and S Yeaman. 2013. "Mandated data archiving greatly improves access to research data." *The FASEB Journal* 27:1304–1308.

Walker, R, and P Rocha da Silva. 2015. "Emerging trends in peer review—a survey." *Frontiers in Neuroscience* 9:169.

Yank, V, and D Barnes. 2003. "Consensus and contention regarding redundant publications in clinical research: Cross-sectional survey of editors and authors." *Journal of Medical Ethics* 29:109–114.

Young, RA, MJ Dehaven, C Passmore, and JG Baumer. 2006. "Research participation, protected time, and research output by family physicians in family medicine residencies." *Family Medicine* 38:341–348.

Chapter 5

Data Science

NEW LIBRARIAN ROLES FOR A NEW FIELD OF RESEARCH

Lisa Federer, National Institutes of Health Library

In 2014, a researcher named Nathan Han presented findings from his research on how mutations in tumor suppressor genes lead to cancer. Specifically, he developed a computer program that could look at mutations in cancer-related genes and determine whether they would be benign or induce cancer. What makes this story most interesting, though, is not what Nathan discovered, but the fact that he was fifteen years old and accomplished all of it using publicly available data.[1] The availability of a vast amount of biomedical research data, combined with new technologies that make it easier, cheaper, and faster to analyze data than ever before, have revolutionized the way that science is practiced and led to a new field of research termed data science. This chapter will provide an overview of data science, including its goals and methods, and discuss how librarians can support researchers conducting data science.

What Is Data Science?

In the 2009 collection *The Fourth Paradigm: Data-Intensive Scientific Discovery*, computer scientist Jim Gray argues that advanced computational technologies have substantively changed the practice of scientific research. Whereas the world's first scientists took an empirical approach, attempting to explain how and why the world works by observing natural phenomena, today's researchers rely on computers to capture, create, and analyze data. Gray suggests that the "techniques and technologies for such data-intensive science are so different that it is worth distinguishing data-intensive science from computational science as a new, *fourth paradigm* for scientific exploration," which he terms "eScience."[2]

It would be difficult to argue with Gray's claim that technology has changed science. Indeed, much of the scientific research conducted today simply couldn't be done without computers and other technology. When it comes to biomedical research in particular, it's hard to imagine research without computers. Despite this reliance on new technologies, by and large, modern researchers still use the same scientific method that the earliest researchers followed: they form a hypothesis, they gather data to test that hypothesis, they analyze the data, and they come to a conclusion about the hypothesis based on the results.

I argue that data science is distinct from what Gray calls eScience in that it differs from traditional science in other significant ways. Data science does follow the traditional scientific method in many regards and relies on the type of sound statistical methods that are the hallmark of good science in general. However, in practice, data science differs from other types of research in several key ways. Many data scientists do not gather or generate their own data; instead, they leverage a wealth of existing data from a variety of sources. Indeed, data science is only possible because we are generating data at an unprecedented rate. These data are often gathered for reasons entirely unrelated to the purposes for which data scientists eventually use them, yet the availability of such data makes it possible for data scientists to query and analyze the data to make new discoveries.

Another distinction of data science is that data scientists may not have developed a specific hypothesis a priori. Instead of forming a hypothesis and making observations that will either prove or disprove that hypothesis, data scientists may start with a dataset of interest and analyze it with the purpose of discovering what knowledge the data may hold. For example, a data scientist may have epidemiologic data about many thousands of patients and analyze the data to identify patterns of similarity that may yield information about disease mechanisms or prognostic factors, without necessarily knowing in advance what those patterns might be.

Because of these differences, training for data scientists differs from the course of education that other types of researchers may follow. In addition, data science researchers have unique information needs because they conduct their research and interact with data in such different ways than their more traditionally grounded peers. Understanding these needs is essential for librarians who aim to support this type of research.

The Era of Big Data

Data science, of course, requires data—and a great deal of it. The term "big data" is frequently tossed around as a buzzword with little in the way of clear meaning or definition, intended to refer to a large amount of data without necessarily specifying just *how* big data have to be in order to be considered "big data." However, meaningful definitions do exist and can be helpful in thinking about how and why big data must be addressed using different strategies than "small data." Big data is frequently described by the three V's: volume, velocity, and variety.[3]

Volume refers to the amount or size of data, though there is no single agreement on the exact size that distinguishes big data. Rather, data can be considered big when it is "beyond the ability of traditional relational databases to capture, manage, and process the data."[4] The Library of Congress's (LC) Twitter archive provides a useful example of why volume matters in terms of our technological capacity to deal with data. In 2010, LC announced it would begin archiving all tweets posted to the social media site Twitter.[5] Though tweets themselves are only up to 140 characters, nearly half a billion tweets are posted each day, resulting in a massive dataset of billions upon billions of tweets. Three years into the project to archive tweets, LC could not yet allow researchers to access the archive because existing technologies could not yet handle such a vast amount of data; a single search of the archive could take days to complete. As LC's report on the project notes, "technology to allow for scholarship access to large data sets is not nearly as advanced as the technology for creating and distributing that data."[6]

Velocity refers to the speed at which data are generated or collected. Big data can be defined as data that are generated much more quickly than they can be analyzed. For example, the Large Hadron Collider, a particle accelerator used for physics experimentation, generates about 25 GB of data per second.[7] The data generated by a single experiment can take months to analyze and involves the work of scientists around the world. At present, our capability to generate data frequently far outpaces the rate at which we can analyze it.

Finally, variety refers to the diverse types and sources of data that comprise big data. Datasets aren't just spreadsheets containing rows and columns of numbers, but may comprise images, video, audio, unstructured free text, results from sensors—indeed, it is now possible to gather information about the world around us to an almost infinite extent. As sensors have grown smaller and cheaper, we are surrounded by them every day in the form of our smartphones, wearable devices such as Fitbits, and monitoring devices such as city traffic cameras. Taken together, all of these diverse streams of data provide a complex and rich view of the world, but finding ways to easily combine and leverage so many different types of data into one meaningful message can be challenging.

The opportunities and challenges that big data presents are especially evident in the world of biomedical research. Genome sequencing technology has significantly contributed to the amount and types of data available for researchers to analyze. By the time the first human genome was sequenced in 2003, it took more than ten years and nearly $3 billion to accomplish the task;[8] today, the cost of sequencing a human genome is in the thousands of dollars,[9] and it can be done in just over a day.[10] In addition, the widespread adoption of electronic health records (EHRs) means that a vast amount of patient data now exists in digital form, with potentially significant implications for research.[11] However, while EHRs represent a valuable data source, the challenges of using such data ethically and with adequate safeguards in place to protect patients' privacy currently limit researchers' ability to use such data in practice.[12]

Biomedical big data has given rise to several fields of study referred to collectively as the omics; researchers in these fields aim to understand the overall structure and function of molecules in organisms. For example, genomics entails the study of an organism's entire genetic sequence, with the goal of elucidating how variations in the sequence outwardly manifest themselves in the organism, while proteomics involves the analysis of proteins' structure and function. These and other omics fields necessarily call for large amounts of data; many individuals must be studied in order to draw conclusions that can be generalized across an entire species. In order to facilitate omics research, a number of large data repositories exist for researchers to share the data they have gathered and locate other data that may be useful for their analysis. The National Center for Biotechnology Information (NCBI), a branch of the National Library of Medicine (NLM) administers a variety of such repositories containing genomic and other omics-related data.[13]

Biomedical big data also makes it possible to conduct research in precision medicine, which involves study of how genetic variations contribute to human health and disease. Once the genetic mechanisms of an illness or condition are understood, targeted therapies can be developed and delivered to patients based on their individual genetic profile. For example, the drug Herceptin (trastuzumab) binds to human epidermal growth factor receptor 2 (HER2), so it is used in the treatment of breast cancer when the tumors overexpress the HER2 gene.[14] As with the omics, precision medicine research relies on big data, requiring information from many thousands of patients.

These examples hint at the many possible applications of data science in the biomedical realm. As we continue to generate more and more data through the course of biomedical research, data science methods and techniques can help generate additional knowledge from these existing data. Especially as data sharing becomes more common, data scientists will have more and more opportunities to leverage publicly available data for their research.

The Data Science Pipeline

Though there are a variety of different specific data science methods, data scientists typically follow a common set of procedures regardless of their end goal, often referred to as the data science pipeline. Just as there are many different ways of visualizing and explaining the research data life cycle, there are also different ways of describing the process and methodology for data science. One useful model is a pipeline that includes five steps: data ingestion, data munging and wrangling, computation and analysis, modeling and application, and reporting and visualization.[15] This pipeline describes the full process of applying data science, from obtaining data to describing one's findings. As with research data life-cycle models, scientists do not always follow the steps in this process in a linear fashion; frequently the process is iterative.

DATA INGESTION

Data exist in many places in a variety of diverse forms, and finding and obtaining the data that will be the raw input of the data science process can be a challenging task. Data scientists working in some settings may be supplied with the data that their employer has collected and wishes for them to analyze. However, for biomedical data scientists, it is rarely the case that they are provided the data they need. Instead, they must locate a dataset that is appropriate to their needs. Just as clinical scientists must ensure they enroll enough patients in their study to achieve adequate statistical power to draw conclusions about the whole population and not just the sample, data scientists must likewise locate a dataset (or combine multiple datasets) with an adequate number of observations or data points to make it possible to draw statistically significant and generalizable results. While a great deal of data is freely available to the public, datasets that contain potentially sensitive patient information may be available only upon request and only once the requestor has demonstrated that their methods and data storage plans will adequately protect the subjects of the data. Even finding a dataset on the topic of interest to the data scientist may be challenging, given that there is no method at present for easily searching across multiple repositories or data sources.

Once an appropriate data source is located, the necessary data must then be acquired, a process referred to as "ingestion." For small datasets, acquiring the data may be as simple as downloading a single spreadsheet or database, but acquiring larger and more complex data is not a trivial task. When downloading large or multiple datasets, it is often possible to obtain the files through a web application processing interface (API), rather than downloading individual files manually. When data sources have an API, a researcher can write a simple program that will connect to the API, request the desired data, download it, and ingest it into a local database or directly into the program that will be used for analysis. Using an API can be especially useful when data acquisition will be an ongoing process, as in cases where data are still being actively collected. Rather than manually downloading new data every time the dataset is updated, the program can automatically retrieve new data and add it to the dataset for ongoing analysis. When sites do not have an API, it may still be possible to obtain data through web scraping, which involves writing programs to automatically find, harvest, download, parse, and save data. These methods are only a few of the many ways that data can be acquired either manually or through automated processes; techniques may vary depending on the type and source of the data.

DATA MUNGING AND WRANGLING

Even when a data scientist has been able to find and acquire data that address a question of interest, those data are typically not in the form necessary for the data scientist to complete his or her analysis. Data collectors arrange their data in a way that makes sense to them, based on their reasons for collecting and using the data, the programs they use, and their personal preferences. Data scientists typically intend to use the data for an entirely different reason and in a different context than the original data collector, so they should expect that it will be necessary to modify the data, sometimes in significant ways, to arrive at a dataset that meets their needs. Indeed, this step of the data science pipeline is usually the most time- and labor-intensive, often comprising around 80 percent of the entire process.

Many different terms are used, often interchangeably, for describing the variety of processes involved in preparing the data for analysis. The data munging or wrangling process can be defined as "chang[ing], in a series of well-specified and reversible steps, a piece of original data to a completely different (and hopefully a more useful) one."[16] Put another way, this process is about "taking a messy or unrefined source of data and turning it into something useful."[17] This process may involve changing file formats (for example, changing an Excel file to the more easily parsed comma separated value or CSV format); merging or combining multiple datasets; finding and removing duplicate, outlier, or erroneous data; standardizing data, particularly when multiple datasets are merged (such as converting measurements in feet to meters); or subsetting data in order to work only with specific data of interest. The steps and processes necessary depend highly on the state of the original data and the format needed for analysis.

COMPUTATION AND ANALYSIS

Data analysis involves the use of statistical techniques and tests to make inferences and conclusions about the dataset. Frequently analysis involves hypothesis testing. For example, a data scientist analyzing a dataset containing demographic, diagnostic, and prognostic data about cancer patients, such as the Surveillance, Epidemiology, and End Result (SEER) dataset,[18] may hypothesize that older age is negatively correlated with survival time after diagnosis. Depending on characteristics of the data (such as whether or not it follows a normal distribution) and the types of hypotheses being tested, the data scientist would select an appropriate statistical test and analyze the data accordingly.

MODELING AND APPLICATION

A major goal of data science is to draw useful and actionable conclusions using data. Once data have been analyzed, models can be generated to use the data to make predictions or understand patterns. For example, a researcher may wish to determine whether a drug will be beneficial to patients based on specific characteristics of their genetic sequence. By considering how other patients have responded to the drug and analyzing their genetic sequences, the researcher can predict other patients for whom the drug may be helpful (or conversely, those for whom the drug may actually be deleterious). It may also be possible to locate patterns in data that help explain mechanisms behind disease, such as identifying that cancer incidence is higher in populations living in areas with high levels of air particulate pollution. A variety of statistical models exist to help scientists understand relationships among variables, find patterns in data, and make predictions about the future based on past data.

REPORTING AND VISUALIZATION

As with any scientific field, data scientists report their findings, often in the form of peer-reviewed articles in journals either specific to statistics and analysis or in journals specifically related to the topic of their analysis (such as biomedical journals, in the case of biomedical data science). Because of the data-intensive nature of this science, visualizations are often employed to more easily demonstrate the findings of an analysis or model. Data visualization can be an effective means of conveying information about big data, particularly when it involves complex relationships or large datasets (see chapter 10 for further discussion of data visualization).

Tools of the Trade

A wide variety of computational tools exist to enable data scientists to accomplish the techniques described above. Most data scientists rely on one or more programming languages to accomplish their work, rather than point-and-click programs, as programming has a variety of advantages over such programs. Many analytic software packages are very expensive, with licenses costing thousands or even tens of thousands of dollars. On the other hand, the software needed to run programming languages is usually free and open source. Conducting analyses with a programming language also means that every step of the process is completely documented in code. If point-and-click software is used, no such documentation is created, unless the user does so by hand. For example, if a variable needs to be recoded, such as from "no" to 0, in order to facilitate analysis, it's possible to use the find and replace function in Excel to do so. However, the user must write documentation to note that this change has been made and that the value of 0 is equivalent to "no." Writing a script to make this change is also very easy, and all that's needed to document this change is saving the code. Because code can be easily saved, it's also easy to reproduce or repeat whatever wrangling or analyses were done. This repeatability is especially helpful when the same functions will be repeated multiple times. For example, if the same wrangling processes need to be done across multiple datasets, code can be written once and deployed multiple times across all the datasets, whereas in a point-and-click program, it would be necessary to manually make all the changes to all the datasets.

Many programming languages are available and frequently used in the data science community. The choice of which programming language to use can depend on a variety of factors, such as the types of analyses to be conducted (some programming languages may have better developed features or be faster for certain applications), the specific field of research (some disciplines may tend to favor one programming language), the size of the data (some programming languages struggle to handle extremely large datasets), and simple personal preference. While there are many options, R[19] and Python[20] are the most frequently used languages in the context of data science, with Julia[21] also gaining some popularity.

While it may seem intimidating to learn a programming language at first, especially to people who don't have a significant background or formal training in computer science, the programming languages used in the data science community are very approachable for beginners. Because they are used by a large and active open-source community, these languages are well documented and frequently updated. In addition to the thousands of books available on both general learning and highly specific applications of these languages, many free, online learning resources are available (see the Recommended Resources at the end of this chapter).

The Librarian's Role in Data Science

As described throughout this entire book, librarians have a wide variety of skills and expertise that make them excellent collaborators and assistants to researchers engaged in data-intensive science. These skills also make them very useful to data scientists. Because data science is a relatively new and emerging field, many opportunities exist for librarians to help data scientists develop their skills and potentially partner with them to help them accomplish their research objectives.

Data Management and Curation

Though data scientists are typically trained in the techniques to wrangle and analyze their data, they may not have extensive experience in best practices for data management and curation. As its name implies, data science involves keeping track of a great deal of data, in addition to the code and scripts used to wrangle and analyze it, the visualizations created as part of the research process, and other data and files. Many data scientists could benefit from assistance with devising workflows for organizing all of these research materials in a manageable and efficient manner. In addition, data scientists may also need advice about long-term curation of their data.

Many librarians have also learned one or more programming languages in order to provide more in-depth assistance to their users, especially with the wrangling stage of the process. While being proficient in a programming language is not completely essential for supporting data science research, librarians who have these skills can be a valuable resource to researchers, able to provide training, consultations, and other support. Just as it is helpful, though not essential, for a subject specialist librarian to be conversant in the research techniques and methodologies employed by the researchers they support, librarians who support data science research may find that learning a programming language will further enhance their ability to provide meaningful assistance to their users.

Finding Data for Reuse and Analysis

As described above, finding the raw data needed to conduct data science analyses can be difficult because of the lack of a single federated search resource for searching across multiple data repositories. Especially for data scientists who are trained in computational methods, but do not have an extensive background in the biomedical sciences, figuring out where to locate data can be frustrating and time consuming. Just as librarians become familiar with the bibliographic databases that will be most relevant to their user group, librarians who anticipate working with data scientists may wish to familiarize themselves with the repositories that contain data that could be of use to these users. In the absence of a federated repository search, sources that provide information about available repositories, such as re3data.org (the Registry of Research Data Repositories) can be helpful for at least narrowing down the search to a repository that is likely to contain the type of data a user needs.[22]

Facilitating Data Sharing

While data scientists typically do not generate their own data, relying instead on existing datasets, they often create new, aggregated datasets that could be of use to other researchers. Data scientists frequently combine multiple datasets for their analyses, drawing on several different data sources to find new meaning in previously unconnected datasets. Creating these new datasets can require a great deal of time and effort, so sharing the combined data can be of great benefit to the research community. Like other researchers, many data scientists are not familiar with the mechanisms for sharing data and may be unaware of how best to make their data publicly available. Librarians who have expertise in preparing data for sharing, familiarity with appropriate repositories and other sharing mechanisms, and experience in working with researchers on sharing data can be a valuable resource to data scientists who have data to share.

Conclusion

With the dawn of the age of big data and the greater public availability of those data, researchers have access to more raw data than at any other time in history. Though data science is still relatively new, the existing methods have the potential to allow researchers to draw knowledge out of that big data, and new methods hold the promise of even more powerful tools for finding meaning. As this nascent field continues to progress, librarians have exciting opportunities to work with data scientists to facilitate their work.

Pearls

- While similar to traditional science and other types of data-intensive science, data science is unique in its processes and methods.
- Most data science research follows an iterative process of data ingestion, wrangling, analysis, modeling, and visualization and reporting.
- Data science techniques can be used to identify patterns in data and make predictions about how similar populations will behave in the future.
- Data scientists can benefit from the assistance of librarians, particularly with regard to data management, finding data, and sharing their newly created datasets.

Recommended Reading and Resources

The following courses and resources may be useful for librarians interested in learning more about data science methods and processes:

- Data Science specialization: this ten-course specialization series offered through Coursera uses the programming language R and provides an overview of multiple data science processes, including statistical analysis, modeling, and visualization. Available at https://www.coursera.org/specializations/jhu-data-science
- Data Carpentry: though intended to be delivered through in-person instruction, several lesson modules are available online for self-study. Available at http://www.datacarpentry.org/lessons/.
- Code Academy: free, interactive resource for learning to code in a variety of languages, including Python. Available at https://www.codecademy.com

Notes

1. Student Science, "Teen's Cancer Research Scores Big at Intel ISEF Competition," https://student.societyforscience.org/article/teen%E2%80%99s-cancer-research-scores-big-intel-isef-competition.
2. Jim Gray, "Jim Gray on Escience: A Transformed Scientific Method," in *The Fourth Paradigm: Data-Intensive Scientific Discovery*, ed. Tony Hey, Stewart Tansley, and Kristin Tolle (Redmond, WA: Microsoft Research, 2009).
3. Greg Laney, "3d Data Management: Controlling Data Volume, Velocity, and Variety," in *Application Delivery Strategies*, ed. META Group (2001).
4. IBM Software, "IBM—Big Data Analytics," http://www-01.ibm.com/software/data/infosphere/hadoop/what-is-big-data-analytics.html.
5. Matt Raymond, "Twitter Donates Entire Tweet Archive to Library of Congress," *News from the Library of Congress*, April 15, 2010, https://www.loc.gov/today/pr/2010/10-081.html.
6. Graeme McMillan, "Huzzah! Library of Congress' Useless Twitter Archive Is Almost Complete . . . but You Can't Read It Yet," http://www.digitaltrends.com/social-media/library-of-congress-useless-twitter-archive-is-almost-complete/.
7. CERN, "Processing: What to Record," http://home.cern/about/computing/processing-what-record.
8. National Human Genome Research Institute, "The Human Genome Project Completion: Frequently Asked Questions," https://www.genome.gov/11006943.
9. Erika Check Hayden, "Is the $1,000 Genome for Real?," *Nature*, January 15, 2014, http://www.nature.com/news/is-the-1-000-genome-for-real-1.14530.
10. Claire Maldarelli, "We Can Now Sequence a Whole Human Genome in 26 Hours," *Popular Science*, September 30, 2015, http://www.popsci.com/scientists-can-now-sequence-whole-genome-in-26-hours.
11. A. Shabo, "The Implications of Electronic Health Record for Personalized Medicine," *Biomed Pap Med Fac Univ Palacky Olomouc Czech Repub* 149, no. 2 (2005).
12. C. Weng et al., "Using EHRs to Integrate Research with Patient Care: Promises and Challenges," *J Am Med Inform Assoc* 19, no. 5 (2012).
13. National Center for Biotechnology Information, "All Resources," http://www.ncbi.nlm.nih.gov/guide/all/.
14. J. Baselga et al., "Adjuvant Trastuzumab: A Milestone in the Treatment of HER-2-Positive Early Breast Cancer," *Oncologist* 11 Suppl 1 (2006).
15. Tony Ojeda et al., *Practical Data Science Cookbook* (Birmingham, UK: Packt Publishing, 2014).
16. Luca Massaron and Alberto Boschetti, "Data Munging," in *Python Data Science Essentials* (Birmingham, UK: Packt Publishing, 2015), 33.

17. Jacqueline Kazil and Katharine Jarmul, *Data Wrangling with Python* (Sebastapol, CA: O'Reilly Media, Inc, 2016), xii.
18. National Cancer Institute, "Surveillance, Epidemiology, and End Results Prorgram," http://seer.cancer.gov.
19. R Core Team, *R: A Language and Environment for Statistical Computing* (Vienna, Austria: R Foundation for Statistical Computing, 2015).
20. Guido van Rossum and Fred L. Drake, *Python Reference Manual* (Virginia: PythonLabs, 2015).
21. Jeff Bezanson et al., " Julia: A Fast Dynamic Language for Technical Computing," *arXiv* (2012).
22. re3data.org Team, "re3data: Registry of Research Data Repositories," http://www.re3data.org/.

Bibliography

Baselga, J., E. A. Perez, T. Pienkowski, and R. Bell. "Adjuvant Trastuzumab: A Milestone in the Treatment of HER-2-Positive Early Breast Cancer." *Oncologist* 11 Suppl 1 (2006): 4–12.

Bezanson, Jeff, Stefan Karpinski, Viral B. Shah, and Alan Edelman. " Julia: A Fast Dynamic Language for Technical Computing." *arXiv* (2012).

CERN. "Processing: What to Record." http://home.cern/about/computing/processing-what-record.

Check Hayden, Erika. "Is the $1,000 Genome for Real?" *Nature*, January 15, 2014, http://www.nature.com/news/is-the-1-000-genome-for-real-1.14530.

Gray, Jim. "Jim Gray on Escience: A Transformed Scientific Method." In *The Fourth Paradigm: Data-Intensive Scientific Discovery*, edited by Tony Hey, Stewart Tansley and Kristin Tolle. Redmond, WA: Microsoft Research, 2009.

IBM Software. "IBM—Big Data Analytics." http://www-01.ibm.com/software/data/infosphere/hadoop/what-is-big-data-analytics.html.

Kazil, Jacqueline, and Katharine Jarmul. *Data Wrangling with Python*. Sebastapol, CA: O'Reilly Media, Inc, 2016.

Laney, Greg. "3d Data Management: Controlling Data Volume, Velocity, and Variety." In *Application Delivery Strategies*, edited by META Group, 2001.

Maldarelli, Claire. "We Can Now Sequence a Whole Human Genome in 26 Hours." *Popular Science*, September 30, 2015, http://www.popsci.com/scientists-can-now-sequence-whole-genome-in-26-hours.

Massaron, Luca, and Alberto Boschetti. "Data Munging." In *Python Data Science Essentials*. Birmingham, UK: Packt Publishing, 2015.

McMillan, Graeme. "Huzzah! Library of Congress' Useless Twitter Archive Is Almost Complete . . . but You Can't Read It Yet." http://www.digitaltrends.com/social-media/library-of-congress-useless-twitter-archive-is-almost-complete/.

National Cancer Institute. "Surveillance, Epidemiology, and End Results Prorgram." http://seer.cancer.gov.

National Center for Biotechnology Information. "All Resources." http://www.ncbi.nlm.nih.gov/guide/all/.

National Human Genome Research Institute. "The Human Genome Project Completion: Frequently Asked Questions." https://www.genome.gov/11006943.

Ojeda, Tony, Sean Patrick Murphy, Benjamin Bengfort, and Abhijit Dasgupta. *Practical Data Science Cookbook*. Birmingham, UK: Packt Publishing, 2014.

R Core Team. *R: A Language and Environment for Statistical Computing*. Vienna, Austria: R Foundation for Statistical Computing, 2015.

Raymond, Matt. "Twitter Donates Entire Tweet Archive to Library of Congress." *News from the Library of Congress*, April 15, 2010. https://www.loc.gov/today/pr/2010/10-081.html.

re3data.org Team. "re3data: Registry of Research Data Repositories." http://www.re3data.org/.

Shabo, A. "The Implications of Electronic Health Record for Personalized Medicine." *Biomed Pap Med Fac Univ Palacky Olomouc Czech Repub* 149, no. 2 (Dec 2005): suppl 251–58.
Student Science. "Teen's Cancer Research Scores Big at Intel ISEF Competition." https://student.societyforscience.org/article/teen%E2%80%99s-cancer-research-scores-big-intel-isef-competition.
van Rossum, Guido, and Fred L. Drake. *Python Reference Manual*. Virginia: PythonLabs, 2015.
Weng, C., P. Appelbaum, G. Hripcsak, I. Kronish, L. Busacca, K. W. Davidson, and J. T. Bigger. "Using EHRs to Integrate Research with Patient Care: Promises and Challenges." *J Am Med Inform Assoc* 19, no. 5 (Sep–Oct 2012): 684–87.

Chapter 6

Data 101

LEARNING AND KEEPING CURRENT IN DATA MANAGEMENT SKILLS

Abigail Goben and Rebecca Raszewski, University of Illinois-Chicago Health Sciences Library

Most librarians are responsible for developing their own skill sets in order to prepare themselves for providing new services at their institution, and data management has become a new area where librarians can retool. While many of the skills needed directly correlate to library skills, data management offers unique challenges and a new vocabulary to master. This chapter provides overviews of the impetus for data management education and of self-directed learning theories. Application of these theories and recommended resources are reviewed for five areas of research data management self-education: foundational material, hands-on experience, data instruction and information literacy, community awareness and engagement, and looking beyond the library. By identifying their learning style and also the type of material sought, librarians can more effectively target their self-education data management activities.

Driving Policy and Background Literature

For many libraries in the United States, the impetus for developing research data management support came from a new trend emerging from federal funder policies. While biomedical librarians will be familiar with the National Institutes of Health (NIH) Public Access Policy[1] that was set forth in 2008, which requires NIH-funded researchers to deposit finished copies of their articles into PubMed Central, the policy does not address research data as a separate or additional object.

The primary policy change bringing this to the fore came from the National Science Foundation (NSF) two years later,[2] when the various directorates began to universally require a two-page data management plan with all grant applications. This policy was followed by the Office for Science and Technology (OSTP) Memorandum,[3] which instructed federal agencies to expand access to the research they funded, including data. During 2014–2015, responses from many federal agencies to the OSTP have been published.[4] Many expand upon their present data policies and practices, like the NIH response.[5]

While these policies can be identified as specific drivers, the interest and focus in research data and the increasing role for librarians has been emerging over the past decade in response to overall changes in research and the scholarly communication landscape. Christine Borgman's book,

Scholarship in the Digital Age: Information, Infrastructure, and the Internet,[6] is a foundational work in this area, providing a thorough overview and evaluating how research has been changing in the twenty-first century. Borgman's audience, which includes librarians, other information professionals, and the general research community, is confronting changing policies and social issues surrounding the research enterprise. Her book provides a framework of policies and practices around research that are evolving and what changes will need to be adopted.

Anna Gold and Dorothea Salo provide the librarian's perspective and identify emerging opportunities to engage with the framework Borgman has established. Gold's two-part article[7] identified a rising focus on cyberinfrastructure and big data, and outlines emerging areas for librarians' skills to be applied including bioinformatics, archival datasets, social science, and geographic information systems (GIS). Salo[8] approached the topic from the reskilling perspective—shifting librarian mindsets from carefully curated digital collections in the face of a poorly managed research data onslaught. While raising concerns regarding staffing and funding models, as well as the cultural shift, Salo is emphatic that these are roles librarians can and should embrace.

An Overview of Self-Directed Learning

Librarians who need to develop their data management skills will be practicing aspects of self-directed learning (SDL), an adult education learning theory. SDL has been described as both a learner attribute and as a process. This learning process is usually controlled by the individual, as opposed to an instructor guiding the individual through formalized instruction. SDL is not an all-or-nothing process; every learner will experience different degrees of SDL, whether they are in a traditional lecture-style course led by an instructor or a self-paced module. SDL is also not done in isolation, as self-directed learners may share or discuss what they have learned with others, including an instructor or their peers.[9] SDL is unlike academic learning, which typically moves from the introductory to the more complex in "a systematic stepwise fashion."[10]

The earliest SDL models were linear in design, assuming the learner went through a series of steps to achieve goals. Tough offered the first comprehensive description of SDL and referred to it as "self-planned learning."[11] His study on sixty-six individuals' learning projects found that learners planned 70 percent of all their learning projects. These learners also used thirteen steps that presented key decision-making points about their learning. These steps included decision making on what detailed knowledge and skills to learn; the specific activities, methods, or equipment needed; when to begin the actual learning activities; estimating current level of knowledge, skill, or progress; and taking steps to increase motivation for learning.[12]

Knowles, who is known for the adult learning theory andragogy theory, based his assumptions about adult learners on SDL.[13] The adult learner's maturity would guide the individual into being self-directed. Knowles's principles of andragogy also focused on SDL by involving the adult learners in planning and evaluating their instructions. This is because adult learning is usually problem centered rather than content oriented, which means instead of learning content in a particular subject area, their learning is more skills focused. Their experience provides the basis for their learning activities, and adults are mostly interested in subjects that are relevant to their job or personal life. His description of self-directed learning had six steps: climate setting, diagnosing learning needs, formulating learning goals, identifying human and material resources for learning, choosing and implementing appropriate learning strategies, and evaluating learning outcomes.[14]

Interactive models about SDL developed later and primarily focused on the learning process. Spear and Mocker interviewed seventy-eight self-directed learners, who had not completed high school requirements, about their self-education experiences.[15] Spear and Mocker discovered that instead of SDL being preplanned, it came from opportunities from the learner's own environment, past or new knowledge, or chance occurrences. SDL usually took place based on circumstances that may have influenced how they organized their learning. These SDL projects may occur from information gathered from one activity that may apply to another.[16] Unlike the linear theories presented in this chapter, Spear thought that a successful learning project would involve taking different learning activities and putting them together to determine what is the most important to what has been learned.[17]

Another example of an interactive SDL model is by Brockett and Hiemstra, whose framework for understanding self-directed learning has been modified over time.[18] The Personal Responsibility Orientation (PRO) model was "designed to recognize both the differences and similarities between SDL as an instructional method and learner self-direction as a personality characteristic."[19] The model both distinguishes between the SDL process and the individual learner and acknowledges how they are used together in SDL. Personal responsibility is seen as the model's central concept, and individuals are viewed as owning their thoughts and actions. Although the individual may not have control of the environment, the individual has control of her response as a learner and the responsibility for accepting the consequences of the actions as a learner. In 2012, Brockett and Hiemstra reconfigured and updated their framework, renaming it the Person Process Context (PPC) Model.[20] In the PPC model, the person, process, and context intersect with self-directed learning being in the middle, making sure all three are equally important, even if one of these will have a greater role in the individual's self-education. The context refers to the environment and sociopolitical climate. Making the context equivalent to the process and the person makes the PPC model distinct from the PRO model.

The last example is Garrison's Model, which has three overlapping dimensions: self-management (task control), self-monitoring (cognitive responsibility), and motivation (entering and task). Self-management situates the learners within the social context and is the degree to which the learners assume control of the environment so they can meet their goals. It also involves the learners' management of their learning materials. Self-management is not done in isolation; it is seen as a collaborative experience between the teachers and learners. Self-monitoring is the ability of the learners to monitor their cognitive and metacognitive processes associated with reflective practice and critical thinking. They are taking responsibility for their learning, integrating their new-found skills with their previous knowledge. Motivation is what keeps learners engaged in self-directed learning. Within the learners' motivations, Garrison differentiates "between the process of deciding to participate (entering motivation) and the effort required to stay on task and persist (task motivation)."[21] Learners should internalize the tasks and goals that are given to them for their own needs.

SDL has also been specifically studied in the workplace. One example is Clardy's research on vocationally oriented SDL projects (VO SDLP).[22] These projects could be influenced by either the employee's motivation or organizational factors. Clardy interviewed fifty-six employees from six different kinds of organizations. Out of the 109 learning projects that were mentioned, 90 projects met the criteria of a VO SDLP. Four types of projects were identified: induced, synergistic, voluntary, and scanning. An induced VO SDLP occurs due to performance job standards, such as needing to learn a new system to do one's job. Voluntary VO SDLPs are based on the employee's own initiative instead of a work requirement. Synergistic VO SDLPs can happen from a combination of the employee's motivation to learn and the workplace's influence. A scanning VO SDLP is defined as ongoing searching for information as a way to keep current.

It is advantageous for librarians to identify the style that is most closely aligned with their preferred learning method in order to most successfully engage in self-education. Once they have identified their style, librarians can choose from the formats and resources mentioned below and determine the learning opportunities that will best meet their needs.

Foundational Data Management Skills

For many librarians, a broad overview and introduction to data management is necessary to help frame future self-education. A number of introductory opportunities exist for librarians. While the majority of opportunities in this section are freely available, ideas for those seeking to develop a formalized, data management specialization will also be covered. The opportunities covered in this section can apply to either linear or interactive SDL models.

Several curricula have been developed as educational tools for librarians seeking self-education, as well as lesson plans in a more classroom-type structure for background and foundational information. These resources provide an introduction to the data life cycle, data management plans, and best practices. It should be noted that these curricula were originally developed several years ago, and there has been a large amount of change in funding agency and institutional policies in the interim. While updated material has been added to some curricula, such as additional case studies, the efficacy of these curricula is slightly lessened in this respect. The NIH-funded New England Collaborative Data Management Curriculum (NECDMC)[23] and the NSF-funded DataOne Curriculum[24] both grew in response to the NSF data management plan requirement. Another excellent curriculum is MANTRA from the UK.[25]

The Lamar Soutter Library at University of Massachusetts Medical School, which cocreated and manages the NECDMC, has become a leader in educating librarians on data management and training librarians in teaching data management. Additionally, since 2009, they have sponsored the University of Massachusetts and New England Area Librarian e-Science Symposium[26] and hosted the e-Science Portal. The symposium's goal is for librarians to understand federal research funding agencies' data management policies, help them gain skills for managing human research data, and see examples of how universities developed their institutional data repositories. Archived presentation materials and videos are available.[27] The Lamar Soutter Library also hosts an e-Science Portal,[28] which draws together subject experts to provide a curated compilation of resources across data management and the research environment. Librarians who prefer to be self-motivated in their SDL may find that these types of resources and curricula will meet their needs.

Librarians who need more formal data management education should consider a post-baccalaureate or post-master's certificate in data management. Data science certificates are available at schools such as Indiana University, but these types of programs may be geared toward librarians with a background or interest in programming rather than data management. Librarians could also consider contacting a library school to see if they can audit a data management course. These more structured educational opportunities will be appropriate for those who prefer something like Tough's linear model for their SDL.

Those who are seeking a more structured educational opportunity but not a certificate could consider training at the Inter-university Consortium for Political and Social Research, (ICPSR), a unit of the Institute for Social Research at the University of Michigan. ICPSR hosts a fee-based workshop on Curating and Managing Research Data for Re-use.[29] This five-day workshop uses ICPSR social science and United Kingdom Data Archive data collections for case studies, tracking the datasets through data assessment, review, processing, and curation. Attendees also learn about data review and preparation, confidential data management, digital repository requirements, and more.

The Medical Library Association (MLA)[30] has offered several data management continuing education opportunities either for individuals or in a group setting. These opportunities usually provide continuing education credits for those interested in earning Academy of Health Information Professional (AHIP) points. The MLA annual meeting usually has fee-based, continuing education data management courses that may be held before or after the annual meeting. Those who cannot attend the annual meeting may also find data management offerings at MLA chapter meetings. MLA has also sponsored data management webinars that can be viewed at libraries that offer to host the webinars for free. Those who cannot attend in person can view the recordings for a fee. Those seeking group educational activities at their institutions or planning chapter meetings should browse the MLA Educational Clearinghouse,[31] which lists several current data management courses. Librarians may also find additional educational opportunities at conferences held by the Association of College and

Research Libraries (ACRL),[32] the American Library Association (ALA),[33] and the Special Libraries Association (SLA).[34] There may also be regional, data-themed conferences for librarians who cannot attend a national conference.

Learners looking for other online continuing education or who cannot travel for this type of education might consider Library Juice Academy.[35] This vendor offers online professional development courses for librarians that allow them to earn continuing education units. Library Juice Academy offers an asynchronous research data management course that can be completed within a month. When the course is not being offered during a given month, the course can be offered as a special session for a group. This course could meet the needs of a variety of self-directed learners, from those who want a structured class to those who want more of an interactive engagement with their classmates.

Hands-On Data Management

As outlined in the SDL interactive models, part of SDL will lie in participating with research data management actively. This may be accomplished through learning to use tools for data management activities or going through the workflow, which would apply in Clardy's article on VO SDLP. However, what may be most impactful is curating a dataset. Self-educators may find it useful to find a dataset that is particularly meaningful to them to curate and use as their sample through the data life cycle and their self-education process. For librarians, this may mean looking at patron interaction statistics, circulation and electronic resources' usage statistics, or other administrative data that has lasting value and may not presently be regularly analyzed past a routine report. As we have outlined in a recent case study,[36] it is valuable to work through the data life cycle with a library dataset because the librarian has immediate context with the data.

By examining a familiar dataset, librarians are able to engage more confidently with the research data management aspect of the new material and identify with the challenges and questions researchers may face. Using library data can also make it easier to explore software tools without having to also potentially struggle with understanding the context of the data. For librarians learning together in a group with a variety of different areas of subject matter expertise, working with a dataset from the library field creates common ground and helps prevent confusion. Finally, using library data may result in the unexpected benefit of improved workflows for the library staff— librarians who learn from using their own data may be able to improve capture or handling of the data, implement data management far earlier in the pipeline, and prevent inconsistencies or other data analysis issues.

Data Instruction and Information Literacy

During the self-education process or after gaining foundational knowledge, librarians may wish to teach data literacy and research data management skills to students, staff, and faculty. Data Information Literacy (DIL) shares many similarities to information literacy skills that librarians are already using in their teaching. The primary DIL resource is the Data Information Literacy Project,[37] which was developed by librarians at Purdue, the University of Minnesota, the University of Oregon, and Cornell. Their work, funded by the Institute of Museum and Library Services (IMLS), was targeted at creating resources for librarians teaching primarily graduate students and researchers about best practices in both creating and consuming data. The book of case studies that has emerged from the project[38] may be of particular interest to librarians determining what audiences to target or those looking for curriculum ideas. This volume also includes recommendations for assessing DIL instruction.

The Data Management Plan Tool (DMPTool), created consortially and hosted by the California Digital Library, may also be helpful to librarians who are preparing for data instruction.[39] The software was designed to guide researchers through creating a DMP that would meet the new NSF requirements. To that end, it has specific templates for each NSF directorate and also continues to be updated to include templates for the NIH, IMLS, and several other funders and foundations as new policies are adopted. Each template guides the researcher through areas to consider and points out questions they may wish to answer prior to grant submission. Updates including the ability to have multiple authors on a DMP, technological capability to allow universities to link to the DMPTool in order to allow researchers to use their institutional log in, and improved opportunities to share and read DMPs have further enhanced this tool both for researchers and for education. Because there is no limit to the type or number of DMPs that can be created, students can work through examples for different kinds of datasets in a controlled environment and identify areas where further exploration or answers may be needed before tackling formal grant applications.

Engaging with the Community

The data librarian community offers the self-educator the opportunity to participate with literature, societies, conferences, and social media. After gaining foundational knowledge through curriculum or literature, librarians are prepared to engage with current trends, identify new opportunities, and collaborate (or commiserate) with other data librarians about the challenges of working with research data management in the library setting.

Presently, there is no one specific peer-reviewed journal identified as the leader for research data management as a subject of study. Instead, research, case studies, editorials, and book reviews are published in a variety of journals that target science, technology, engineering, and mathematics (STEM) librarians and also scholarly communication librarians. Table 6.1 includes a selection of journals that may be of particular interest to biomedical librarians interested in working with research data management.

A number of professional library organizations have increased their focus on data management as the topic has grown in popularity and importance to the profession. Many host conference sessions, online and in-person education, and listservs or other communication channels that allow the community to engage with each other and collaborate to develop new resources. Among these organizations, the most targeted toward research data management is the Research Data, Access, and Preservation (RDAP)[40] subsection of the Association for Information Science and Technology (ASIS&T). RDAP holds a two-day conference each spring, specifically addressing the needs, emerging opportunities, and challenges for librarians and information professionals focused on research data. The listserv is the other primary outlet for this group. As previously mentioned, MLA also continues to provide continuing education for biomedical librarians working with research data. Other library organizations with groups that address research data management include ACRL, SLA, and the Association of Research Libraries (ARL).[41]

While traditional types of professional engagement like conference attendance and participation in listservs has helped create community, engagement in the data librarian community has also grown through different forms of social media. As these platforms are frequently subject to change, it is challenging to provide a specific list of users or accounts to follow. On Twitter, searching the *#datalibs* hashtag will assist in identification of who is presently discussing this topic. Another project built recently to bring the community together is the DataQ project, which describes itself as "a collaborative platform for answering research data questions in academic libraries."[42] Also sponsored by IMLS, this project brings both common and unusual topics together for review by interested librarians and provides a forum for advice from experts in the field.

Beyond the Library

Though most librarians will be focused on serving their library, the expanding interest in data brings new opportunities for librarians to develop new skillsets and take on new roles working with research

Table 6.1. Journals of Potential Interest

Title	Publisher	Publication Schedule	Publication Model	Website
College & Research Libraries (CRNL)	Association of College and Research Libraries	Bimonthly	Open access	http://crl.acrl.org/site/misc/about.xhtml
D-Lib Magazine	Corporation for National Research Initiatives	Bimonthly	Open access	http://www.dlib.org/
Evidence Based Library and Information Practice (EBLIP)	University of Alberta Learning Services	Quarterly	Open access	http://ejournals.library.ualberta.ca/index.php/EBLIP
International Journal of Digital Curation (IJDC)	University of Edinburgh	Biannually	Open access	http://www.ijdc.net/
Issues in Science & Technology Librarianship (ISTL)	Science & Technology Section of the Association of College and Research Libraries	Quarterly	Open access	http://www.istl.org/
Journal of Academic Librarianship (JAL)	Elsevier	Bimonthly	Subscription	http://www.journals.elsevier.com/the-journal-of-academic-librarianship/
Journal of eScience Librarianship (JESLIB)	University of Massachusetts Medical School	Irregular	Open access	http://escholarship.umassmed.edu/jeslib/
Journal of Librarianship and Scholarly Communication (JLSC)	Pacific University Library	Quarterly	Open access	http://jlsc-pub.org/jlsc/about.html
Journal of the Medical Librarian Association (JMLA)	Medical Library Association	Quarterly	Open access	https://www.mlanet.org/publications/jmla
Medical Reference Services Quarterly	Taylor and Francis	Quarterly	Subscription	http://www.tandfonline.com/loi/wmrs20#.VZQOnflViko
Practical Academic Librarianship	Special Libraries Association Academic Division	Quarterly	Open access	https://journals.tdl.org/pal/index.php/pal/index
Science and Technology Librarianship	Taylor and Francis	Quarterly	Subscription	http://www.tandfonline.com/toc/wstl20/current#.Vct_rbWvHKE

data. Data science (further discussed in chapter 5 of this book) can be broadly defined as an interdisciplinary field that is seeking to identify answers to myriad questions drawing on the increasing amounts of available data. Data visualization (further discussed in chapter 10 of this book) seeks to present data in charts, graphs, and images that provide impact and are easily understood. These fields have specific degree and certificate programs and a defined skill set beyond the research data management targeted in this chapter. However, basic familiarity will be beneficial for those interested in going beyond academia and further understanding the vocabulary of the field.

A librarian looking for a transitional text between librarianship and data science could consider reading *The Accidental Data Scientist.*[43] Working within the framework of librarianship, Affelt identifies the relationship between the two fields and outlines the opportunities for librarians who are interested in further engagement. She also provides vocabulary to clarify the topic. O'Neil and Schutt's text *Doing Data Science: Straight Talk from the Frontline*[44] is another helpful book that provides further foundation in data science. It provides an in-depth outline of the field including practical applications from fields where data science is most heavily used, including finance, engineering, journalism, and data visualization.

After reviewing the literature but perhaps before seeking out a formal program, free or low-cost self-education in the area of Massive Open Online Courses (MOOCs) can provide a bridge between librarianship and data science. Coursera[45] provides free MOOCs on data-related topics from universities, with the fee-based option to receive a certificate upon successful completion of the course. A MOOC like Johns Hopkins's data science specialization[46] may be a consideration for those who want a free or low-cost option outside of formal library education. The specialization, which can be taken for a certification, includes a series of nine monthlong courses, ending with a capstone project. Other course providers include Lynda[47], a fee-based learning website many academic institutions use, and Udacity.[48] These online courses often assume a higher level of statistical knowledge or coding capability than most library-targeted education, so introductory courses in those areas may be needed first.

Finally, as with library professional organizations, there are a number of data-focused professional organizations for engaging with the community and the research. While RDAP, described above, is primarily made up of data librarians, its parent organization ASIS&T spans information science, computer science, technologists, linguists, and educational specialists. The Research Data Alliance (RDA)[49] is an international organization that promotes the cross-disciplinary sharing of data and has Libraries for Research Data Interest Group.

Conclusion

As librarians continue to develop data management services, self-education and continuing education will be important aspects of preparation. Fortunately, traditional library skills will still serve librarians doing this work, and there are many resources that can aid learners who want to gain new skills. After exploring their self-education style and finding the best resources to meet their individual needs, librarians can become part of a rich network of data-interested and or data-supporting librarians.

Pearls

- Identify the best learning style for you as the self-directed learner. This will help you to choose resources that will best meet your needs.
- Choose a combination of both foundational and current/networking.
- Educational opportunities for learning about data management exist in several different formats. These can be taken in person or online.

Recommended Reading and Resources

Borgman, Christine L. 2012. "The Conundrum of Sharing Research Data." *J Am Soc Inf Sci Technol* 63 (3): 1059–78. doi:doi: 10.1002/asi.22634.

Borgman, Christine L. 2015. *Big Data, Little Data, No Data: Scholarship in the Networked World*. Cambridge, MA: MIT Press.

Briney, Kristin. 2015. *Data Management for Researchers: Organize, Maintain and Share Your Data for Research Success*. Exeter, United Kingdom: Pelagic Publishing.

Goben, Abigail, and Rebecca Raszewski. 2015. "The Data Life Cycle Applied to Our Own Data." *Journal of the Medical Library Association: JMLA* 103 (1): 40.

Gold, A. 2007a. "Cyberinfrastructure, Data, and Libraries, Part 1: A Cyberinfrastructure Primer for Librarians." *D-Lib Magazine* 13 (9/10). doi:doi:10.1045/september20september-gold-pt1.

———. 2007b. "Cyber Infrastructure, Data, and Libraries, Part 2." *D-Lib Magazine* 13 (9/10). doi:doi:10.1045/july20september-gold-pt2.

Goodman, Alyssa, Alberto Pepe, Alexander W. Blocker, Christine L. Borgman, Kyle Cranmer, Merce Crosas, Rosanne Di Stefano, et al. 2014. "Ten Simple Rules for the Care and Feeding of Scientific Data." *PLoS Comput Biol* 10 (4): e1003542. doi:10.1371/journal.pcbi.1003542.

Salo, Dorothea. 2010. "Retooling Libraries for the Data Challenge." *Ariadne*, no. 64. http://www.ariadne.ac.uk/issue64/salo.

Notes

1. National Institutes of Health, "Revised Policy on Enhancing Public Access to Archived Publications Resulting from NIH-Funded Research."
2. National Science Foundation, "Dissemination and Sharing of Research Results."
3. Holdren, "Memorandum for the Heads of Executive Departments and Agencies: Increasing Access to the Results of Federally Funded Scientific Research."
4. Whitmire et al., "A Table Summarizing the Federal Public Access Policies Resulting from the US Office of Science and Technology Policy Memorandum of February 2013."
5. National Institutes of Health, "National Institutes of Health Plan for Increasing Access to Scientific Publications and Digital Scientific Data from NIH Funded Scientific Research."
6. Borgman, *Scholarship in the Digital Age*.
7. Gold, A., "Cyberinfrastructure, Data, and Libraries, Part 1: A Cyberinfrastructure Primer for Librarians"; Gold, A., "Cyber Infrastructure, Data, and Libraries, Part 2."
8. Salo, "Retooling Libraries for the Data Challenge."
9. Merriam and Bierema, "Self-Directed Learning."
10. Spear, "Beyond the Organizing Circumstance: A Search for Methodology for the Study of Self-Directed Learning."
11. Tough, *The Adult's Learning Projects: A Fresh Approach to Theory and Practice in Adult Learning*.
12. Merriam and Bierema, "Self-Directed Learning"; Ellinger, "The Concept of Self-Directed Learning and Its Implications for Human Resource Development."
13. Knowles, *The Adult Learner : A Neglected Species*.
14. Spear, "Beyond the Organizing Circumstance: A Search for Methodology for the Study of Self-Directed Learning."
15. Spear and Mocker, "The Organizing Circumstance: Environmental Determinants in Self-Directed Learning."
16. Spear, "Beyond the Organizing Circumstance: A Search for Methodology for the Study of Self-Directed Learning."
17. Merriam, Caffarella, and Baumgartner, "Self-Directed Learning."

18. Brockett and Hiemstra, "A Conceptual Framework for Understanding Self-Direction in Adult Learning."
19. Ibid., 26.
20. Hiemstra and Brockett, "Reframing the Meaning of Self-Directed Learning: An Updated Model."
21. Garrison, "Self-Directed Learning: Toward a Comprehensive Model," 26.
22. Clardy, "Learning on Their Own: Vocationally Oriented Self-Directed Learning Projects."
23. Lamar Soutter Library–University of Massachusetts Medical School, "New England Collaborative Data Management Curriculum."
24. DataONE, "DataONE Education Modules."
25. University of Edinburgh, "MANTRA: Research Data Management Training."
26. "University of Massachusetts and New England Area Librarian E-Science Symposium."
27. University of Massachusetts and New England Area Librarians, *eScience Symposium Channel*.
28. University of Massachusetts Medical School, "E-Science Portal for New England Librarians: A Librarians Link to E-Science Resources."
29. Inter-university Consortium for Political and Social Research, "Course Descriptions."
30. Medical Library Association, "MLA : Home Page."
31. Medical Library Association, "MLA Educational Clearinghouse."
32. American College of Research Libraries, "Association of College & Research Libraries."
33. American Library Association, "American Library Association."
34. Special Libraries Association, "Special Libraries Association."
35. Library Juice Academy, "Library Juice Academy Courses."
36. Goben and Raszewski, "The Data Life Cycle Applied to Our Own Data."
37. "Data Information Literacy."
38. Carlson and Johnston, *Data Information Literacy*.
39. California Digital Library, "Data Management Planning Tool."
40. RDAP, "RDAP: Research Data Access & Preservation Summit."
41. Association of Research Libraries, "Association of Research Libraries."
42. DataQ, "Welcome to DataQ."
43. Affelt, Amy, *The Accidental Data Scientist*.
44. *Doing Data Science*.
45. Coursera, "Coursera—Free Online Courses from Top Universities."
46. Johns Hopkins University, "Launch Your Career in Data Science."
47. Lynda.com, "Lynda.com."
48. Udacity, "Udacity."
49. Research Data Alliance, "RDA-Research Data Sharing without Barriers."

Bibliography

Affelt, Amy. *The Accidental Data Scientist: Big Data Applications and Opportunities for Librarians and Information Professionals*. Medford, NJ: Information Today, Inc., 2015.

American College of Research Libraries. "Association of College & Research Libraries," 2015. http://www.ala.org/acrl/.

American Library Association. "American Library Association," 2015. http://www.ala.org/.

Association of Research Libraries. "Association of Research Libraries." Accessed September 29, 2015. http://www.arl.org/.

Borgman, Christine L. *Scholarship in the Digital Age: Information, Infrastructure, and the Internet*. Cambridge, MA: MIT Press, 2010.

Brockett, Ralph G., and Roger Hiemstra. "A Conceptual Framework for Understanding Self-Direction in Adult Learning." In *Self-Direction in Adult Learning: Perspectives on Theory, Research, and Practice*, 18–33. London: Routledge, 1991.

California Digital Library. "Data Management Planning Tool," 2015. https://dmptool.org/.

Carlson, Jake, and Lisa R. Johnston, eds. *Data Information Literacy: Librarians, Data and the Education of a New Generation of Researchers*. West Lafayette, IN: Purdue University Press, 2015.

Clardy, Alan. "Learning on Their Own: Vocationally Oriented Self-Directed Learning Projects." *Human Resource Development Quarterly* 11, no. 2 (2000): 105–25. doi:10.1002/1532-1096(200022)11:2<105::AID-HRDQ2>3.0.CO;2-5.

Coursera. "Coursera -Free Online Courses from Top Universities," 2015. https://www.coursera.org/.

"Data Information Literacy." Accessed September 29, 2015. http://www.datainfolit.org/.

DataONE. "DataONE Education Modules," November 12, 2012. https://www.dataone.org/education-modules.

DataQ. "Welcome to DataQ," 2015. http://researchdataq.org/.

Ellinger, Andrea D. "The Concept of Self-Directed Learning and Its Implications for Human Resource Development." *Advances in Developing Human Resources* 6, no. 2 (2004): 158–77. doi:10.1177/1523422304263327.

Garrison, D. R. "Self-Directed Learning: Toward a Comprehensive Model." *Adult Education Quarterly* 48, no. 1 (1997): 18–33. doi:10.1177/074171369704800103.

Goben, Abigail, and Rebecca Raszewski. "The Data Life Cycle Applied to Our Own Data." *Journal of the Medical Library Association: JMLA* 103, no. 1 (2015): 40–44. doi:10.3163/1536-5050.103.1.008.

Gold, A. "Cyberinfrastructure, Data, and Libraries, Part 1: A Cyberinfrastructure Primer for Librarians." *D-Lib Magazine* 13, no. 9/10 (2007). doi:10.1045/september20september-gold-pt1.

———. "Cyber Infrastructure, Data, and Libraries, Part 2." *D-Lib Magazine* 13, no. 9/10 (2007). doi:10.1045/july20september-gold-pt2.

Hiemstra, R., and R. G. Brockett. "Reframing the Meaning of Self-Directed Learning: An Updated Model," 155–61. Saratoga Spring, NY: SUNY Empire State College, 2012.

Holdren, John P. "Memorandum for the Heads of Executive Departments and Agencies: Increasing Access to the Results of Federally Funded Scientific Research." *Office of Science and Technology Policy, Executive Office of the [US] President, The White House*, February 22, 2013. http://www.whitehouse.gov/sites/default/files/microsites/ostp/ostp_public_access_memo_2013.pdf.

Inter-university Consortium for Political and Social Research. "Course Descriptions." Accessed September 21, 2015. http://www.icpsr.umich.edu/icpsrweb/content/sumprog/courses.html.

Johns Hopkins University. "Launch Your Career in Data Science," 2015. https://www.coursera.org/specializations/jhudatascience.

Knowles, Malcolm S. *The Adult Learner : A Neglected Species*. 4th ed. Building Blocks of Human Potential. Houston: Gulf Publishing Co, 1990.

Lamar Soutter Library–University of Massachusetts Medical School. "New England Collaborative Data Management Curriculum," 2015. http://library.umassmed.edu/necdmc/index.

Library Juice Academy. "Library Juice Academy Courses." Accessed September 21, 2015. http://libraryjuiceacademy.com/courses.php.

Lynda.com. "Lynda.com," 2015. http://www.lynda.com/.

Medical Library Association. "MLA Educational Clearinghouse." Accessed September 21, 2015. http://cech.mlanet.org/.

———. "MLA : Home Page," 2015. http://mlanet.org/.

Merriam, Sharan B., and Laura L. Bierema. 2014. Adult *Learning: Linking Theory and Practice*. The Jossey-Bass Higher and Adult Education Series. San Francisco: Jossey-Bass.

Merriam, Sharan B., Rosemary S. Caffarella, and Lisa Baumgartner. "Self-Directed Learning." In *Learning in Adulthood: A Comprehensive Guide*. San Francisco: Jossey-Bass, 2007.

National Institutes of Health. "National Institutes of Health Plan for Increasing Access to Scientific Publications and Digital Scientific Data from NIH Funded Scientific Research," February 2015. http://grants.nih.gov/grants/NIH-Public-Access-Plan.pdf.

———. "Revised Policy on Enhancing Public Access to Archived Publications Resulting from NIH-Funded Research," January 11, 2008. http://grants.nih.gov/grants/guide/notice-files/NOT-OD-08-033.html.

National Science Foundation. "Dissemination and Sharing of Research Results." *US NSF—About*, November 30, 2010. http://www.nsf.gov/bfa/dias/policy/dmp.jsp.

O'Neil, Cathy, and Rachel Schutt. *Doing Data Science: Straight Talk from the Frontline*. Sebastopol, CA: O'Reilly Media, 2013.

RDAP. "RDAP: Research Data Access & Preservation Summit," 2015. https://www.asis.org/rdap/.

Research Data Alliance. "RDA-Research Data Sharing without Barriers." Accessed September 21, 2015. https://rd-alliance.org/.

Salo, Dorothea. "Retooling Libraries for the Data Challenge." *Ariadne*, no. 64 (2010). http://www.ariadne.ac.uk/issue64/salo.

Spear, George E. "Beyond the Organizing Circumstance: A Search for Methodology for the Study of Self-Directed Learning." In *Self Directed Learning: Application and Theory*, edited by H. G. Long, 199–222. Athens: University of Georgia Press.

Spear, George E., and Donald W. Mocker. "The Organizing Circumstance: Environmental Determinants in Self-Directed Learning." *Adult Education Quarterly* 35, no. 1 (1984): 1–10. doi:10.1177/0001848184035001001.

Special Libraries Association. "Special Libraries Association." *Special Libraries Association*, 2015. http://www.sla.org/.

Tough, Allen M. *The Adult's Learning Projects: A Fresh Approach to Theory and Practice in Adult Learning*. Austin, TX: Ontario Institute for Studies in Education, 1979. http://ieti.org/tough/books/alp.htm.

Udacity. "Udacity," 2015. https://www.udacity.com/.

University of Edinburgh. "MANTRA: Research Data Management Training," September 10, 2014. http://datalib.edina.ac.uk/mantra/.

"University of Massachusetts and New England Area Librarian E-Science Symposium." Accessed September 17, 2015. http://escholarship.umassmed.edu/escience_symposium/.

University of Massachusetts and New England Area Librarians. *eScience Symposium Channel*, n.d. https://www.youtube.com/user/UMeScienceSymposium.

University of Massachusetts Medical School. "E-Science Portal for New England Librarians: A Librarian's Link to E-Science Resources," 2015. http://esciencelibrary.umassmed.edu/index.

Whitmire, Amanda, Kristin Briney, Amy Nurnberger, Margaret Henderson, Thea Atwood, Margaret Janz, Wendy Kozlowski, Sherry Lake, Micah Vandegrift, and Lisa Zilinski. "A Table Summarizing the Federal Public Access Policies Resulting from the US Office of Science and Technology Policy Memorandum of February 2013," April 9, 2015. http://figshare.com/articles/A_table_summarizing_the_Federal_public_access_policies_resulting_from_the_US_Office_of_Science_and_Technology_Policy_memorandum_of_February_2013/1372041.

Part II

Data Management across the Research Data Life Cycle

More than 90 percent of the R01 grants (the primary funding mechanism for research projects) funded by the National Institutes of Health (NIH) in 2012 were awarded for a period of four or five years.[1] In other words, the vast majority of biomedical researchers who receive NIH funding will be actively working with their project's data for up to five years. Moreover, the NIH's current NIH Grants Policy Statement stipulates that data must be retained for at least three years following the end of grant funding.[2] As new data sharing policies emerge from journals and funders, it is increasingly likely that researchers will have to retain and share data for an even longer period. Thus, a researcher who begins a project is taking on a commitment to care for their data for close to a decade—or more.

Especially for researchers who do not have extensive experience or training in data management, the thought of having to steward their data for such a long period of time can be intimidating. As part I of this collection demonstrates, librarians have skills and expertise that can make them invaluable partners for researchers who need guidance on how to manage, curate, preserve, and share their data. Part II provides examples from librarians who have developed and provided services meeting a diverse range of researcher needs.

In thinking about the many tasks that must be done to successfully maintain a dataset for a decade or more, it can be useful to break down the process into its various parts. Research data life cycle models are helpful for understanding what tasks must be conducted at various stages in the research process. Many different models exist, and though all differ slightly in how they describe the various stages of the life cycle process, most begin with a pre-project planning stage, then follow the data from its creation or collection through the analysis phase, ending with the disposition of data after the active research phase is complete. The typical model includes the following phases and activities (or variations thereof):

- Pre-project planning: writing a data management plan (DMP); devising data workflows; determining whether data already exist and can be reused; identifying appropriate standards for data format and description; planning for how the data will eventually be archived or stored, including determining costs of long-term preservation

- Data collection or generation: gathering, locating, or creating data; ensuring that data are adequately documented and described using an accepted metadata standard; organizing data and files; maintaining security and privacy of data
- Data analysis and visualization: conducting statistical and other analyses of data; documenting analyses, such as by writing scripts or code; creating exploratory and publication-ready visualizations; producing documentation of findings, such as peer-reviewed journal articles or presentations
- Data sharing: anonymizing or de-identifying sensitive data; depositing data in a suitable repository, such as a subject-specific, institutional, or general repository; publishing data in a data journal; producing persistent unique identifiers to facilitate data citation, such as digital object identifiers (DOIs) or Archival Resource Keys (ARKs)
- Data preservation: migrating formats as file types and physical storage media become obsolete; conducting ongoing curation to ensure data accessibility; ensuring long-term data security

Though many of the models display these stages in some sort of a linear or circular fashion, in practice, the process is often iterative, with researchers conducting activities from multiple stages of the life cycle at the same time, or following the progression of stages in a different order than what a model may demonstrate.

It is also important to emphasize that most data life cycle models do not end when active collection and analysis is complete. In light of new data management and sharing requirements, researchers cannot simply put their data aside and forget about them. In today's research ecosystem, the expectation exists that data will be available, discoverable, and accessible well after the project is done. Long-term preservation of data is an active process, and one with which researchers may need significant assistance.

Data life cycle models can be useful not only in conceptualizing the tasks that must be done throughout a research project, but also in helping libraries determine how to strategically develop a program of support for data management. When planning for new services, it may be helpful for librarians to consider what activities in the data life cycle are already supported, and where needs are going unmet in the institution. For example, some institutions have robust institutional repositories where researchers can share and store data; in such cases, libraries might wish to focus on other stages of the data life cycle that are not as well supported. Thinking about services through the lens of the data life cycle model can also help libraries promote their services and find appropriate partners at their institution, such as the Office of Sponsored Research (or the institution's equivalent).

Many libraries anchor their data services on support for writing DMPs. In many ways, DMP support is the low-hanging fruit of data services; researchers are required to write DMPs and are likely to need assistance in interpreting new DMP policies and complying with them, so providing this support is a logical first step for libraries. The DMP writing stage may also be the ideal phase of the research process at which to provide services, helping researchers determine how best to organize and manage their data before they collect it, not after. Melissa Ratajeski, Carrie Iwema, and Andrea Ketchum discuss their library's DMP services in chapter 7, as well as sharing common themes in library DMP services from their interviews with other librarians providing such support.

In many libraries, DMP support is only one of an entire suite of services offered in support of research data management. Researchers often need support across the entire research data life cycle, not just in the pre-project planning stage. In chapter 8, Lisa Zilinski, Abigail Goben, and Kristen Briney describe how librarians can provide a variety of services and offer training for researchers that will help them work more effectively with their data at every step of the research process.

In designing a comprehensive suite of services to support research data management, it is important for librarians to consider not only the entirety of the research data life cycle, but also to remember that data may come in many different shapes and sizes. While a great deal of attention is paid to "big data," researchers who work with smaller and less complex datasets also have data management needs and could benefit from the support of library services. In his discussion of data services in chapter 9, Steven Braun describes the concept of "scholarship at scale," emphasizing that one-size-fits-all approaches may not adequately address the varied needs of the research community at a given institution, where researchers may have a wide range of unique and specialized needs. Of course, it would be impossible to provide highly customized services for every researcher's special case, but careful planning of services can ensure support for a range of different needs that is still sustainable and scalable.

Given the broad range of services that libraries may provide in support of their researchers' unique needs, librarians may be called upon to put their skills to use in new and unexpected ways. In chapter 10, Marci Brandenburg and Justin Joque provide a brief background on data visualization and describe how libraries can provide support for data visualization. Though researchers may not think of the library as a place to look for help with data visualization, or even data management in general, librarians often have a great deal of expertise and can provide valuable assistance and services in this and other areas.

As the chapters in this section demonstrate, librarians have a wealth of opportunities to engage with researchers in new and exciting ways. The authors of these chapters exemplify how librarians can successfully work with researchers throughout the entire research data life cycle, providing services in support of a wide variety of needs. Depending on a librarian's specific expertise and interests, and the needs of researchers at the institution, the possibilities for supporting research data management are broad.

Notes

1. Sally Rockey to Rock Talk, 2013, https://nexus.od.nih.gov/all/2013/11/07/how-long-is-an-r01/.
2. National Institutes of Health, "NIH Data Sharing Policy and Implementation Guidance," http://grants.nih.gov/grants/policy/data_sharing/data_sharing_guidance.htm.

Bibliography

National Institutes of Health. "NIH Data Sharing Policy and Implementation Guidance." http://grants.nih.gov/grants/policy/data_sharing/data_sharing_guidance.htm.

Rockey, Sally. "How Long Is an R01?" In *Rock Talk*, 2013.

Chapter 7

Library Support for Data Management Plans

Carrie L. Iwema, Melissa A. Ratajeski, and Andrea M. Ketchum, Health Sciences Library System, University of Pittsburgh

As more funders begin to require data management plans (DMPs), libraries are stepping up to assist researchers with creating them. This chapter briefly defines and discusses DMPs, including the benefits of creating one (even when not specifically required to do so), why they are necessary components of grant proposals both currently and in the near future, the availability of an online tool that guides the generation of DMPs, and insights from fourteen academic/biomedical libraries that currently provide DMP support services. This information is intended to spark ideas and provide practical approaches as librarians develop or enhance DMP services at their home institutions.

What Is a DMP?

Definition

A Data Management Plan (DMP) is a formal document that outlines how the researcher will handle the research output, in the form of data, both *during* the data collection phase and *after* the research project is completed. The term "data" is quite broad, covering multiple types of sources and formats including:[1]

- Observational: captured in real time, usually outside of a lab, and irreplaceable. Examples include surveys and study types such as case-control, cohort, cross-sectional, and longitudinal.
- Experimental: data from clinical trials or lab equipment, often expensive to reproduce. Examples include magnetic field readings and double-blind or randomized control trials.
- Simulation: generated from test models and metadata, where input is often more critical than output. Examples include disease spread, climate, or economic models.
- Derived/Compiled: created from existing data, time-consuming and expensive to reproduce. Examples include 3D models and text/data mining.
- Formats: text, audiovisual, numeric, computer code, which may be instrument-specific and discipline-specific.

DMP Mandates

The White House Office of Science and Technology Policy (OSTP) issued a six-page memorandum on February 22, 2013, directing each federal agency with over $100 million in annual research and development expenditures to develop a Public Access Plan to increase the access to results of federally funded scientific research.[2] Among other requirements, each federal agency's plan must

> ensure that all extramural researchers receiving Federal grants and contracts for scientific research and intramural researchers develop data management plans, as appropriate, describing how they will provide for long-term preservation of, and access to, scientific data in digital formats resulting from federally funded research, or explaining why long-term preservation and access cannot be justified.

This memorandum will significantly increase the number of researchers required to write a data management plan for grant submissions, as many agencies currently have no such requirements. The National Science Foundation (NSF) is one of the few major funders to do so, having required a two-page DMP for full proposals since January 18, 2011.[3] Recently, several agencies are starting to release their own Public Access Plans.[4] Particularly noteworthy is the National Institutes of Health (NIH); this major granting agency for biomedical research released its access plan in February 2015.[5] It states that NIH will "ensure that all NIH-funded researchers prepare data management plans and that the plans are evaluated during peer review."

While all federal agencies were expected to finalize their requirements by the end of 2015, as of publication of this chapter, no date for implementation has been set for the NIH's plan. Current data-related requirements mandated by the NIH include a Data Sharing Policy from 2003[6] requiring that researchers awarded $500,000 or more a year must submit a data sharing plan explaining how the research data will be shared or why it cannot be shared. The Genomic Data Sharing Policy from 2014[7] requires that researchers receiving NIH funding for genomic research develop data sharing plans and submit their data to a central repository to facilitate sharing.

DMP Components

Components typically included in a DMP are:

- types, formats, methods, and amount of data collected;
- documentation of process and coding sheets or data dictionaries needed for interpretation; and
- policies for storage, access, use and distribution, preservation, and archiving of data.

A DMP should clearly describe how data will be created or captured, as well as any standards applied, such as metadata used to describe data; software used to create or analyze the data; and any other information necessary for file accessibility, interoperability, and reproducibility. Coordinating these details in advance saves time and effort and avoids unforeseen complications during the data submission process for a journal or into a repository. Additional consideration must be given to human subject data, including de-identification, management of consent forms, and secure archival processes.[8]

DMP Benefits

Whether or not a DMP is required for grant submission, it is best practice to write one for each project. Doing so benefits the research group, collaborators, and potentially the scientific community at large.[9] Although writing a DMP requires time and energy up front, ultimately making plans can save researchers time in the long run by providing an outline and strategy for handling data management concerns before they become impediments. DMPs simplify research, facilitate data sharing and preservation, decrease the chances of data loss, promote replicability, and extend the life of research. From the perspective of the researcher, crafting a DMP also prevents duplication of effort in terms of saving time, resources, and energy, as each member of the research team is clear on their role in managing, documenting, and protecting the data.[10]

How Libraries Can Help with DMPs

According to an Online Computer Library Center (OCLC) report on university-wide research data management policy[11] libraries "may be the most appropriate place on campus for safe, sustained, and trusted stewardship of research data," thanks to librarians' experience with information management, archiving and preservation, metadata, copyright and privacy issues, storage and preservation, managing repositories, and controlled/open access. In a survey on the effect of data management requirements of research and teaching faculty, sponsored programs office staff, and institutional repository librarians, Diekema and colleagues report there is "an important knowledge gap that libraries appear to be well positioned to fill."[12]

Since data management is a new and emerging role for many libraries,[13] we contacted librarians working in academic institutions known to be actively providing data management services to discover their current practices, specifically in terms of DMP support. These librarians were asked to provide answers to the following five questions:

1. Who is your target audience?
2. Briefly describe your service.
3. What worked?
4. What didn't work?
5. What would you change?

We asked respondents to focus their answers specifically on DMP-related practices, rather than the myriad additional data management services profiled elsewhere in this book.

Responses were received from librarians who provide data management support for academic and health sciences researchers at fourteen different institutions. These included Brown University, James Madison University, National Institutes of Health (NIH), Oregon Health Sciences University (OHSU), Oregon State University, University of California-Los Angeles (UCLA), University of Massachusetts, University of Michigan, University of Minnesota, University of Oregon, University of Tennessee-Knoxville, University of Virginia, and Virginia Commonwealth University (VCU). A full list of the librarians who responded is available in the acknowledgment section at the conclusion of this chapter. In the following sections, we describe the experiences of these librarians as well as our own work at the University of Pittsburgh. We quote the contributing librarians as much as possible in order to capture their experience and expertise in their own words.

Target Audience

It can be difficult to generalize the target audience in a large academic research community, as there are many varieties of patrons, hierarchies, and research types, requiring broad communication skills and flexibility. The majority of respondents indicated that DMP support tends to be focused on faculty and principle investigators (PIs) who are required to write DMPs as part of grant submissions, typically in an academic medical center or health sciences institution. For example, L. Johnston (U Minnesota) noted that current support is primarily for PIs writing DMPs for NSF grants, although the library is "monitoring the changes at other agencies with intentions to expand," which reinforces that keeping track of grant requirements is an active process, since there are numerous granting agencies and therefore numerous requirements that can change over time. Y. Shorish (James Madison U) expressed hope that working on data management issues with faculty members will result in a "'trickle down' to their instruction in their classrooms." A few respondents mentioned that postdoctoral fellows, students, and staff may also require DMP assistance, and that DMPs can be written not just as part of a grant, but also as a standard data management practice.

DMP-specific Library Services

Academic and health sciences libraries are offering a great deal of support for DMPs, as indicated by the variety of service descriptions we received. These services fell under five broad themes: DMPTool Customization, Online Guides, Consultations, DMP Reviews, and Instruction.

DMPTOOL CUSTOMIZATION

The DMPTool is a freely available online resource that assists researchers with creating DMPs and provides links to sample plans for researchers to review.[14] The original tool was created in January 2011 by the University of California Curation Center (UC3) of the California Digital Library in partnership with seven contributing institutions. The project was undertaken in direct response to funding agencies requiring plans for managing research data. The second version of the tool was released in 2014 and offers ready-to-use templates to guide researchers through the process of generating a comprehensive plan tailored to the specific requirements of agencies, including NIH, NSF, and the United States Department of Energy. New templates are added and modifications made to existing templates as agencies create or change their policies.

Institutions can become DMPTool Partners in order to create templates and provide other customizations to meet the needs of the specific institution. There is no cost to become a partner; institutions simply agree to the Partner Principles as outlined on the DMPTool website, plus complete at least one of the following:

- establish institutional authentication with the DMPTool (Shibboleth, LDAP, etc.);
- customize the tool with resources, help text, suggested answers, or other information specific to their institution; or
- contribute to the maintenance and enhancement of the DMPTool codebase.

Librarians from two administratively separate library systems at the University of Pittsburgh, the University Library System and Health Sciences Library System (HSLS), partnered to initiate the process of their institution becoming a DMPTool Partner in January of 2015. As a result, researchers from the institution can create a personal account and log in with their University of Pittsburgh computing account username and password. Creating an account allows researchers to create and save customized DMPs, add co-owners and editors to their plans, and share their DMPs with others at the University of Pittsburgh or even the general public. Institution-specific resource links and contact information for the librarians appear on every template for everyone logged into DMPTool from the University of Pittsburgh, allowing researchers to quickly access customized help. For example, librarians at HSLS customized the NIH Genomic Data Sharing Policy template with specific guided language for University of Pittsburgh researchers. Partnership also allows the librarians to view institution-specific DMPTool statistics and administer, review, and edit both templates and DMPs.

Respondents from other institutions have also become DMPTool Partners in order to provide their own customizations. DMPTool customizations at Virginia Commonwealth University include pointing to "a few of the system-wide services the university has available (Google Drive, IR [institutional repository])" (M. Henderson). If an existing DMPTool template is not available, DMPTool editors may create a new one that is visible only to users from their home institution. This feature was used by librarians at the University of Virginia for researchers submitting grants to the American Heart Association (A. Horne Denton) and at Virginia Commonwealth University, in collaboration with the Rice Center for Environmental Life Science, to create a new template with "GIS coordinates for all research taking place at the center."[15] It is possible for local administrators who create customized DMPTool templates to require approval from a designated institutional reviewer before allowing users to export the DMP they create using the template. This reviewer role could be filled by a librarian who would provide feedback or play an advisory role to researchers working on their plans.

ONLINE GUIDES

By far the most common service offered among our respondents is a website or online guide to data management. Most of these cover the various aspects of data management, such as the research life cycle, metadata, and storage concerns, and almost all provide specific information on crafting a DMP. Our Data Management Group at the University of Pittsburgh provides support not only through a LibGuide but also via articles written on a bimonthly basis for the online library newsletter.

When developing a strategy to support a new research data management service, Virginia Commonwealth University determined that the creation of a web presence and communication plan was a high priority,[16] and emphasized the development of "guides and web pages to explain research data management and . . . services, and a guide to using DMPTool." A University of Oregon team comprised of a data service librarian, electronic records archivist, head of digital library services, and representatives from various university offices of research and technology/information services worked together to create a guidance website for formulation of DMPs.[17] Three engineering librarians and one postdoctoral fellow at the University of Michigan were charged by their director of research data services to provide a Web-based NSF DMP guide and resources, using the popular LibGuide platform.[18] Links to data management and DMP websites for all libraries that contributed information may be found in the Library Guides section at the end of this chapter.

CONSULTATIONS

Another common service offered by libraries is consultations to help researchers as they begin writing their DMPs. Librarians can discuss the best practices for each of the DMP components, available institutional resources, or point researchers to sample plans that others have shared through resources like the DMPTool. Pinfield and colleagues interviewed library practitioners regarding library-based data management services and found that a DMP advisory service with accompanying advice regarding compliance with funder requirements is of particular interest to faculty researchers.[19] Similarly, McLure and colleagues found that a consult service that included discussions of discipline-specific metadata standards and how they should be incorporated into DMPs would be useful.[20] The Advanced Core Technologies Initiative (ACTI) Data Management Working Group advises appointing at least one dedicated data management consultant to support researchers, as it foresees an expansion of time-sensitive data life cycle service points.[21]

Although many librarians have extensive experience with conducting consultations in the context of library services like literature searches, they may be unfamiliar with the most appropriate questions to ask researchers about their data practices. Garritano and Carlson nevertheless note that "the classic reference interview, used to identify and interpret the information needs of patrons, still has an important place when dealing with researchers that produce and work with large amounts of data."[22] To help design reference interview skills to include discussions about data, the Purdue Libraries developed a Data Curation Profile Toolkit.[23] This toolkit covers background information about different types of research, including the types of data researchers in these fields typically collect, how data management is often handled, and other information to help librarians gain essential knowledge to guide their discussions with researchers.

Consults are often arranged through typical library reference support channels (phone call, chat, ask-a-librarian), by specific data management contact forms, via liaisons, or from referrals. L. Johnston (U Minnesota) shared that "we respond to user requests for consultations on DMPs. There is a contact form on our website and requests come in through liaisons. We have performed a SIPOC analysis (from Six Sigma) on this service to understand the relevant workload and we have trained liaison librarians to respond to requests."

Though numerous needs assessments have demonstrated that researchers are interested in consulting with an expert regarding their DMPs,[24] comments from many of our respondents make it clear that consultations are not frequently requested, despite attempts to promote such services. The offering of DMP consulting "is a low-traffic activity," according to A. Horne Denton (U Virginia). J. Wirz (OHSU) lamented "we had a small grant to try and bribe students to come in for research data management services, and we have found that it isn't really very effective!"

DMP REVIEWS

A small proportion of respondents describe extending their services beyond providing information about how to write a DMP to also reviewing DMPs. A. Whitmire (Oregon State U) reported reviewing "DMPs prior to submission (via e-mail or in DMPTool)." B. Myers (UCLA) is responsible for DMP review in partnership with a data curation analyst, which demonstrates an opportunity for collaboration. L. Johnston (U Minnesota) shared that they "review the DMPs submitted to successful NSF grants to better understand the [researcher] needs," which is an insightful method for gathering data on data management practices that can in turn be used to assist additional researchers. Librarians at the University of Illinois also took this approach, enabling them to clearly identify common data repositories and storage solutions used by researchers and then share this information in future DMP consultations.[25] A project funded by the Institute of Museum and Library Services (IMLS) titled "Analysis of Data Management Plans as a Means to Inform and Empower Academic Librarians in Providing Research Data Support" (referred to as DART) aims to create an "analytic rubric to standardize the review of data management plans as a means to inform targeted expansion or development of research data services at academic libraries."[26] This rubric will be a very useful tool to librarians, and is a further example of how the review of DMPs can help guide library services and support.

INSTRUCTION

Offering instruction on data management planning, either hands-on or lecture style, is well within the academic librarian's toolkit. These may be one-shot sessions held in the library, by request for a specific department or school, as part of a class curriculum, or as a webinar. The Data Management Group at the University of Pittsburgh provides instruction for researchers and support staff on data management topics such as data sharing, file naming conventions, file organization, and how to craft a data management plan. Instruction is offered at the library, through the Responsible Conduct of Research office within our Clinical and Translational Science Institute (CTSI), and upon request. Regarding data literacy instruction, L. Federer (NIH) shared, "I teach an introduction to data management class that looks broadly at data management across the life cycle. Even though my researchers don't write DMPs because that's not an NIH requirement yet, I talk about DMPs as a useful way of thinking about what will be needed in terms of data management down the road when the project gets started. A lot of people don't really think about these kinds of things at the start of the project and then they end up with really messy data sets that are hard for them to use, and very difficult to share."

For librarians just starting a DMP instruction service, the New England Collaborative Data Management Curriculum[27] is a very useful resource that includes lesson plans and case-based activity questions.

What Worked/What Didn't?

According to our respondents, several different approaches to providing DMP-related support through the library have been successful to varying degrees. This seems to be institution-dependent, which suggests that discovering what will work best at your home institution is an empirical exercise. In the following sections, we provide quotes from our respondents on what approaches worked, as well as what didn't work based on their unique experiences.

COLLABORATIONS

Across an institution, there are many stakeholders interested in and concerned about data management and the creation of DMPs. Identifying and engaging with these stakeholders is often imperative for a successful service. Erway offers a list to help librarians decide with whom they should meet when planning new data services, as well as topics to include in the conversation.[28] Stakeholders include the University/Institution, Office of Research, Research Compliance Office, information technology department, researchers, academic units, and of course the library.

When asked about their DMP-related services, a striking number of librarians noted their collaborations with not only researchers, but also other institutional entities such as their Clinical and Translational Science Institute (CTSI), Offices of Research, computing services, statistical support services, graduate student and postdoctoral organizations, and additional libraries both within and outside of the institution. J. Carlson noted that it can take some time and experimentation to find the right campus partners; at the University of Michigan, they "started too high with [the] IT group, so went to departmental people, which took longer but has been worthwhile." Partnering to provide workshops can be a useful approach and perhaps lend more credibility, particularly with offices that, as A. Creamer describes, "have missions for developing research skills and sharing research." At the University of Pittsburgh, we found that partnering with groups outside the library, such as the CTSI, has helped increase the visibility of our workshops and therefore achieve larger attendance than is typical of those held within the library.

Collaboration can also be useful in helping to connect researchers to the entire suite of services that are available across the institution. Libraries are not able to provide all of the services that researchers need to access in the process of writing and carrying out their DMP. For example, libraries can refer researchers to resources like the information technology department that provide services outside of the library's purview, such as backup and storage of data. In turn, these other offices can refer researchers to the library for help with writing their DMPs, reference management, and other library services. B. Westra successfully used this "referral structure" with the University of Oregon's Office of Research to "incorporate a notification option within their grant proposal management system [that] provides information about our services, and form fields through which proposal writers can request our help with a DMP."

DMPTOOL CUSTOMIZATION

As discussed above, the DMPTool is a free and easy first step for librarians to provide highly customized guidance and assistance for researchers at their institution. Such a tool is a helpful way for researchers to approach data management, which can be somewhat "large and nebulous" as L. Federer described it, and overwhelming to researchers who have never had to write a DMP before. However, the librarians who responded to us had mixed success with using the DMPTool. L. Johnston found that "outreach and getting the word out is difficult," and A. Whitmire similarly commented that DMPTool usage was low at Oregon State University, and that they were "not sure how to boost these numbers." Even offering customization may not guarantee that researchers using the DMPTool will find their way to the library; B. Myers noted that she had yet to receive a plan for review through the DMPTool, despite having reviewer status in UCLA's DMPTool customization.

CONSULTATIONS/DMP REVIEWS

As mentioned previously, consultations are offered by a number of libraries with varying degrees of success. Though uptake of such services tended to be low across many of the institutions, researchers who had taken advantage of such consultations generally expressed satisfaction and considered the service worthwhile. Y. Shorish found that getting larger uptake for such services may be a long-term process, noting that "I'm going into my fourth year of doing this work and I think that I am just now getting broad buy-in."

Some librarians who have had success with consultations emphasized the need to provide pragmatic assistance at the point when it was most needed by researchers. B. Myers was able to assist a researcher whose original DMP had been rejected by the NSF, and J. Carlson suggested that librarians "find a way to become a part of the grants administration office workflow." However, at the University of Oregon, where the proposal management system automatically notifies the library when a researcher is applying for a grant with a DMP requirement, attempts to proactively contact researchers to offer help with DMPs were unsuccessful; B. Westra said that "in most cases they do not want help unless they have specifically requested it, so we no longer contact researchers unless they request a consultation." Although we have argued here that writing a DMP can be useful and practical even when not required for a grant, J. Wirz found that OHSU found little uptake by "trying to sell RDM as a 'good thing to do', 'accelerate science broadly', etcetera," and suggested that librarians would have better luck in supporting researchers if they were "practical" about the assistance they provided.

INSTRUCTION

Instruction is an important component of DMP services and a way to reach a large number of researchers at one go, though our respondents did not have universal success with such classes. C. Eaker at the University of Tennessee-Knoxville notes that "offering one-off workshops in the library for graduate students hasn't worked well . . . the attendance is low." The Data Management Group at the University of Pittsburgh teaches the class "Crafting a Data Management Plan" as a live webinar, a format that has increased the number of registrants in comparison to in-person offerings. Making DMP classes part of a larger data management event can also be a helpful way to draw participants, as M. Henderson found when offering a DMPTool session at the January 2015 Virginia Data Management Bootcamp.

Even when researchers do take advantage of training, providing appropriate support for all attendees may be difficult. L. Federer suggested that such classes "would work really well if people truly did attend before the start of a project and thought about these things from the beginning. Realistically, that's almost never the case, and people are midway through a project, so they don't have the benefit of thinking about a DMP before the project, when it would really be helpful." In addition, open enrollment workshops often draw researchers working in widely varied disciplines with different needs and practices, making it difficult to provide content that is useful to all. "While you could argue it could be valuable to expose people to other disciplines and situations," A. Horne noted, "one-on-one consultations would have been much more efficient and successful."

What Would You Change?

As with all library services, it is critical for libraries to reflect upon the DMP services they offer to assess whether they are successful or unsuccessful. Libraries need to iteratively evaluate the success they are having and periodically revisit how to best achieve their goals. Even a service or approach that works for a few years may need to be phased out or ramped up as practices and needs change. This is especially true with DMP services, as funder policies emerge and change. Librarians potentially have a role to help shape the future of DMP requirements and guidance through "broader collaboration of libraries and data curators with funding agencies, disciplinary societies and others," as B. Westra points out. A. Horne suggests, "I think the lesson for us from the NIH Open Access Policy is that until a more robust data sharing plan is required in NIH grant submissions, that busy researchers will, understandably, not concern themselves with documenting more than is needed. When the changes are made in response to the OSTP memo, we will be ready to assist." In other words, once there is a mandate for DMPs, researchers may be more inclined to seek assistance with creating them. Librarians should be strategic and gain expertise and skills to be prepared for this likelihood.

Evaluating and modifying DMP services is especially important in the context of instruction. When developing DMP instruction sessions, librarians must keep in mind that they may not always go as planned. Topics might not be of interest or fill an information need, or the delivery method might not prove to be the most effective. Workshops that are interactive can be especially helpful, and librarians want to think about what slides can be deleted and replaced with specific examples or an activity. Asking for feedback on specific questions, like "'what topics would you like to see included in future data management classes' or 'how would you change this DMP session for the future' is good practice," particularly when attendees have the opportunity to answer anonymously.[29] As researchers start to become more familiar with DMPs, they may need more in-depth instruction on specific topics within data management planning, as L. Federer did when she began "breaking the data management class up into distinct parts and getting more in-depth into topics in their own standalone courses."

Promotion of new library services, such as those described here, is essential to increase awareness of available resources. Several respondents noted the need to be proactive and start reaching out to more individuals as opposed to waiting for them to come to the library. Increased collaboration and integration of DMP services with librarians who provide liaison services to departments may provide an opportunity to market these services more broadly. Y. Shorish hopes that it will be possible "to distribute these services more holistically across the library, so it becomes seen as a natural complement to the other research support that the library offers."

Libraries may need to consider hiring new staff or appointing one or more librarians to provide full-time support for DMPs and data management more generally. As L. Johnston points out, "DMPs are just the beginning of the process. We need a full-service approach for grant support that continues year after year." However, like many respondents, M. Henderson felt that "as only one person doing this job, it is hard to do everything." She adds, "if I had help, I would go out to more faculty meetings to talk about research data management and encourage DMPs for their own sake, and I would teach graduates and undergraduates the value of having a plan." Increasingly, libraries are hiring librarians for positions like "data librarian" or "digital scholarship librarian." While appointing additional staff to these positions may stretch already thin library budgets, libraries may wish to consider operating such services on a cost-recovery model; at the University of Oregon, B. Westra says they "are working on defining pricing structures for data curation services."

Conclusion

There are as many ways for libraries to support DMPs as there are types and formats of data. Typical services at academic/biomedical libraries include providing online guides, one-on-one consultations, hands-on and lecture-style workshops, review of DMPs prior to submission, and customization of the freely available online DMPTool. However, services that are successful at one institution might not be as well utilized at another, so librarians should consider how best to support their research communities and experiment with different approaches. It is useful, encouraging, and perhaps even comforting to learn about what worked and did not work at another library in terms of data management support. The key is to generate thoughtful strategies and to go ahead and begin implementation; if one service is underutilized, try another.

Pearls

- There is a growing need for DMP support, and libraries are perfectly poised to be of assistance.
- To facilitate researcher and institutional buy-in, partner with other stakeholders such as the Clinical and Translational Science Awards group and/or Responsible Conduct of Research group, Office of Research, IT/Computing Services, Statistical Support Services, graduate student and postdoctoral organizations, and additional libraries both within and outside of the institution.
- Recognize that is it not uncommon for outreach to researchers and potential institutional partners to be challenging; it may take time to develop successful collaborations.
- Customization of the DMPTool is free and easy to do with minimal effort.
- Development of an online resource to provide information on DMPs is also easy to do with minimal effort and cost; consider usability of the resource and how to promote it.
- It is not necessary to create DMP resources from scratch; instead refer to the numerous preexisting resources others have created (with proper attribution of course).
- You do not have to be a full-time data management specialist or be working in a team to provide useful DMP services.

Library Guides

- Brown University: http://libguides.brown.edu/data-curation
- James Madison University Libraries: http://guides.lib.jmu.edu/data
- National Institutes of Health Library: http://nihlibrary.campusguides.com/dataservices/
- Oregon Health Sciences University Library: http://www.ohsu.edu/xd/education/library/data/plan-and-organize/index.cfm
- Oregon State University Libraries: http://guides.library.oregonstate.edu/friendly.php?s=dmp
- University of California–Los Angeles Library: http://www.library.ucla.edu/support/publishing-data-management/scholarly-communication-services/data-management-curation-services/data-management-plans
- University of Massachusetts Medical School Lamar Soutter Library: http://libraryguides.umassmed.edu/content.php?pid=496368
- University of Michigan Library: http://www.lib.umich.edu/research-data-services/data-management-plan-review-service-pilot
- University of Minnesota Libraries: https://www.lib.umn.edu/datamanagement
- University of Oregon Libraries: https://library.uoregon.edu/datamanagement/dmp.html
- University of Pittsburgh Health Sciences Library System: http://hsls.libguides.com/datamanagement/DMP
- University of Tennessee–Knoxville Libraries: http://www.lib.utk.edu/scholar/data-management/
- University of Virginia Library: http://data.library.virginia.edu/data-management/dmp-support/
- Virginia Commonwealth University Libraries: http://guides.library.vcu.edu/dmptool

Acknowledgments

The authors wish to acknowledge the following librarians who responded to our request for information about their DMP services.

- Jake Carlson, University of Michigan
- Andrew Creamer, Brown University
- Chris Eaker, University of Tennessee-Knoxville
- Lisa Federer, National Institutes of Health Library
- Margaret Henderson, Virginia Commonwealth University
- Andrea Horne Denton, University of Virginia
- Lisa Johnston, University of Minnesota
- Elaine Martin, University of Massachusetts
- Bethany Myers, University of California-Los Angeles
- Yasmeen Shorish, James Madison University
- Brian Westra, University of Oregon
- Amanda Whitmire, Oregon State University
- Jackie Wirz, Oregon Health Sciences University

Notes

1. DMPTool, "Data Management General Guidance," https://dmptool.org/dm_guidance#types.
2. Executive Office of the President Office of Science and Technology Policy, "Increasing Access to the Results of Federally Funded Scientific Research," https://www.whitehouse.gov/sites/default/files/microsites/ostp/ostp_public_access_memo_2013.pdf.
3. National Science Foundation, "Dissemination and Sharing of Research Results," http://www.nsf.gov/bfa/dias/policy/dmp.jsp.
4. Research Data Services University of Wisconsin-Madison, "Federal Funding Requirements," http://researchdata.wisc.edu/resources/federal-funding-requirements/.
5. National Institutes of Health, "Plan for Increasing Access to Scientific Publications and Digital Scientific Data from NIH Funded Scientific Research," http://grants.nih.gov/grants/NIH-Public-Access-Plan.pdf.
6. "NIH Data Sharing Policy," http://grants.nih.gov/grants/policy/data_sharing/.
7. "NIH Genomic Data Sharing Policy," http://gds.nih.gov/03policy2.html.
8. Michael Fary, Kim Owen, and ACTI Data Management Working Group, "Developing an Institutional Research Data Management Plan Service," *Educause*, January 8, 2013).
9. Carly Strasser et al., "Primer on Data Management: What You Always Wanted to Know," www.dataone.org/sites/all/documents/DataONE_BP_Primer_020212.pdf.
10. A. T. Creamer, E. R. Martin, and D. Kafel, "Research Data Management and the Health Sciences Librarian," in *Health Sciences Librarianship*, ed. M. S. Wood (Lanham, MD: Rowman & Littlefield, 2014).
11. Ricky Erway, "Starting the Conversation: University-Wide Research Data Management Policy," (Dublin, Ohio: OCLC Research 2013).
12. Anne R. Diekema, Andrew Wesolek, and Cheryl D. Walters, "The NSF/NIH Effect: Surveying the Effect of Data Management Requirements on Faculty, Sponsored Programs, and Institutional Repositories," *Journal of Academic Librarianship* 40, nos. 3–4 (2014), 328.
13. Karen Antell et al., "Dealing with Data: Science Librarians' Participation in Data Management at Association of Research Libraries Institutions," *College & Research Libraries* (2013); I. D. Cooper and J. A. Crum, "New Activities and Changing Roles of Health Sciences Librarians: A Systematic Review, 1990–2012," *J Med Libr Assoc* 101, no. 4 (2013).

14. University of California Curation Center of the California Digital Library, "Data Management Planning Tool," https://dmptool.org/.
15. M. E. Henderson and T. L. Knott, "Starting a Research Data Management Program Based in a University Library," *Med Ref Serv Q* 34, no. 1 (2015), 6.
16. Margaret Henderson et al., "Research Data Management on a Shoestring Budget," *ASIS&T Bulletin* 40, no. 6 (2014).
17. B. Westra, "Developing Data Management Services for Researchers at the University of Oregon," in *Research Data Management. Practical Strategies for Information Professionals*, ed. Joyce M. Ray (West Lafayette, IN: Purdue University Press, 2014).
18. Natsuko H. Nicholls et al., "Resources to Support Faculty Writing Data Management Plans: Lessons Learned from an Engineering Pilot," *International Journal of Digital Curation* 9, no. 1 (2014).
19. S. Pinfield, A. M. Cox, and J. Smith, "Research Data Management and Libraries: Relationships, Activities, Drivers and Influences," *PLoS One* 9, no. 12 (2014).
20. Merinda McLure et al., "Data Curation: A Study of Researcher Practices and Needs," *portal: Libraries and the Academy* 14, no. 2 (2014).
21. Fary, Owen, and ACTI Data Management Working Group, "Developing an Institutional Research Data Management Plan Service."
22. Jeremy R. Garritano and Jake R. Carlson, "A Subject Librarian's Guide to Collaborating on E-Science Projects," *Issues in Science and Technology Librarianship* (2009).
23. J. Carlson, "Demystifying the Data Interview: Developing a Foundation for Reference Librarians to Talk with Researchers about Their Data," *Reference Services Review* 40, no. 1 (2012).
24. McLure et al., "Data Curation: A Study of Researcher Practices and Needs"; Susan Wells Parham, Jon Bodnar, and Sara Fuchs, "Supporting Tomorrow's Research: Assessing Faculty Data Curation Needs at Georgia Tech," *College & Research Libraries News* 73, no. 1 (2012).
25. William Mischo, Mary Schlembach, and Megan O'Donnell, "An Analysis of Data Management Plans in University of Illinois National Science Foundation Grant Proposals," *Journal of eScience Librarianship* 3, no. 1 (2014).
26. DART Project Team, "Data Management Plans as a Research Tool," http://dmpresearch.library.oregonstate.edu/.
27. Lamar Soutter Library at the University of Massachusetts Medical School, "New England Collaborative Data Management Curriculum," http://library.umassmed.edu/necdmc/index.
28. Erway, "Starting the Conversation: University-Wide Research Data Management Policy."
29. Christopher Eaker, "Planning Data Management Education Initiatives: Process, Feedback, and Future Directions," *Journal of eScience Librarianship* 3, no. 1 (2014).

Bibliography

Antell, Karen, Jody Bales Foote, Jaymie Turner, and Brian Shults. "Dealing with Data: Science Librarians' Participation in Data Management at Association of Research Libraries Institutions." *College & Research Libraries* (2013).

Carlson, J. "Demystifying the Data Interview: Developing a Foundation for Reference Librarians to Talk with Researchers about Their Data." *Reference Services Review* 40, no. 1 (2012): 7–23.

Cooper, I. D., and J. A. Crum. "New Activities and Changing Roles of Health Sciences Librarians: A Systematic Review, 1990-2012." *J Med Libr Assoc* 101, no. 4 (Oct 2013): 268–77.

Creamer, A. T., E. R. Martin, and D. Kafel. "Research Data Management and the Health Sciences Librarian." In *Health Sciences Librarianship*, edited by M. S. Wood, 252–74. Lanham, MD: Rowman & Littlefield, 2014.

DART Project Team. "Data Management Plans as a Research Tool." http://dmpresearch.library.oregon state.edu/.

Diekema, Anne R., Andrew Wesolek, and Cheryl D. Walters. "The NSF/NIH Effect: Surveying the Effect of Data Management Requirements on Faculty, Sponsored Programs, and Institutional Repositories." *Journal of Academic Librarianship* 40, nos. 3–4 (2014): 322–31.

DMPTool. "Data Management General Guidance." https://dmptool.org/dm_guidance-types.

Eaker, Christopher. "Planning Data Management Education Initiatives: Process, Feedback, and Future Directions." *Journal of eScience Librarianship* 3, no. 1 (2014): 1.

Erway, Ricky. "Starting the Conversation: University-Wide Research Data Management Policy." Dublin, Ohio: OCLC Research 2013.

Executive Office of the President Office of Science and Technology Policy. "Increasing Access to the Results of Federally Funded Scientific Research." https://www.whitehouse.gov/sites/default/files/microsites/ostp/ostp_public_access_memo_2013.pdf.

Fary, Michael, Kim Owen, and ACTI Data Management Working Group. "Developing an Institutional Research Data Management Plan Service." *Educause*, January 8, 2013.

Garritano, Jeremy R., and Jake R. Carlson. "A Subject Librarian's Guide to Collaborating on E-Science Projects." *Issues in Science and Technology Librarianship*, no. 57 (Spring 2009): http://www.istl.org/09-spring/refereed2.html.

Henderson, M. E., and T. L. Knott. "Starting a Research Data Management Program Based in a University Library." *Med Ref Serv Q* 34, no. 1 (2015): 47–59.

Henderson, Margaret, Regina Raboin, Yasmeen Shorish, and Steve Van Tuyl. "Research Data Management on a Shoestring Budget." *ASIS&T Bulletin* 40, no. 6 (2014).

Lamar Soutter Library at the University of Massachusetts Medical School. "New England Collaborative Data Management Curriculum." http://library.umassmed.edu/necdmc/index.

McLure, Merinda, Allison V. Level, Catherine L. Cranston, Beth Oehlerts, and Mike Culbertson. "Data Curation: A Study of Researcher Practices and Needs." *portal: Libraries and the Academy* 14, no. 2 (2014): 139–64.

Mischo, William, Mary Schlembach, and Megan O'Donnell. "An Analysis of Data Management Plans in University of Illinois National Science Foundation Grant Proposals." *Journal of eScience Librarianship* 3, no. 1 (2014).

National Institutes of Health. "NIH Data Sharing Policy." http://grants.nih.gov/grants/policy/data_sharing/.

———. "NIH Genomic Data Sharing Policy." http://gds.nih.gov/03policy2.html.

———. "Plan for Increasing Access to Scientific Publications and Digital Scientific Data from NIH Funded Scientific Research." http://grants.nih.gov/grants/NIH-Public-Access-Plan.pdf.

National Science Foundation. "Dissemination and Sharing of Research Results." http://www.nsf.gov/bfa/dias/policy/dmp.jsp.

Nicholls, Natsuko H., Sara M. Samuel, Leena N. Lalwani, Paul F. Grochowski, and Jennifer A. Green. "Resources to Support Faculty Writing Data Management Plans: Lessons Learned from an Engineering Pilot." *International Journal of Digital Curation* 9, no. 1 (2014): 242–52.

Parham, Susan W., Jon Bodnar, and Sara Fuchs. "Supporting Tomorrow's Research: Assessing Faculty Data Curation Needs at Georgia Tech." *College & Research Libraries News* 73, no. 1 (2012): 10–13.

Pinfield, S., A. M. Cox, and J. Smith. "Research Data Management and Libraries: Relationships, Activities, Drivers and Influences." *PLoS One* 9, no. 12 (2014): e114734.

Research Data Services University of Wisconsin-Madison. "Federal Funding Requirements." http://researchdata.wisc.edu/resources/federal-funding-requirements/.

Strasser, Carly, Robert Cook, William Michener, and Amber Budden. "Primer on Data Management: What You Always Wanted to Know." http://www.dataone.org/sites/all/documents/DataONE_BP_Primer_020212.pdf.

University of California Curation Center of the California Digital Library. "Data Management Planning Tool." https://dmptool.org/.

Westra, B. "Developing Data Management Services for Researchers at the University of Oregon." In *Research Data Management. Practical Strategies for Information Professionals*, edited by Joyce M. Ray, 375–91. West Lafayette, IN: Purdue University Press, 2014.

Chapter 8

Going Beyond the Data Management Plan

SERVICES AND PARTNERSHIPS

Abigail Goben, Library of the Health Sciences, University of Illinois at Chicago
Lisa Zilinski, Carnegie Mellon University
Kristin Briney, University of Wisconsin-Milwaukee

As reviewed in the previous chapter, data management plans (DMPs) have provided an excellent gateway for librarians seeking ways to collaborate with researchers. However, the DMPs frequently capture only initial plans for data at the end of a grant application, often written just hours before the submission deadline. Researchers may also have data captured from a previous pilot project, a project already underway, or a project that is already completed. Further, once the grant is received or a plan has been completed, the researcher may realize she needs something entirely different halfway through the process; may run into intellectual property, patent, or privacy issues; or may encounter an unexpected publisher or university mandate regarding data.

These myriad experiences provide a variety of points for librarian-researcher collaboration that require the librarian to consider a broader array of research data management activities in order to best meet the needs across the data life cycle. Considering a panoply of services also allows librarians to anticipate questions that may be referred to them. Before launching any data management services, it is important for librarians to understand the purpose of each service in order to select the services they are prepared to offer, identify library staff and funding needed to support these efforts, and have advance communication with relevant campus partners. To assist with this, we have outlined services and grouped those that require progressive levels of time and effort, as well as identified the primary campus partners with whom the library will wish to communicate when launching these services. By identifying appropriate service levels, librarians can expand their collaborations in stages without feeling overwhelmed or unable to appropriately direct researchers. When investigating research data services for your library, it is best to start small, investigate research data needs locally, and develop strategies to build services over time.

Background

Library literature on research data management activities recommends librarians consider opportunities beyond the data management plan, although researchers are quick to qualify that one size won't fit all libraries. Tenopir and colleagues surveyed college and research librarians in 2012 and asked them to identify services that they were currently offering or were planning to offer.[1] At that time, only helping users find datasets and creating guides to finding data had greater than 50 percent current or planned uptake in the following two years. In that same year, Raboin and colleagues described three universities with different approaches to research data management.[2] All identified the need for a broader variety of activities, but each identified unique opportunities at their institutions. Speaking from experience at his institution, Westra outlines embedded approaches to offering data management guidance, support, and collaboration.[3] He discusses the notion that subject specialist liaisons need to incorporate data management responsibilities into their roles, while data librarians need to improve their skills in areas of science research, research and data analysis tools, metadata, and curation and preservation workflows to support the subject specialists. More recently, Henderson and Knott[4] describe the process of establishing data services, which starts with collaborating on and reviewing DMPs and then branching out. This paper is particularly useful as it shows what can be done by an institution that is only able to employ one person to focus on data services.

Researchers examined more emerging roles with science librarians and noted that the publications on research data management have focused on individual, institution-based case studies.[5] Antell and colleagues identify the relatively new nature of research data management as the reasoning behind seeing this lower level of evidence.[6] However, it is important that librarians continue to move their research beyond case studies to more authoritative research levels.

With the National Science Foundation (NSF) DMP mandate now in its fifth year and responses to the Office of Science and Technology Policy mandates having been released throughout 2015, librarians are better positioned to understand the emerging funder requirements surrounding data and target services at their institutions.[7] This expertise will allow for more targeted services as well as improved assessment and research in order to determine the effectiveness and sustainability of library services in research data management.

Internal Preparation

Before embarking on the development of research data services in the library, it is important for libraries to assess their capabilities and outline their planned services, as well as how they will be staffed and evaluated. Adding data management into the library's strategic plan and creating a specific strategic plan for the identified data services provides a framework for structuring these services. Education of internal staff, including librarians and front-line support, is integral to successful and sustainable research data services.

Strategic Planning

Beyond individual services, librarians can collaborate in mapping out an institutional vision for the development of data services based on local researcher needs. These efforts will allow the librarian to work with administration to identify partnerships, be aware of particular challenges with unique areas of research, and create action plans toward meeting community needs. An excellent example comes from Oregon State University Libraries & Press. This Strategic Agenda for Research Data Services outlines different phases of goals and activities, and lists partners and timelines.[8] Any library wishing to strategically build its data offerings over time is likely to benefit from at least an informal strategic plan.

Data Management Education (Internal)

In order to promote data services and fully support researchers, it is essential that liaison librarians and those working with researchers become familiar with the vocabulary of research data management.

Preliminary education may provide data life cycle overview, guidance in locating datasets for reuse, a review of current funding mandates, and explanations of resources being supported by the library and their uses. Further education may include performing initial data management interviews, providing external data management education, and collaborating with research teams. One example of librarian-focused data management education is the Data Scientist Training for Librarians program created and led by Christopher Erdmann in Boston.[9] Data librarians or an internal committee focusing on improving library data management awareness are best positioned to lead this internal training, although support and time must be offered by library management. Chapter 6 of this book provides further information on internal education and self-education opportunities.

Library Data Management Services

The concept of offering "data management services" may seem nebulous and too large a target for a solo librarian or a library committee for whom data management is only one of many responsibilities. The following services are defined with key examples from libraries currently offering these services and from the case study literature, with suggestions of who could provide the service and the target audience. These services should be considered in addition to the DMP assistance described in the previous chapter.

As libraries are developing their research data management service portfolio, it would be unsustainable to attempt to provide all services immediately without bringing in multiple librarians and staff. Additionally, the cultures of different institutions will likely not allow for all of these library services to develop, nor relationships to grow. It will be up to the individuals involved at each library to determine what additional workload can be absorbed and which services will best meet the needs of their institution.

While reviewing these services, librarians should consider what resources may be allocated to research data management and how data management aligns with the library mission. New data services must also align with other library strategic goals and current services so as not to exist in a vacuum. A suggested level of staff support is included for many service descriptions; however, this may vary depending on the library and external campus partners who can lend their support, whether in terms of time, money, or personnel. Though the majority of services primarily need library staff time, several of them require greater financial commitment.[10]

Finding Data

Just as librarians are experts with assisting patrons in locating appropriate literature, so too can they become facile in locating datasets for use in coursework and research. Due to the increasing amount of data available, particularly from open government initiatives and funder sharing requirements, patrons will need increasing assistance in locating appropriate data and navigating reuse requirements. Columbia University Libraries' Digital and Social Science Center (DSCC) leads their "Services to Users" list with helping to identify datasets both within and externally to the library collections.[11] While a data librarian may be of assistance, liaison librarians can also be helpful thankful to their subject matter expertise. One specific resource to explore is Re3data.org, which is a repository registry of research data that can be explored and shared with students, faculty, and researchers.[12] As of this publication, the registry held over fourteen hundred repositories, with nearly three hundred fifty in medicine alone.

Purchasing Data

Allowing patrons to request datasets easily aligns with collection development responsibilities. However, it may come with some new challenges. Many datasets are purchased by individuals or labs, and the dataset owner may not have procedures for institutional purchase or access. As most libraries do not purchase materials solely for an individual or small group's use, this can cause challenges in licensing. Datasets may also include material with unique storage and security requirements. Consultation with library or campus information technology (IT) departments to ensure discoverability without privacy violations may be necessary prior to purchase. An example of a data purchasing program is available from the University of Illinois at Urbana-Champaign, where purchase requests were solicited from faculty, academic professionals, and graduate students with the goals of meeting smaller needs (>$5,000) and improving the datasets available to the campus.[13]

Data Citation

While matters of intellectual property and copyright surrounding data as an object continue to evolve, a best practice for those reusing or referring to another's data is to provide a citation. Data and liaison librarians have the opportunity to assist faculty, researchers, students, and their peers in teaching how to cite a dataset. In their article on creating a metadata scheme for the DataCite consortium, Starr and Gastl describe suggested core pieces of a data citation that are used by DataCite and other organizations.[14]

A library may also be interested in setting up a service to create digital object identifiers (DOI) for researchers who are releasing data and who would like it to be cited and accessible. The advantage of using a DOI is that it can remain persistent over time, where websites are more likely to change or go unmaintained. One service that libraries can work with to offer DOIs and other unique identifiers is EZID from the California Digital Library. This service is likely to be managed by a specific data librarian, though education and referrals from liaison librarians will be essential.

Data Management Education (External)

While it is unlikely that a librarian could be assigned to work one-on-one with every research team at an institution, the library can offer education about research data management. Graduate and doctoral level students and faculty supervising them are often interested in this education, as these skills may not be taught elsewhere in the curriculum. Full curricula such as the New England Collaborative Data Management Curriculum (NECDMC) and the DataONE Curriculum, developed with grant support from the NIH and NSF respectively, are available for librarians to use as a starting point to develop their instructional offerings.[15] Muilenburg provides insight into using the NECDMC curriculum and identifies areas where the framework may need to be adapted for individual institutions.[16] External data management instruction may take the form of workshops, video series, webinars, and tutorials and may be offered by the data librarian alone or in collaboration with the liaison librarians. Jake Carlson and Lisa R. Johnston provide additional information in their edited volume about planning instruction.[17]

Data Management Consultations

Individual or group consultations for research data management are a natural opportunity for data librarians and liaison librarians to offer assistance. Such consultations may be either the product of or impetus to create additional services focusing on education, workflow creation, embedded librarians, or other data-related services. With a target of reaching faculty, students, and lab groups in particular, these consults are an opportunity to provide guidance, support, and resources on implementing data management, as well as providing a preliminary assessment of current data workflows for managing, curating, and publishing data. Carlson describes the Data Curation Profile (DCP) Toolkit as "the means for librarians to conduct data interviews with an individual research or small lab group."[18] The DCP can be used as a starting point in conducting data management consultations and can be customized to serve a number of purposes or disciplines.

Developing Data Workflows

Data librarians may also provide more targeted consultations by collaborating with lab staff or a lab manager in order to improve data workflows; example workflows include intra-lab data transfer or the evolution of naming conventions across the analysis process. Workflows may be established at the grant, project, or lab level with the goal of ensuring that data is captured in process rather than in backfill. As outlined by Tina Griffin, developing workflows will entail finding the difficult points within a lab group—whether that be tied to individuals, processes, or equipment, and determining needs from there to improve behavior.[19] This service relies on the librarians providing an outside perspective on information organization and metadata, which are areas of librarian expertise. Workflow improvement may include organization changes, developing new lab policies or procedures, and data curation touch points for quality deposits and preservation. As this process is time-intensive, cost recovery for the librarians' efforts may be required.

Embedded Librarian

Even more in-depth than consultations and workflow development is being embedded within the lab itself. This entails being an information manager for aspects of an entire research project. Medical librarians have participated in other forms of embedded librarianship, engaging in curriculum, clinical rounds, and other activities as described by Florance and Davidoff; here, however, "embedded" refers specifically to being in a research laboratory.[20] Several examples of the embedded librarian in a grant come from the NIH Administrative Supplements for Information Services in NIH-Funded Research Projects.[21] Supplement Awards, paired with R01 and other large grants, have been given in 2012 and 2014, and are anticipated for 2016.

The goal of this grant funding is to enhance the research process by adding an information specialist as an active and ongoing member of the research team. Previous awards have been used to develop online communication tools, create databases and warehouses, develop input tools, introduce best practices at the laboratory level, improve collaboration between multiple research groups, assist with GIS data, and perform literature searches and facilitate bibliographic management. While embedding has allowed data and liaison librarians to engage deeply with a research team, uncertainty remains about the sustainability of the efforts after the end of the funding cycle and the difficulties in scaling this level of service to other researchers who do not have similar funding.

Metadata Services

Another area of expertise that may be offered by the library is metadata services. Metadata librarians in particular have the opportunity to assist in contextual description and documentation in standard formats. As metadata standards vary widely across disciplines, there are many schemas, ontologies, and taxonomies that researchers may need to refer to or work within. Medical librarians may be most familiar with the NLM Metadata Schema used for materials published by the National Library of Medicine,[22] which incorporates Medical Subject Headings (MeSH) into standard Dublin Core elements. A metadata service, as defined by the CalTech Metadata Services Group, may include helping researchers use metadata in order to find data, apply descriptive and technical metadata to identify what a dataset is about, identify rights metadata to assist with legal reuse, and create preservation and administrative metadata to document the data and its workflows over time.[23]

Promoting Open Data

In examining whether shared data will be reused, Wallis affirmed the gift culture of scholarship, where data is shared between colleagues and friends based on personal relationship.[24] This has a great potential effect on access to data across institutions. As arbiters of information access, librarians have a unique opportunity to promote open data access. In much medical research this must, of course, be balanced with protecting research subject privacy, but librarians can assist in finding ways to share data subsets or appropriate metadata to facilitate awareness that a dataset exists that allows other researchers to discover it and consider going through their institutional review board to petition for access. This is best done in collaboration with the scholarly communications librarian or other open access advocates.

Preparing Datasets for Deposit

While ideally a researcher would have consulted with the library early in the grant process and created a data management plan, researchers may approach the library only after the completion of data gathering and as they are preparing datasets for deposit. The degree to which the library is willing and able to provide this service is likely to vary based on factors such as time needed to prepare the dataset, homogeneity of the data, cleanliness, dataset complexity, and repository requirements. The data librarian should have some capacity to provide consultations for data deposit preparation in a subject or other noninstitutional repository. The Inter-University Consortium for Political and Social Research provides a data preparation guide with overarching guidelines.[25]

Collaborative Data Management Services

Some services and activities are more resource intensive than an individual campus unit can frequently support. In addition to librarian expertise, they may require technical systems, physical space, or further commitments from administration and faculty to ensure success. Despite requiring more resources, these services can meet a specific campus need, and they should be considered when strategizing the best data offerings.

Data Policy

Policies surrounding data, including ownership, access, and sharing are evolving quickly. Researchers may encounter policies from funders, institutions, and journals, and these policies may vary across disciplines. Until recently, the NIH required a data management plan only for research with greater than $500,000 requested in any grant year and expressed particular concern for maintaining protection of human subject data.[26] The February 2015 response to the OSTP mandate described a planned requirement that all NIH-funded researchers have data management plans for peer review. However, at the time of publication, this new policy has not been fully implemented.[27] A table summarizing the federal public access policies resulting from the US Office of Science and Technology Policy memorandum of February 2013, compiled by a collaboration of data librarians around the country, is updated regularly and attempts to collect and consolidate the guidelines and policies from federal agencies related to their plans for facilitating public access to results from the research each agency funds.[28] Along with becoming familiar with external policies, librarians can collaborate to create or update institutional policies surrounding data.

Collaborating on policy development offers a different avenue than many data services for the library: the opportunity to work with administration and the research office. While education efforts to assist with compliance will continue to focus on students and faculty, policy creation provides an opportunity for a data librarian to work alongside campus research support personnel and administration. Briney reviews the current institutional policy environment and identifies further opportunities for librarians to engage with data policy.[29]

Data Repositories

As part of promoting open data and preparing datasets for deposit, librarians may connect patrons with subject data repositories such as GenBank or general data repositories like Figshare. However, a library may also wish to explore providing a data repository at their institution to meet the needs of their researchers, faculty, and students. The purpose of a repository is to provide preservation and access to datasets, allowing researchers to meet funding agency requirements or to gain further citations and awareness of the research. One example of institutional data repositories is the Purdue University Research Repository (PURR), which provides all faculty, students, and staff with a collaborative working space and data sharing platform, as well as DOIs for datasets.[30] PURR also allows inter-institutional collaboration, as long as one member of the team is at Purdue. Because of the hardware, software, and storage space required for a dedicated data repository, creating a repository will require collaboration with the library IT department and possibly the campus IT department, as well as potentially significant financial investment. Further details on creating an institutional data repository can be found in an article by Michael Witt and a chapter by D. Scott Brandt, which describe the Purdue experience.[31]

For those interested in focusing on small data, or the long tail as described by Borgman, adding datasets to what is accepted into existing institutional repositories—which typically focus primarily on articles—may prove a more reasonable option.[32] Some libraries may also wish to explore collecting data corresponding to the electronic theses and dissertations in their institutional repositories. Any such data collection should involve collaboration between the repository manager and the data librarian. Library policies should be established early to clarify what data are appropriate for deposit in either a dedicated data repository or an institutional repository, as well as the formats accepted and how data must be prepared for ingest.

Data Analysis Support

Data analysis support should not be taken to mean that the library is taking on the responsibilities of the researcher to perform research data analysis. Rather, the focus of this service is to teach the tools for performing analysis. These tools may fall into a number of categories: statistical analysis such as SPSS or SAS, qualitative software such as NVivo, programming languages such as Python, documentation software such as Colectica, or other analysis tools such as OpenRefine. A data librarian will need awareness of these tools in order to understand where processed data may be coming from.

Library offerings may include teaching introductory webinars, coordinating access to webinars on these tools offered by professional organizations or the vendors, or going further to establish a digital scholarship center in the physical library. More expensive software may be loaded on dedicated computers in the library for greater access among students and researchers who are not able to purchase individual subscriptions for a small or unfunded project. One example of such a center can be found at Notre Dame, which provides assistance with GIS, data use, text mining, digitization, data management, and referral.[33] If such services are offered, it is important that more than one member of the library staff be able to perform basic troubleshooting on the software.

Data Visualization

As with data analysis, the purpose of library data services in visualization comes more in terms of instruction, opportunities for experimentation, and collaboration than in providing end services themselves. Data visualization is defined here as transforming data into visual representations including a map, bar chart, timeline or an artistic rendering and these services have a target audience of faculty, researchers, and students. The library could specialize in teaching a couple of specific tools, such as GeoCommons or Tableau, which allow for easy interactive maps that could be used for public health projects. A visualization space, with dedicated workstations and loaded software such as Duke University offers, also allows for collaboration and experimentation outside of dedicated program-specific computer labs.[34] The library also has an opportunity to serve as a location where visualizations may be shared. If there is a Biomedical Visualization program at the institution, class samples may be displayed with permission in the library on a dedicated computer or in a gallery space. Chapter 10 provides further discussion of library-based data visualization services.

Secure Data Room

Institutions and university security offices are faced with the challenge of allowing researchers to use sensitive secondary data while maintaining appropriate precautions. This may include educational, personal, health, financial, or other kinds of data from outside sources. The library has the opportunity to become a location for secure data access on campus by setting aside a locked space containing a secure, non-networked computer. The library can also provide boilerplate information on secure access for grant applications. Such a space allows security checks to be centralized and prevents duplication of secure rooms in multiple departments.

Creating a secure space in the library will require collaboration with the IT department and may require extra staff to monitor the room. Though this solution is not necessarily scalable for the entire campus, there may be opportunities to partner with high-performance computing centers. For example, the Pittsburgh Supercomputing Center (PSC) is a joint effort of Carnegie Mellon University and the University of Pittsburgh.[35] PSC provides researchers with access to their Data Supercell to enable storage, transfer, and access services for all sizes of datasets.

Identifying Campus Partners

In order to best develop these services, it will be important for libraries to develop relationships across the institution.[36] Partners can provide services that the library cannot presently tackle, as well as augmenting services the library does provide with their resources and expertise. Campus partners also have the opportunity to refer researchers, faculty, and students to the library for data management services at different points in their research. By collaborating, the library prevents service duplication across different units on campus. For the purposes of this chapter, campus partners will be considered external to the library, as it is assumed that all departments in the library have been engaged as partners and stakeholders in relevant services.

CAMPUS IT

Researchers frequently work with campus IT when they are trying to find storage space for their research data. Campus IT often provides data storage and infrastructure during the life of the project and will also have an interest in data security. Their concerns are not necessarily focused on what happens after a research grant is done or in describing the data, and they may have limited interest in sharing the data. At the very least, data librarians should communicate with local IT to learn local best practices and storage offerings to recommend during consultations with researchers.

OFFICE OF RESEARCH AND/OR SPONSORED PROGRAMS

The Office of Research and/or Sponsored Programs is likely to work with all researchers at some point, whether in an oversight or grant reviewing capacity. Researchers who are applying for external funding and those who have received funding will work with this office on fulfilling the terms of application and compliance for their grant. As such, this office has a strong interest in ensuring that researchers have data management plans where required and that these meet minimum expectations of grant review boards. They further have an interest in ensuring compliance with data requirements and that any required data sharing is done to prevent delay in receiving renewal or new grants. This office can refer researchers who are struggling with research data management as it relates to the grant process and would be integral partners in determining needs of the campus for the strategic plan of the library.

In addition, this office is likely able to contact all graduate students and to encourage them to attend educational programs. Some offices even run programming themselves, such as a Responsible Conduct of Research series, in which data librarians can take part as core instructors. The Association of Research Libraries' SPEC Kit on 336: Responsible Conduct of Research Training provides examples of what these workshops may entail and opportunities for librarians to offer instruction.[37] The research office is also likely to know about campus funding opportunities, as well as more significant research that may not be receiving external funding, particularly in subspecialties like history of medicine.

INSTITUTIONAL REVIEW BOARD (IRB) / ANIMAL CARE COMMITTEE (ACC)

Anyone working with human subjects or animals should have contact with the IRB or ACC to ensure compliance with federal regulations for safety and ethics. In this capacity, the review boards are particularly well placed to refer questions about workflow and data sharing plans back to the library for consultation, workflow review, and similar services. Where possible, a librarian sitting on these committees could serve as a contact point.

FACULTY SENATE

As a body, the faculty senate has a particular interest in the intellectual property produced by the university researchers and will likely have opinions about research data. As libraries are advocating for policy development or changes, the senate can provide insight and direction and serve as a conduit to the faculty as a whole. Because their focus is different from other administrations, they are likely to identify other services and needs that may not be readily apparent from the infrastructure side.

OFFICE OF TECHNOLOGY MANAGEMENT/INTELLECTUAL PROPERTY/BUSINESS DEVELOPMENT

While faculty are often primarily focused on the generation of new knowledge and moving science, medicine, and scholarship forward, saleable intellectual property may also be an outcome of research. This office has the responsibility of taking ideas created by researchers at the institution to the point of sale for private business. They will be engaged in filing for patents, developing businesses, or marketing patents to companies. Because patent filing has specific data retention requirements and sharing restrictions, this office may influence data storage and sharing policies and practices that the library is implementing.

Selecting the Right Services

Selecting the right data services for a library depends primarily on three factors: staffing, funding, and the library's goals. On the staffing side, the library must decide if data support will be the purview of a single librarian or if it will take a group approach. While a skilled librarian may be able to deliver very specialized services, it is often more sustainable to have several individuals providing at least low-level data support. A group approach also enables data support to be a normalized part of the total library offerings. Additionally, partnering with other campus offices could allow for resource sharing of both personnel and budget.

Each of the services described in this chapter also requires a different level of staff support. This is exemplified by the three consultation services—data management consultations, developing workflows for a project, and embedded librarians—which require increasing levels of staff time and therefore may be more or less feasible, depending on the library. Staff time devoted for a project should be balanced against staff skills. For example, metadata services and data repositories both require specialized skills or coordination with librarians who work in these areas. Finally, librarians' interests should be taken into consideration, especially when services are provided by a group. Leveraging individual librarians' existing interests is a great way to more quickly establish services in a new area.

The other consideration for staffing services is identifying personnel outside the library who can act as partners in support. As has been discussed, a wide range of potential campus partners may be able to assist libraries. While not critical for every potential service, working with campus stakeholders can make services stronger and more far-reaching. Wherever they exist, partnerships with other campus groups should be leveraged and new relationships cultivated to prove the best data support.

Staff time will be a major resource needed for new services, but additional funding is often necessary, to a greater or lesser degree depending on the service. For example, data purchase programs and providing a secure data room will require more money than advocating for data policy or providing training. The library may also need to dedicate resources to technical solutions, such as when building a data repository or providing DOIs. As several of the described services are not scalable for the whole campus, the library should consider the scale of the project as well as the tradeoff between staff time and money when deciding on offerings. At least one of the two resources will be required for any service.

The ultimate goal is to find the right service portfolio to meet the library's mission. For example, a library that is a strong advocate for openness may wish to support open data and a data repository, whereas a library that is more focused on information literacy might adopt a data management training curriculum. Reviewing the library's strategic plan and developing a coordinating strategic plan for data services will be of benefit.

Conclusion

Libraries have a considerable number of options for providing data support beyond consulting on data management plans. This chapter describes an array of possible services that different libraries are already offering. While it is rarely feasible to provide every service listed, libraries should take advantage of their staff skills, their goals, and existing partnerships on campus to provide a level of data support that is right for their campus. When in doubt, start small, examine local researcher data needs, and create a plan for how to grow data support over time.

Pearls

- A wide variety of research data management services are needed beyond data management plans for grants.
- Services can be targeted at different audiences and rolled out over time or as staffing is available.
- Funding for resources or staff will be necessary for a successful service launch.
- Collaborating with other campus partners will help with alerting researchers to the services available and prevent duplication of effort.

Notes

1. Tenopir et al., "Academic Libraries and Research Data Services."
2. Raboin et al., "Forging New Service Paths: Institutional Approaches to Providing Research Data Management Services."

3. Westra, "Developing Data Management Services for Researchers at the University of Oregon."
4. Henderson, and Knott, "Starting a Research Data Management Program Based in a University Library."
5. Westra, "Developing Data Management Services for Researchers at the University of Oregon."; Henderson, and Knott, "Starting a Research Data Management Program Based in a University Library"; Antell et al., "Dealing with Data: Science Librarians' Participation in Data Management at Association of Research Libraries Institutions."
6. Antell et al., "Dealing with Data: Science Librarians' Participation in Data Management at Association of Research Libraries Institutions."
7. National Science Foundation, "Dissemination and Sharing of Research Results."; Burwell et al., "Memorandum for the Heads of Executive Departments and Agencies"; Holdren "Memorandum for the Heads of Executive Departments and Agencies: Increasing Access to the Results of Federally Funded Scientific Research"; Whitmire et al., "A Table Summarizing the Federal Public Access Policies Resulting from the US Office of Science and Technology Policy Memorandum of February 2013."
8. Sutton et al., "Oregon State University Libraries and Press Strategic Agenda for Research Data Services."
9. Guillette and Damon, "Data Scientist Training for Librarians: A Course and a Community."
10. Jones et al., *How to Develop RDM Services—a Guide for HEIs.*
11. Columbia University Libraries, http://library.columbia.edu/locations/dssc/data/service.html.
12. re3data, Registry of Research Data Repositories, http://www.re3data.org/.
13. "Data Purchase Program." http://www.library.illinois.edu/sc/datagis/purchase/description2014.html.
14. Starr and Gastle, "A Metadata Scheme for DataCite."
15. "New England Collaborative Data Management Curriculum," http://library.umassmed.edu/necdmc/index; "Education Modules," https://www.dataone.org/education-modules.
16. University of Washington, Muilenburg et al., "Lessons Learned from a Research Data Management Pilot Course at an Academic Library."
17. Carlson and Johnston, *Data Information Literacy: Librarians, Data and the Education of a New Generation of Researchers.*
18. Carlson, "Demystifying the Data Interview: Developing a Foundation for Reference Librarians to Talk with Researchers about Their Data," 8.
19. Griffin, "How Data Management Issues Manifest: Using Concept Mapping to Discover the Information Network in a Laboratory Environment."
20. Davidoff and Florance, "The Informationist: A New Health Profession?"
21. National Library of Medicine, "NLM Administrative Supplements for Informationist Services in NIH-Funded Research Projects (Admin Supp)." http://www.nlm.nih.gov/ep/AdminSupp.html.
22. National Library of Medicine, "NLM Metadata Schema," http://www.nlm.nih.gov/tsd/cataloging/metafilenew.html.
23. Metadata Services Group https://library.caltech.edu/metadata/.
24. Wallis et al., "If We Share Data, Will Anyone Use Them? Data Sharing and Reuse in the Long Tail of Science and Technology."
25. "Guide to Social Science Data Preparation and Archiving: Introduction," http://www.icpsr.umich.edu/icpsrweb/content/deposit/guide/index.html.
26. National Institutes of Health, "NIH Data Sharing Information," http://grants.nih.gov/grants/policy/data_sharing/.
27. "National Institutes of Health Plan for Increasing Access to Scientific Publications and Digital Scientific Data from NIH Funded Scientific Research," http://grants.nih.gov/grants/NIH-Public-Access-Plan.pdf.

28. Whitmire et al., "A Table Summarizing the Federal Public Access Policies Resulting from the US Office of Science and Technology Policy Memorandum of February 2013."
29. Briney et al., "Do You Have an Institutional Data Policy? A Review of the Current Landscape of Library Data Services and Institutional Data Policies."
30. "What Is PURR?," https://purr.purdue.edu/.
31. Witt, "Defining and Deploying an Institutional Data Repository Service at Purdue (PURR)"; Brandt, "Purdue University Research Repository: Collaborations in Data Management."
32. Borgman, "Big Data and the Long Tail: Use and Reuse of Little Data."
33. Center for Digital Scholarship, http://library.nd.edu/cds/.
34. "The Brandaleone Lab for Data and Visualization Services," http://library.duke.edu/data/about/lab.
35. Pittsburgh Supercomputing Center, "PSC Data Supercell," https://www.psc.edu/index.php/major-initiatives/data-supercell
36. Erway and OCLC Research, *Starting the Conversation University-Wide Research Data Management Policy*.
37. Leonard and Bennett, "Responsible Conduct of Research Training, SPEC Kit 336."

Bibliography

Antell, K., J. B. Foote, J. Turner, and B. Shults. "Dealing with Data: Science Librarians' Participation in Data Management at Association of Research Libraries Institutions." *College & Research Libraries* 75, no. 4 (2014): 557–74. doi:10.5860/crl.75.4.557.

Borgman, Christine. "Big Data and the Long Tail: Use and Reuse of Little Data." *Oxford eResearch Centre Seminar*. March 2013. http://works.bepress.com/borgman/269.

Brandt, D. Scott. "Purdue University Research Repository: Collaborations in Data Management." In *Research Data Management: Practical Strategies for Information Professionals*, edited by Joyce M. Ray, 325–45. West Lafayette, IN: Purdue University Press, 2014.

Briney, Kristin, Abigail Goben, and Lisa Zilinski. "Do You Have an Institutional Data Policy? A Review of the Current Landscape of Library Data Services and Institutional Data Policies." *Journal of Librarianship and Scholarly Communication* 3, no. 2 (2015).

Burwell, Sylvia, Steven VanRoekel, Todd Park, and Dominic Mancini. "Memorandum for the Heads of Executive Departments and Agencies." Office of Management and Budget, May 9, 2013. http://www.whitehouse.gov/sites/default/files/omb/memoranda/2013/m-13-13.pdf.

Caltech Library. "Metadata Services Group." Accessed May 31, 2015. https://library.caltech.edu/metadata/.

Carlson, Jake. "Demystifying the Data Interview: Developing a Foundation for Reference Librarians to Talk with Researchers about Their Data." *Reference Services Review* 40, no. 1 (2012): 7–23.

Carlson, Jake, and Lisa R. Johnston, eds. *Data Information Literacy: Librarians, Data and the Education of a New Generation of Researchers*. West Lafayette, IN: Purdue University Press, 2015.

Center for Digital Scholarship. Accessed June 1, 2015. http://library.nd.edu/cds/.

Columbia University Libraries. "DSSC Data Service." Accessed May 31, 2015. http://library.columbia.edu/locations/dssc/data/service.html.

DataONE. "Education Modules." Accessed June 12, 2015. https://www.dataone.org/education-modules.

Davidoff, Frank, and Valerie Florance. "The Informationist: A New Health Profession?" *Annals of Internal Medicine* 132, no. 12 (2000): 996–98.

Duke University Libraries. "The Brandaleone Lab for Data and Visualization Services." Accessed June 1, 2015. http://library.duke.edu/data/about/lab.

Erway, Ricky, and OCLC Research. *Starting the Conversation: University-Wide Research Data Management Policy*. Dublin, OH: OCLC Research, 2013. http://www.oclc.org/content/dam/research/publications/library/2013/2013-08.pdf.

EZID. "EZID Home." Accessed June 16, 2015. http://ezid.cdlib.org/.
Griffin, Tina. "How Data Management Issues Manifest: Using Concept Mapping to Discover the Information Network in a Laboratory Environment." Presented at the Research Data Access & Preservation Summit, Minneapolis, MN, April 23, 2015.
Guillette, Jeremy, and James Damon. "Data Scientist Training for Librarians: A Course and a Community." *Library Connect*, November 13, 2014. http://libraryconnect.elsevier.com/articles/2014-11/data-scientist-training-librarians-course-and-community.
Henderson, Margaret E., and Teresa L. Knott. "Starting a Research Data Management Program Based in a University Library." *Medical Reference Services Quarterly* 34, no. 1 (2015): 47–59. doi:10.1080/02763869.2015.986783.
Holdren, John P. "Memorandum for the Heads of Executive Departments and Agencies: Increasing Access to the Results of Federally Funded Scientific Research." Office of Science and Technology Policy, Executive Office of the President, The White House, February 2013. http://www.whitehouse.gov/sites/default/files/microsites/ostp/ostp_public_access_memo_2013.pdf.
ICPSR. "Guide to Social Science Data Preparation and Archiving: Introduction." Accessed June 1, 2015. http://www.icpsr.umich.edu/icpsrweb/content/deposit/guide/index.html.
Jones, Sarah, Graham Pryor, and Angus Whyte. *How to Develop RDM Services: A Guide for HEIs*. Edinburgh, UK: Digital Curation Centre, 2013. http://www.dcc.ac.uk/resources/how-guides/how-develop-rdm-services.
Lamar Soutter Library–University of Massachusetts Medical School. "New England Collaborative Data Management Curriculum." Accessed May 31, 2015. http://library.umassmed.edu/necdmc/index.
Leonard, Michelle, and Denise Beaubien Bennett. "Responsible Conduct of Research Training, SPEC Kit 336," ARL Digital Publications, September 2013. http://publications.arl.org/Responsible-Conduct-Research-Training-SPEC-Kit-336/.
National Institutes of Health. "National Institutes of Health Data Sharing Information." Accessed October 21, 2015. http://grants.nih.gov/grants/policy/data_sharing/.
———. "National Institutes of Health Plan for Increasing Access to Scientific Publications and Digital Scientific Data from NIH Funded Scientific Research." February 2015. http://grants.nih.gov/grants/NIH-Public-Access-Plan.pdf.
National Library of Medicine. "NLM Administrative Supplements for Informationist Services in NIH-Funded Research Projects (Admin Supp)." NLM, 2015. Accessed May 31. http://www.nlm.nih.gov/ep/AdminSupp.html.
———. "NLM Metadata Schema." NLM, 2015. Accessed May 31. http://www.nlm.nih.gov/tsd/cataloging/metafilenew.html.
National Science Foundation. "Dissemination and Sharing of Research Results." NSF, November 30, 2010. http://www.nsf.gov/bfa/dias/policy/dmp.jsp.
Pittsburgh Supercomputing Center. "PSC Data Supercell." Accessed May 31, 2015. https://www.psc.edu/index.php/major-initiatives/data-supercell.
Purdue University Research Repository. "What Is PURR?" Purdue University. Accessed May 3, 2015. https://purr.purdue.edu/.
Raboin, Regina, Rebecca Reznik-Zellen, and Dorothea Salo. "Forging New Service Paths: Institutional Approaches to Providing Research Data Management Services." *Journal of eScience Librarianship*. doi:10.7191/jeslib.2012.1021.
re3data, Registry of Research Data Repositories. Accessed June 2, 2015. http://www.re3data.org/.
Starr, Joan, and Angela Gastle. "isCitedBy: A Metadata Scheme for DataCite." *D-Lib Magazine* 17, nos. 1–2 (2011). doi:10.1045/january2011-starr.
Sutton, Shan, David Barber, and Amanda L. Whitmire. "Oregon State University Libraries and Press Strategic Agenda for Research Data Services." Oregon State University, May 30, 2013. http://ir.library.oregonstate.edu/xmlui/handle/1957/38794.

Tenopir, Carol, Ben Birch, and Suzie Allard. "Academic Libraries and Research Data Services." ACRL, 2012. http://www.ala.org/acrl/sites/ala.org.acrl/files/content/publications/whitepapers/Tenopir_Birch_Allard.pdf.

University of Illinois Library. "Data Purchase Program." Accessed June 1, 2015. http://www.library.illinois.edu/sc/datagis/purchase/description2014.html.

University of Washington, Jennifer Muilenburg, Mahria Lebow, and Joanne Rich. "Lessons Learned from a Research Data Management Pilot Course at an Academic Library." *Journal of eScience Librarianship* 3, no. 1 (2014): 67–73. doi:10.7191/jeslib.2014.1058.

Wallis, Jillian C., Elizabeth Rolando, and Christine L. Borgman. "If We Share Data, Will Anyone Use Them? Data Sharing and Reuse in the Long Tail of Science and Technology." Edited by Luís A. Nunes Amaral. *PLoS ONE* 8, no. 7 (2013): e67332. doi:10.1371/journal.pone.0067332.

Westra, Brian. "Developing Data Management Services for Researchers at the University of Oregon." In *Research Data Management: Practical Strategies for Information Professionals*, edited by Joyce M. Ray, 375–91. West Lafayette, IN: Purdue University Press, 2014.

Whitmire, Amanda, Kristin Briney, Amy Nurnberger, Margaret Henderson, Thea Atwood, Margaret Janz, Wendy Kozlowski, Sherry Lake, Micah Vandegrift, and Lisa Zilinski. "A Table Summarizing the Federal Public Access Policies Resulting from the US Office of Science and Technology Policy Memorandum of February 2013." http://figshare.com/articles/A_table_summarizing_the_Federal_public_access_policies_resulting_from_the_US_Office_of_Science_and_Technology_Policy_memorandum_of_February_2013/1372041.

Witt, Michael. "Defining and Deploying an Institutional Data Repository Service at Purdue (PURR)." Purdue University, 2014. http://docs.lib.purdue.edu/lib_fspres/44/.

Chapter 9

Library Infrastructures for Scholarship at Scale

Steven Braun, University of Minnesota Libraries

In the past decade, the word "data" has burrowed its way into nearly every aspect of our daily lives. As has been quipped in popular media, "data is the new oil,"[1] and indeed, it is difficult to ignore the ways in which data are manifest in almost everything we do. Even in our personal lives, data seem ubiquitous as we are ensnared in an ever-growing Internet of Things,[2] with each electronic device we own collecting some form of data about our daily behaviors. The data economy continues to build in step with the advancement of technology, and there is no shortage of supply or demand to stifle its growth.[3]

If this sounds clichéd, it is for good reason. The effects of this data surplus have been far-reaching in social and cultural dimensions, even fostering new language to describe the ways in which our relationships with data are changing over time. Metaphors like "big data," "data deluge," and "the exabyte age" abound not only in scholarly literature, but also popular journalism, where such expressions are often dramatic, bringing to the imagination a crisis of almost mythic proportions. The *New York Times*, heralding the "Age of Big Data," has devoted many columns over the past several years to exploring how the evolving nature of data has permeated all levels of academia, industry, and society;[4] likewise, the *Economist* has examined both the challenges and opportunities that big data usher into the economic sphere, suggesting that no aspect of daily life is left untouched.[5] By such standards, managing the data all around us can feel like an impossible endeavor, especially considering growing concerns over the implications that our devices and the trail of data they leave behind—the so-called "data exhaust"—have for the commodification of information and individual privacy.[6]

The language of big data that is used in these spheres is often mixed with an air of prophecy and even dire portent, depicting a future in which we are unprepared for how data will radically transform our daily lives. However provocative it may be, though, this tenor of exigency oversimplifies the fact that a breadth of responses to deal with the coming changes has already emerged, particularly in realms beyond the corporate sector alone. Academe is a prime example of this and has been keenly attuned to the winds of change for many years, although perhaps not always expressed in the exact same terms. At academic institutions, the measure of change has been focused less exclusively on data, which can mean different things in different disciplines, and more broadly on the changing cultures and practices of scholarship writ large, including scholarly communication, data sharing, and data discoverability.[7] Even so, it is not uncommon to hear these changes being measured through a framework that is oriented primarily around the language of big data; to many researchers, for whom data are plentiful but the requisite skills (or confidence) to manage them sometimes are not,[8] the notion that "data is the new oil" resonates close to home.

In this context, the expression "big data" can indeed be useful for describing the new challenges that many academics face in managing the scholarship they produce. Yet for many others, such language must be used with caution, balanced with an awareness of its assumptions and limitations. Certainly not all researchers identify their work as involving big data, and developing services to support researchers based on the presumption that they do can result in alienation and neglect. Many of these assumptions originate in the term's variable meaning across scholarly literature and the media, an examination of which reveals a vastness of territory with unclear boundaries. Indeed, "big data" connotes a wide range of interpretations that cannot be easily collapsed into a single definition, and scholars do not always agree on what forms of scholarship should and should not be classified as big data.[9] For example, Edd Dumbill, technology analyst for O'Reilly Radar,[10] offers one interpretation of the term in the inaugural issue of the journal *Big Data* that focuses on measures of size and management, stating "Big data is data that exceeds the processing capacity of conventional database systems. The data is too big, moves too fast, or doesn't fit the strictures of your database architectures."[11] Meanwhile, in their review of its variable definitions, Hashem et al. offer another one that integrates conceptions of big data in terms of both commodities and methodologies, proposing "Big data is a set of techniques and technologies that require new forms of integration to uncover large hidden values from large datasets that are diverse, complex, and of a massive scale."[12]

Given the range of definitions proposed, "big data" is thus better understood as an umbrella term applied generically to any data that quickly outgrow the infrastructure currently in place to support them, measured in whatever dimensions are most relevant. One useful conceptual framework that has been broadly adopted in both academe and industry distinguishes big data from other conventions by three particular characteristics: big data are large in their file size, produced at a high speed, and diverse in their formats.[13] Also known as the "three Vs," this triad is central to a definition provided by Gartner Research, who describe big data as "high-*volume*, high-*velocity* and high-*variety* information assets that demand cost-effective, innovative forms of information processing for enhanced insight and decision making" (emphasis added).[14] More recent models extend these signatures further, adding that big data are characterized by their low *veracity* (limited authority) and high *value*.[15] The term thus describes not only data but also the technologies that are needed to work with and manage them, which can be as diversified across disciplines and data types as the data themselves.

Lack of consensus on a precise definition lends the language of big data a great amount of flexibility, which can be beneficial in opening broad dialogue about the challenges data bring across diverse populations and practices of research. At the same time, however, it can turn such language into a semantic dumping ground, a net cast widely across many different understandings of data that may be only tangentially related. When this ambiguity serves as the fundamental motivation in designing services or technologies to support the needs of researchers, the result can be a hotbed of assumptions that reduces highly variable needs down to a one-size-fits-all solution. Therein persists a hidden danger; when researchers are unable to see how their own needs fit into the broader climate of conversation around data, "big data" can foster a sense of alienation, especially when that climate hyper-focuses on conceptions of data at the highest end of the complexity spectrum. Even more importantly, subconsciously framing data management around the kinds of data most immediately noticeable at our institutions—those that take up the most space in our workflows, language, and policy—can make it easy to neglect the more specialized needs of other researchers at the eponymous long tail of scholarship, those for whom our approaches to data management are still nascent.[16] With a framework based exclusively on big data, thus, we romanticize a problem that both circumvents as well as misrepresents a more fundamental reality: the nature of scholarship and researchers' relation to it are changing in ways that are more adequately measured in many dimensions beyond size alone.

In response to this, a more sophisticated linguistic and theoretical schema is needed to capture the nuances of what "big data" means for researchers across academe, including its constituent assumptions about scholarship and scale. As a field, academic librarianship is well-poised to provide the foundation for such a schema; in their many roles of support, librarians have an experiential understanding of the needs of their researchers as they navigate their scholarship amid the complexities of the research life cycle. When building infrastructure to support researchers in managing their scholarship, libraries would be amiss to neglect leveraging this unique understanding at all stages in the research life cycle and across all spectra of needs. It is thus perhaps more appropriate to think not in the terms of "big data" but rather in language that reconceptualizes the meanings of both "big" and "data" in ways that reflect the complexities therein: *scholarship at scale,* where scholarship is all encompassing and scale is relative to the frame of reference.

In this chapter, we will explore the implications that thinking about researchers' needs in terms of scholarship at scale has for librarianship's understanding of data management in the design and deployment of library infrastructures. We will survey infrastructure at three levels in which libraries are increasingly demonstrating authority, including systems (in other words, technological platforms for enabling the practice, management, and discoverability of scholarship); library services for research support; and policy defining responsibilities around data management between researchers, institutions, granting agencies, and the federal government. Using case studies from the University of Minnesota, we will consider how challenges manifest differently at each level, and in the process, what those challenges mean for designing infrastructure with sustainability in mind.

Language, Researcher Identity, and Discipline-Agnosticism

Academic libraries are well known for the suite of services they provide to support researchers at all points in the research life cycle. The exact nature of these services can vary, but their design is generally motivated by the specific needs of the institutional environment they serve, whether small or large. At the University of Minnesota, where the faculty population is large and the spread of needs they have is vast, the University Libraries have built a constellation of services and resources that focus on different aspects of scholarship and scholarly communication. Central to these is data management, which is the cornerstone of the Libraries' Data Management and Curation Initiative (DMCI). Convened in 2014, DMCI has been heavily steeped in ongoing efforts around user needs assessment, user education about best practices in data management, and the creation of an institutional data repository (the Data Repository for U of M, or DRUM[17]) that provides specialized curation services to help researchers document and share their research data in compliance with federal and grant agency requirements.

University of Minnesota Libraries staff have expertise across the natural sciences, social sciences, and arts and humanities, resulting in close relationships with researchers of many different backgrounds. As this diversity continues to grow, so does the awareness that much of librarians' ability to provide research support is heavily dependent upon the design of services and technologies that are scalable across disciplines and capable of growing with changing practices. At the same time, however, there is also awareness that this diversity is a double-edged sword; while it may serve as a major impetus for shifting the focus of support, it is also perhaps the most significant challenge to making such support possible and sustainable.

Developing services in this way thus requires a careful balance between the needs of individuals, which may be quite specialized, and the practicality of what can be operationalized to support the greatest breadth of those needs possible. Having a realistic understanding of where the fulcrum sits in the balance is essential to leveraging it effectively, and this can only be achieved by knowing a priori the landscape of needs into which academic librarians must integrate themselves. Recognizing this, the University of Minnesota Libraries have invested a great amount of energy into efforts to identify the specific areas in which researchers need the most support, with DMCI functioning as a major epicenter of activity. One important and enduring approach to this at libraries' disposal is the direct survey of faculty, and accordingly, DMCI has endeavored in this way to programmatically capture a snapshot of researchers' practices throughout the research life cycle.

Beginning in fall of 2013 and continuing through spring of 2015, DMCI collaborated with staff in the College of Liberal Arts Research Support Services to design surveys assessing the data management practices and needs of researchers on campus. These surveys were distributed in four colleges and centers across several disciplines in the arts, humanities, social sciences, and physical/life sciences, and each was adapted to the particular cultures and traditions of scholarship in their respective populations. Respondents were asked to provide information about the scholarly works they produced in the course of their research, including file types and storage sizes, as well as their current practices in managing those products, with particular attention to their documentation, backup and preservation, and sharing. Responses were collected from over seven hundred faculty members in nearly one hundred different departments.[18]

The results of these surveys have revealed important insights about the practices and needs of researchers at the University of Minnesota, and they are being used to inform the development of services the University Libraries provide. One of the most striking of these insights is the dramatic heterogeneity of behaviors and needs among researchers, not only across but also within disciplines. The variety is evident in many domains, including the media and data types produced in research, practices for managing them, and cultures or traditions of collaboration within and outside given disciplines. Perhaps most interestingly, survey results showed that these variations corresponded strongly with differences in terminology; depending on the population being surveyed, respondents identified more or less naturally with different choices in the specific language used to refer to their research.

An illustrative example of this is the choice of language used in the surveys to refer to the scholarly works produced in research, especially the term "data," which highlighted important sensitivities across different disciplines. For many researchers, including those in the physical and health sciences, referring to scholarship using the term "data" elicited responses without resistance; these researchers were likely to naturally refer to their scholarship as data, and thus the term resonated closely with their disciplinary conventions. For researchers in disciplines more firmly rooted in the arts, humanities, and social sciences, however, the term was less appropriate; many of these respondents, who were less likely to refer to the products of their scholarship as exclusively "data," associated the term with predominantly hard scientific (i.e., quantitative) research, thus limiting the language's relevance to them. To adjust for these semantic differences and broaden inclusivity, the term "digital materials" was used instead for these respondents, signifying a deeper awareness of the multimodality of their scholarship, which ranged from media such as photographs and voice recordings to literary works used in textual analyses.

Framing scholarship in a data-centric lexicon can pose difficulties not only across different disciplines but also within them. In another version of the survey, concern was expressed that researchers in public health might feel uniquely alienated by the use of the word "data" because of differences in its interpretation that were not adequately captured in the survey's design. These researchers primarily use population-based data; however, the survey characterized data in only clinical and experimental terms based on definitions from the National Institutes of Health and the National Science Foundation. In addition, the work that many of these researchers produced was not necessarily the outcome of collecting original data, as might be the case with clinical studies or wet lab experimentation, but rather consisted of derivative works resulting from the analysis of existing data. Semantics thus proved to be problematic in two ways, one with respect to the meaning of "data" in terms of *data as practice* and the other with respect to *data as output of research*.

This nontriviality of the word "data" is important and provides one of the critical motivations in our shift from a big data-centric framework to one that focuses on scholarship more broadly. When viewed through the lens of researchers across many different fields and cultures of practice, conceptions of data cannot be taken for granted; as a result, the language librarians use when communicating with different researchers is not just a matter of word choice but more fundamentally a signal of how well they understand researchers' needs. When narrow language is used as a proxy for the wider spectrum of scholarship, the resulting naiveté can stigmatize researchers and cause support to be ineffectively targeted. Thus, an open definition of scholarship—one that moves beyond the confines of "data" and toward reference to any and all modalities of research output, including quantitative or qualitative data, media, creative works, and other materials that are collected in the course of research—enables deeper dialogue and the design of support structures to more robustly facilitate it.

The relationship between language and researcher identity is not accidental, nor is it even anything new to librarians. However, what may be new is the relationship between language and the library infrastructures designed to support researchers in managing their scholarly works, where the meaning of "infrastructure" is understood from several different perspectives. In the first of these, infrastructure is used in a literal sense, referring to the technological capacity that is needed to store, preserve, and manage the digital products of research. This includes, for example, the information technology platforms that make it possible to create, capture, and store the outputs of research, such as server space, institutional repositories that preserve data for the long term, or systems that enable the discoverability of scholarship for reuse by others.

More figuratively, however, the term also describes the collective services, expertise, and conceptual frameworks through which libraries provide support for the *practice* of research, including consultation about best practices in data management, data curation, and user education about options for data sharing. Above those services, it also refers to the policies and standards that shape the research enterprise at the highest level, guiding shifts in cultures of scholarship. In this sense, the meaning of infrastructure articulates the many capacities in which libraries provide support at the levels of systems, services, and policy, which is important for understanding the breadth of roles that librarians serve across the entirety of the research life cycle.

Along with a discussion of infrastructure comes the requisite consideration of the resources needed for that infrastructure to persist over time, which can limit the lifespan of support provided. The subject of sustainability has become particularly salient across the field of academic librarianship, especially as libraries learn how to operationalize services and technologies for the long term with a balanced consideration of the resources available to deploy them. As a result, library infrastructures are challenged to be sustainable in many ways, minimizing their footprint while maximizing their impact at all points in the research life cycle. We will intertwine with the nuances of these challenges ahead, noting how they manifest at each level in the systems-services-policy scaffold.

Designing for Sustainability in Library Infrastructures

The results of the University of Minnesota Libraries' data management surveys have challenged preconceptions of the practices of researchers, helping shift assumptions about the areas in which they are most challenged when managing their scholarship. The outputs of research can extend across many different measures of complexity, and scale in each of those measures may consequently be expressed through different frames of reference. Some of these are more immediately noticeable than others and already built into libraries' support architectures with scalability in mind. For example, storage size needs and the long-term stability of different file formats are common talking points on data management and preservation, and libraries have established approaches for assisting researchers in meeting those needs.[19] Other measures are more specialized and complex, however, and libraries may be lacking in the expertise available to support them. As a result, designing infrastructure to support scholarship at scale requires an understanding of scalability that may change on a case-by-case basis.

We can focus our discussion of scalability down to a select handful of frames of reference that have become particularly salient to libraries' approaches to data management, each of which poses challenges to sustainability at the systems, services, and policy levels. These include the frames of structuredness, modality, temporality, and sensitivity, and each can be expressed in scholarship in nuanced ways. In the first of these, we refer to structuredness as the extent to which a body of scholarship is internally ordered. Low structuredness, for example, tends to be associated with the long tail of research data; these datasets tend to be small, unrelated, and poorly documented, making it difficult to capture them.[20] Artistic or other creative works may also exhibit low structuredness, especially in communities of scholarship where standards for documentation are weak. High structuredness, meanwhile, is a characteristic intrinsic to data stored in relational databases, making them easy to parse and link to other scholarly works. This frame of reference can be influenced by both the specific forms of scholarship produced in research (such as file types or media) as well as researchers' practices in managing, organizing, and documenting those variable outputs.

The next dimension, modality, can be expressed in primarily two senses. In one sense, modality refers to the culture of practice or ethos through which a scholarly work is produced. For instance, the practices of a scholar in the humanities conducting literary analyses, which may be more firmly rooted in a culture that emphasizes discursive inquiry, will differ from those of a physicist who collects instrument data through experiments, shaped by the emphasis on empirical observation enshrined in the scientific method. Modality may also refer to the specific file formats or media in which researchers produce scholarly works. As an example, an ethnographer may produce large quantities of video footage, photographs, and interview transcripts, but a scholar whose research involves nuclear magnetic resonance spectroscopy to elucidate protein structures may produce data in the form of spectral analyses and molecular dynamics simulations. Boundaries between disciplines tend to demarcate differences in modalities as a result of the nature of their work, reflecting the diversity of quantitative, qualitative, and creative works that may result from research. As data management practices can change according to the modality of a scholarly work (such as determining how to most effectively organize data that are collected across several media from a single research project), modality can also be related to measures of structuredness.

If modality refers to the mode of expression of scholarship, temporality describes how scholarly works and the way they are expressed may evolve over time. When designing support for researchers, there is a tendency to treat scholarly works as discrete, independent entities that are created as static and stored as such for the long term. The reality is that scholarship is never truly static, however.[21] This is exemplified, for instance, when considered from a perspective of discoverability and reuse; when a scholarly work is created, it must be documented, organized, and preserved in a way that ensures it can be reused appropriately by researchers in the future. Additionally, when a new project begins, the outputs resulting from that project may be created over variable lengths. Data collection may be irregular and take place over several years, starting and stopping according to the rhythm of research. The result is what Samuel Arbesman calls "long data," or data that extend over massive sweeps of time.[22] This understanding of temporality recognizes that a scholarly work may never truly become complete and thus should not be treated as such.

The final frame of reference we will consider is sensitivity. Here again, the precise interpretation of "sensitivity" can vary across disciplines. In a clinical setting, sensitivity may concern precautions that must be taken when handling protected health information (PHI), whereas in an experimental setting, sensitivity may describe the efforts taken to keep data from being stolen and discoveries from being leaked prematurely. While both of these understandings involve protecting and managing access to scholarly works, their infrastructural implementation can be quite different. Data repositories can be particularly challenged to meet needs around sensitivity, especially when scaled across different standards for handling data that are variably susceptible to misuse.

These measures provide a baseline of heterogeneity that libraries infrastructures are increasingly called upon to support, and they often intersect in complex ways that may not have straightforward solutions. By transforming the volume-velocity-variety model of big data into one that considers scholarship from the perspectives of structuredness, modality, temporality, and sensitivity, we establish a framework that leaves more space for needs arising from different understandings of data. At each level of systems, services, and policy, this heterogeneity entails different principles for sustainable, scalable design, which we will discuss here.

Systems

Systems-level infrastructure can mean many different things, including server space for the storage of research materials, platforms that enable networking between researchers, and institutional repositories that help make scholarship discoverable for posterity. Naturally, the quantity and size of what researchers produce in their work tend to pose the most significant challenges to sustainability, and indeed, many studies have shown that researchers commonly indicate access to more storage space as one of their most important needs.[23] Research will continue to produce new digital materials at an inexorable rate, and one of the first questions to answer will always concern where to store those products for the short term.

Storage space may be the most immediately cited need at the systems level, but it reveals just a fraction of a more complex picture, much of which has been reflected in the results of the University of Minnesota data management surveys. For example, respondents consistently indicated a wide range of data types and media produced in their work as well as variability in how they stored, backed up, and organized those types across platforms and file types. Reported materials included media such as videos and photographs, interview transcripts, written works for textual analyses, spectral analyses, spreadsheets, and protected health information, illustrating that the support researchers need covered a large terrain of scholarship across many measures of structuredness, modality, temporality, and sensitivity.

In light of this, systems to support scholarship at scale depend on several design principles to ensure their ability to sustain the scholarly works of researchers as practices and products of research change. One particularly important principle is interoperability. Information and data rarely stand alone; they often must be passed between different systems, standards, and architectures, and it is often up to researchers themselves to determine how to most effectively facilitate those translations. Researchers and institutions constantly manage a wide variety of platforms that all operate independently but in parallel, including different operating systems, software, instruments, and backup and storage systems. These platforms may all differ in their metadata schemas, file formats, or procedures for collecting and managing data, requiring strategies for communicating across them. As modes of scholarship and scholarly communication continue to diversify, systems will continue to be challenged to grow in ways that overcome these proprietaries and move toward more robust structures for linked data across many different modalities. The advancement of cloud computing has helped accelerate this trend as research becomes increasingly massively parallel in nature[24]; at the same time, however, cloud computing has the potential to engender new challenges in managing the increasingly distributed temporality of scholarship as research materials become more dispersed across many different platforms simultaneously.

Another design principle entails maintaining a high threshold for the quality of the data that systems manage. Although here we may use the term "data quality," we will consider it in the broader context of scholarly works in whatever form, referring to their capacity for long-term preservation and reuse. Data quality has a limiting effect on systems that is actually amplified by interoperability; poor data quality quickly propagates upward and has a ripple effect on other linked systems. Sustainability at the systems level thus relies on designing platforms that integrate practices to maximize preservation and reuse, such as in terms of protections against bitstream-level corruption and migration of file formats. It is also dependent upon architectures that both have a high capacity for handling data with low structuredness as well as encourage high standards of structuredness through clean metadata practices. The discoverability of scholarly works cannot be sustained well into the future if rigorous standards for documentation have not been established or if systems providing those discovery layers are unable to handle highly heterogeneous objects with high fidelity.

A final key principle of design to consider is security, which is critical for scaling support across different measures of sensitivity. Working with sensitive data can be extremely difficult; in the case of protected health information, for instance, it is often easy to overlook information that has the potential to identify individuals, and it takes trained expertise to identify those risks across different disciplines. Systems that are able to maintain rigorous standards for de-identification can be built to scale, and as our procedures for handling such scholarship continue to evolve, so must our technologies that are deployed to do so. At the same time, systems must also be built to provide secure access to sensitive information that has not been de-identified; as needs grow around clinical data, for instance, creating secure platforms that control access to those data while still enabling integration with other systems will be important for advancing scholarship.

Services

Library services provide support at many different points of entry in the research life cycle. From the very beginning, these include assistance with grant writing, the development and execution of data management plans, and scholarly communication. These services can come in many shapes and forms, varying as widely as the specific needs of researchers they are designed to support.[25] This is perhaps the greatest challenge to sustainability in the service domain; while services supporting researchers in the management of their scholarship need to be designed generically to reach the broadest populations possible, they must also retain enough flexibility to grow under the pressure of rapidly changing technologies, research practices, and data sharing requirements. The sustainability of these services is thus fundamentally dependent upon both the technologies and people that exist to steward them. As Geneva Henry states, "Decisions about how best to manage digital content are intricately intertwined with the people and systems available to support the data curation life cycle," and this ethos applies at any service level.[26]

In this domain, the ability to balance that which can be operationalized with that which must be adapted to specialized needs is inevitably informed by the limitations of human resources. Librarians are challenged to economize those limited resources while constantly looking for new directions of growth, often through the cultivation of new skillsets enabling libraries to expand their portfolio of expertise. An example of this is the increased emphasis in recent times on raising librarians' data literacy skills, as libraries try to stay ahead of researchers' needs around software, statistical analysis, and data visualization to support many different modalities of scholarship. Additionally noteworthy is the emergent trend of non-librarians (i.e., those without formal library science degrees) being hired into new "functional specialist" positions to pull forward-looking skills into libraries, such as informaticists, data architects, and business strategists.[27] Expectations of librarians' knowledge and skills continue to rise, and librarians' roles are constantly evolving as a result.[28]

This emphasis on new skills has already begun to practically influence the variety of services libraries are able to provide. One such example is data curation, which requires familiarity with a broad range of subject areas and file types to be carried out effectively. Following suit of other academic institutions, the University of Minnesota Libraries began a program in 2015 to offer curation services to researchers, specifically to those who deposit their data into the Data Repository for University of Minnesota (DRUM). These services include helping researchers organize their data submissions, create clear and thorough documentation to facilitate reuse, and explore alternative preservation-friendly file formats, all with the aim of easing compliance with federal mandates and grant agency requirements on data sharing.

Perhaps once controversial, services for the curation of research scholarship are no longer new or surprising additions to libraries' roles.[29] However, best practices for scaling them across many specialized subject- and data-specific needs are still relatively nascent, ultimately requiring hands-on experience to fully mature. In 2013, the University of Minnesota Libraries made an effort to formulate best practices by holding a "curation sandbox" in which functional and subject specialists from across the libraries were convened to experiment with curation workflows. Participants were given one of five datasets, differing in their disciplinary focus, format, and data-specific considerations, and challenged to create a standardized workflow for curating that dataset for maximum preservation, discoverability, and reuse. After individual workflows were created, participants came together to identify similarities and differences between them, collectively integrating them into a standard procedure that could be applied to any scholarly work.[30]

The outcome of this sandbox demonstrated that while the details of curation workflows can be highly unique to different subject areas or data types, it is possible to develop a high-level procedural template that can be adapted and scaled to the needs at hand. The University Libraries have since leveraged these insights in the design of curation services, federating curation expertise across several staff members with subject- and data-specific knowledge and skills, including informatics and geospatial data specialists. As individual submissions are received through DRUM, they are assigned to specific staff based on a match of expertise, and the assigned staff member then curates submissions following a standard process. This process includes appraising submissions for the preservation-friendliness of file formats, data quality, possible sensitivity, and thoroughness of documentation, and curators collaborate directly with submitters so they can be actively involved throughout.

In the yet early age of these curation services, submissions have spanned many different disciplines and forms of scholarship, including mass spectrometry data, three-dimensional digital models of archaeological artifacts, and quantitative results from a study about the psychology of survey design. All of these have been unique in their complexity (including, of course, in their modalities and extent of structuredness) and attention to detail is required to curate them, yet at the same time, each has fit successfully into the template curation workflow. Here again is an important signature of sustainability: services can persist over time as long as they are provided the space to stretch with new challenges as they emerge.

Policy

We have so far considered library infrastructure at some of the more granular levels of the research life cycle. In terms of the long arc of scholarship, however, these short-scale modes of support may have limited influence on broader cultures of research. To find what engenders the kind of long, persistent, enduring change that moves communities of scholarship forward, we also must consider forces that operate at the highest levels of the research life cycle: the web of policies that define expectations around the ownership, transparency, and management of scholarship.

These policies exist in many layers of the research enterprise, and libraries have established expertise in helping guide researchers through their complicated and confusing implications. Federal mandates now declare rigorous standards for the sharing of research data; likewise, grant funding agencies increasingly require grantees to meet high expectations around data management and preservation. As these policies mature with time, so does the acknowledgment that all stakeholders in the research process jointly bear the onus of maintaining high standards for responsible stewardship of scholarship. This extends well beyond researchers alone and increasingly to academic institutions themselves, which are beginning to shape their own policies in ways that align institutional expectations about the management of scholarly works with those already put forth by grant agencies and the federal government.

The University of Minnesota has taken a decisive step in this direction, enacting two institutional policies in 2015 that more boldly define University standards for how research scholarship is managed and disseminated. The first of these, "Open Access to Scholarly Articles," grants the University a nonexclusive right to make scholarly works produced as the result of research at the University on or after January 1, 2015, openly accessible, such as by depositing them into the University's institutional repository. Researchers retain copyright of their works and are freely granted waivers when requested. This policy advances the University's land-grant mission in public engagement and follows the model of several other academic institutions that have enacted their own policies on open access, including Harvard University, Massachusetts Institute of Technology, and Duke University.[31]

The other policy, "Research Data Management: Archiving, Ownership, Retention, Security, Storage, and Transfer," takes a significant step forward in concretely outlining the roles and responsibilities of University entities in several matters of data governance, including who claims ownership of research data, required procedures for retaining and destroying data, and accountability for adhering to high standards of data management. Responsibility for these matters is shared between several stakeholders, including the Office of the Vice President for Research, the principal investigator, and most importantly here, the University Libraries. More specifically, the policy identifies the Libraries as being jointly responsible with other stakeholders in ensuring that practices and solutions for research data management are maintained at a high level of quality and rigor in accordance with federal, state, funding agency, and University requirements.[32]

The implications of both of these policies are enormous for researchers at the University of Minnesota and reflect important winds of change that are stirring in the broader research community. They decisively shift the responsibility for maintaining rigorous standards for research data management to not only individual researchers but also the many entities with which they interface. As a result, researchers have a vested interest in adhering to standards put forth collectively by federal mandates, sponsor requirements, and University policy, with accountability built in at each level. While the heterogeneity of scholarly works will continue to pose challenges to the research community, stricter guidelines for openness will make it easier to respond to those challenges more quickly. The result is a more robust and sustainable framework for catalyzing the dissemination of scholarly works, propelled forward by cultural shifts toward transparency and sharing in research.

Pressure is growing also around academic journals to take the lead in establishing new policies and guidelines for author submissions, especially in light of recent discoveries of research malpractice. In a June 2015 issue of *Science*, for example, Alberts et al. and Nosek et al. discuss the imbalance between research cultures and standards of accountability that hinder scientific transparency and encourage unethical practices.[33] These authors suggest that openness is poorly incentivized by current pressures in scholarly communication, including emphasis on publishing work that is innovative rather than high quality, that engender problems of irreproducibility and call into question the integrity of science. Recognizing the central role that academic journals play in the communication of research findings, Nosek et al. describe a collection of standards formulated by the Transparency and Openness Promotion (TOP) Committee that seek to change journals' procedures for publishing research results and consequently encourage more openness in the scientific community. These include more rewards for engaging in open research, stricter measures of reproducibility, and more rigorous expectations around the sharing of data through trusted repositories. Reaffirming the responsibility that universities, funding agencies, and academic journals each have in being actively involved in the research life cycle, the authors note that "nudging scientific practices toward greater openness requires complementary and coordinated efforts from all stakeholders."[34]

The emerging policy infrastructure demonstrates a growing awareness that providing support for scholarship at scale requires a long view of the research life cycle, installing checkpoints of accountability at each stage. Data management is not only about the products of research but also the cultures that inform researchers' practices. Sustainability is thus achieved by policy that strives to be continuously forward thinking, holding researchers to new expectations that challenge whole communities of scholarship to evolve. Stricter guidelines for managing research draw attention to the reality that the scholarly works that researchers produce today are unprecedented in their diversity and the challenges they pose, and progress can be made only if all stakeholders assume shared responsibility of the infrastructure required to facilitate it. The new research ecosystem is still relatively uncharted, but policy can provide the clear momentum needed to shape the direction in which that ecosystem grows.

Conclusion

For many years, libraries have been at the vanguard of data management, providing researchers the resources they need to document, store, and share their scholarship. As we have seen, however, roles around data management are changing as the research landscape continues to become more diversified. Understandings of data and research practices are continuously shifting across disciplines, and it is incumbent upon all stakeholders in the research life cycle to acknowledge that current infrastructures may be unprepared for the changes they bring. Equipped with an intimate understanding of researchers, their practices, and the communities of scholarship in which they are cultured, libraries are uniquely poised to play a significant role in formulating the technological, service, and policy infrastructure requisite for sustaining resilience against these shifting needs.

In this chapter, we explored the ways in which libraries can leverage their unique position by considering the implications of working with scholarship at scale in the design of library infrastructure at several different levels. We began by discussing the limitations of a conceptual framework defined in the language of "big data," suggesting that this term provides an unsophisticated view of the nuanced challenges that researchers and their institutions face in data management. Instead, we shifted our discussion toward thinking about these challenges in terms of scholarship at scale, reinforcing the idea that infrastructure to support data management must be guided by a discipline agnosticism that recognizes the many spectra of complexity across which research scholarship can be diversified.

We considered challenges to sustainability and scalability in the design of library infrastructures through a select set of frames of reference, namely structuredness, modality, temporality, and sensitivity. From a systems perspective, we considered technological platforms that preserve scholarly works, facilitate their sharing, and enhance their discoverability, noting that such platforms must be built to sustain highly diversified and dynamic scholarship. Interoperability, data quality, and security were all fundamental principles of design thereof, building robustness against the challenges of heterogeneity. Meanwhile, at the level of library services, we discussed new roles that libraries are beginning to take on to engage with researchers at more points in the research life cycle, including services for the curation of data. We noted that sustainability is best achieved at the services level through a careful balance between what can be operationalized and what can be scaled to specialized needs, which requires a priori an intimate knowledge of what those special needs may be. Finally, we explored these ideas from a policy perspective, considering guidelines that are being established by institutions, funding agencies, and the government to encourage more checkpoints of accountability in research. We saw that sustainability at the policy level requires active participation by all stakeholders in the research enterprise, constantly challenging researchers to meet more rigorous standards in the management, sharing, and transparency of their scholarly works. The implementation of such standards can help change data management practices, leading to more robust responses to the challenges of working with highly diversified scholarship at earlier points in the research process.

Academic librarianship is constantly challenged to sustain relevance in a research ecosystem that evolves constantly and rapidly. To meet this challenge, libraries must continually demonstrate their breadth of expertise in as many ways as possible, striving to meet researchers' current needs while anticipating those yet to come. When libraries take risks in new directions, whether that means the development of new services, piloting new technologies, or hiring new skillsets to advance the field as a whole, they can generate anecdotal evidence of their value. Librarians' relationships with researchers become more deeply symbiotic as a result; as researchers lean into the infrastructures of support libraries provide, libraries themselves can learn how to grow to meet their changing needs. As perceptions of the roles that libraries play in providing research support continue to shift, new opportunities for libraries to sustain authority as a critical stakeholder in the research life cycle will emerge for years to come.

Pearls

- Working definitions of "big data" can provide a narrow and simplistic depiction of the challenges researchers face today in managing their scholarly works.
- To account for different understandings of data across researchers, shifting our language toward *scholarship at scale* provides a more flexible framework for considering how data management needs may manifest uniquely across researchers.
- Libraries have an intimate understanding of researchers' practices and cultures of scholarship and are thus poised to respond quickly to needs as they rapidly evolve.
- Researchers' needs for support in the management of their scholarly works are increasingly complex as scholarship becomes more diversified across several spectra of heterogeneity, including structuredness, modality, temporality, and sensitivity.
- Library infrastructures can provide support for scholarship across these many scales, but they must be designed for sustainability at systems, services, and policy levels.

Recommended Resources and Reading

Hey, Tony, Tansley, Stewart, and Tolle, Kristin, eds. *The Fourth Paradigm: Data-Intensive Scientific Discovery*. Redmond, WA: Microsoft Research, 2009. http://research.microsoft.com/en-us/collaboration/fourthparadigm/.

Notes

1. Perry Rotella, "Is Data the New Oil?" *Forbes*, April 2, 2012, http://www.forbes.com/sites/perryrotella/2012/04/02/is-data-the-new-oil/.
2. Luigi Atzori, Antonio Iera, and Giacomo Morabito, "The Internet of Things: A Survey," *Computer Networks* 54 (2010); Eleonora Borgia, "The Internet of Things Vision: Key Features, Applications and Open Issues," *Computer Communications* 54 (2014).
3. Alexander B. Howard, "Here Comes the Data Economy," *Slate*, September 10, 2012, http://www.slate.com/articles/technology/future_tense/2012/09/brightscope_castlight_new_businesses_built_on_open_government_data_.html; Michael Mandel, "The Data Economy Is Much, Much Bigger Than You (and the Government) Think," *Atlantic*, July 2013, http://www.theatlantic.com/business/archive/2013/07/the-data-economy-is-much-much-bigger-than-you-and-the-government-think/278113/.
4. Steve Lohr, "The Age of Big Data," *New York Times*, February 11, 2012.
5. "Data, Data Everywhere," *Economist*, February 25, 2010, http://www.economist.com/node/15557443.
6. Alasdair Allan, "Tertiary Data: Big Data's Hidden Layer," *O'Reilly Media*, March 19, 2012, http://radar.oreilly.com/2012/03/hidden-data-exhaust-leakage-location.html.
7. Don MacMillan, "Data Sharing and Discovery: What Librarians Need to Know," *Journal of Academic Librarianship* 40 (2014); Carla J. Stoffle, Robert Renaud, and Jerilyn R. Veldof, "Choosing Our Futures," *College & Research Libraries* 76, no. 3 (2015).
8. Li Si et al., "Investigation and Analysis of Research Data Services in University Libraries," *Electronic Library* 33, no. 3 (2015).

9. Matthew B. Hoy, "Big Data: An Introduction for Librarians," *Medical Reference Services Quarterly* 33, no. 3 (2014); Ibrahim Abaker Targio Hashem et al., "The Rise of 'Big Data' on Cloud Computing: Review and Open Research Issues," *Information Systems* 47 (2015).
10. "O'Reilly Radar," O'Reilly Media, Inc., http://radar.oreilly.com/.
11. Edd Dumbill, "Making Sense of Big Data," *Big Data* 1, no. 1 (2013), 1.
12. Hashem et al., "The Rise of 'Big Data' on Cloud Computing: Review and Open Research Issues," 100.
13. Ibid.; Min Chen, Shiwen Mao, and Yunhao Liu, "Big Data: A Survey," *Mobile Networks and Applications* 19 (2014).
14. "Big Data," Gartner Research, http://www.gartner.com/it-glossary/big-data.
15. Xialong Jin et al., "Significance and Challenges of Big Data Research," *Big Data Research* 2 (2015).
16. Jillian C Wallis, Elizabeth Rolando, and Christine L Borgman, "If We Share Data, Will Anyone Use Them? Data Sharing and Reuse in the Long Tail of Science and Technology," *PLoS ONE* 8, no. 7 (2013).
17. "Data Repository for University of Minnesota (Drum)," http://z.umn.edu/drum.
18. Alicia Hofelich Mohr et al., "When Data Is a Dirty Word: A Survey to Understand Data Management Needs Across Diverse Research Disciplines," *Bulletin of the Association for Information Science and Technology 42*, no. 1 (2015): 51–53.
19. Travis Weller and Amalia Monroe-Glick, "Understanding Methodological and Disciplinary Differences in the Data Practices of Academic Researchers," *Library Hi Tech* 32, no. 3 (2014); Katherine Akers and Jennifer Doty, "Disciplinary Differences in Faculty Research Data Management Practices and Perspectives," *International Journal of Digital Curation* 8, no. 2 (2013).
20. Wallis, Rolando, and Borgman, "If We Share Data, Will Anyone Use Them"
21. Ibid.
22. Samuel Arbesman, "Stop Hyping Big Data and Start Paying Attention to 'Long Data,'" *Wired.com*, January 2013, http://www.wired.com/2013/01/forget-big-data-think-long-data/.
23. Akers and Doty, "Disciplinary Differences in Faculty Research Data Management Practices and Perspectives"; Weller and Monroe-Glick, "Understanding Methodological and Disciplinary Differences in the Data Practices of Academic Researchers"; Mohr et al., "Surveying Academic Researchers to Identify Disciplinary-Specific Needs for Research Data Management Services."
24. Dennis Gannon and Dan Reed, "Parallelism and the Cloud," in *The Fourth Paradigm: Data-Intensive Scientific Discovery*, ed. Tony Hey, Stewart Tansley, and Kristin Tolle (Redmond, WA: Microsoft Corporation, 2009).
25. Si et al., "Investigation and Analysis of Research Data Services in University Libraries."
26. Geneva Henry, "Data Curation for the Humanities," in *Research Data Management: Practical Strategies for Information Professionals*, ed. Joyce M. Ray (West Lafayette, IN: Purdue University Press, 2014), 350.
27. Janice Jaguszewski and Karen Williams, "New Roles for New Times: Transforming Liaison Roles in Research Libraries," (Association of Research Libraries, 2013). http://www.arl.org/publications-resources/2893-new-roles-for-new-times-transforming-liaison-roles-in-research-libraries#.VzdasfkrKUk
28. Evgenia Vassilakaki and Valentini Moniarou-Papaconstantinou, "A Systematic Literature Review Informing Library and Information Professionals' Emerging Roles," *New Library World* 116, nos. 1–2 (2015).
29. Merinda McLure et al., "Data Curation: A Study of Researcher Practices and Needs," *portal: Libraries and the Academy* 14, no. 2 (2014).
30. Lisa Johnston, *A Workflow Model for Curating Research Data in the University of Minnesota Libraries: Report from the 2013 Data Curation Pilot* (Minneapolis: University of Minnesota Libraries, 2014).
31. University of Minnesota Board of Regents, "Open Access to Scholarly Articles," 2015, https://policy.umn.edu/research/scholarlyarticles.

32. University of Minnesota Board of Regents, "Research Data Management: Archiving, Ownership, Retention, Security, Storage, and Transfer," 2015, http://policy.umn.edu/research/researchdata.
33. Bruce Alberts et al., "Self-Correction in Science at Work," *Science* 348, no. 6242 (2015); B. A. Nosek et al., "Promoting an Open Research Culture," *Science* 348, no. 6242 (2015): 1422–25.
34. Nosek et al., "Promoting an Open Research Culture," 1422.

Bibliography

Akers, Katherine, and Jennifer Doty. "Disciplinary Differences in Faculty Research Data Management Practices and Perspectives." *International Journal of Digital Curation* 8, no. 2 (2013).

Alberts, Bruce, et al. "Self-Correction in Science at Work." *Science* 348, no. 6242 (2015).

Allan, Alasdair. "Tertiary Data: Big Data's Hidden Layer." *O'Reilly Media*, March 19, 2012. http://radar.oreilly.com/2012/03/hidden-data-exhaust-leakage-location.html.

Arbesman, Samuel. "Stop Hyping Big Data and Start Paying Attention to 'Long Data.'" *Wired.com*, http://www.wired.com/2013/01/forget-big-data-think-long-data/.

Atzori, Luigi, Antonio Iera, and Giacomo Morabito. "The Internet of Things: A Survey." *Computer Networks* 54 (2010).

Borgia, Eleonora. "The Internet of Things Vision: Key Features, Applications and Open Issues." *Computer Communications* 54 (2014).

Chen, Min, Shiwen Mao, and Yunhao Liu. "Big Data: A Survey." *Mobile Networks and Applications* 19 (2014).

Dumbill, Edd. "Making Sense of Big Data," *Big Data* 1, no. 1 (2013): 1–2.

Economist. "Data, Data Everywhere." February 25, 2010. http://www.economist.com/node/15557443.

Gannon, Dennis, and Dan Reed. "Parallelism and the Cloud." In *The Fourth Paradigm: Data-Intensive Scientific Discovery*. Redmond, WA: Microsoft Corporation, 2009.

Gartner Research. "Big Data," http://www.gartner.com/it-glossary/big-data.

Hashem, Ibrahim Abaker Targio, et al. "The Rise of "Big Data" on Cloud Computing: Review and Open Research Issues." *Information Systems* 47 (2015): 98–115.

Henry, Geneva. "Data Curation for the Humanities." In *Research Data Management: Practical Strategies for Information Professionals*, ed. Joyce M. Ray. West Lafayette, IN: Purdue University Press, 2014).

Hofelich Mohr, Alicia, Josh Bishoff, Carolyn Bishoff, Steven Braun, Christine Storino, and Lisa R. Johnston. "When Data Is a Dirty Word: A Survey to Understand Data Management Needs Across Diverse Research Disciplines," *Bulletin of the Association for Information Science and Technology 42*, no. 1 (2015): 51–53.

Howard, Alexander B. "Here Comes the Data Economy," *Slate*, September 10, 2012. http://www.slate.com/articles/technology/future_tense/2012/09/brightscope_castlight_new_businesses_built_on_open_government_data_.html.

Hoy, Matthew B. "Big Data: An Introduction for Librarians," *Medical Reference Services Quarterly* 33, no. 3 (2014).

Jaguszewski, Janice, and Karen Williams, "New Roles for New Times: Transforming Liaison Roles in Research Libraries." Association of Research Libraries, 2013. http://www.arl.org/publications-resources/2893-new-roles-for-new-times-transforming-liaison-roles-in-research-libraries#.VzdasfkrKUk

Jin, Xialong, et al., "Significance and Challenges of Big Data Research." *Big Data Research* 2 (2015).

Johnston, Lisa. *A Workflow Model for Curating Research Data in the University of Minnesota Libraries: Report from the 2013 Data Curation Pilot*. Minneapolis: University of Minnesota Libraries, 2014.

Lohr, Steve. "The Age of Big Data." *New York Times*, February 11, 2012.

MacMillan, Don. "Data Sharing and Discovery: What Librarians Need to Know." *Journal of Academic Librarianship* 40 (2014).
Mandel, Michael. "The Data Economy Is Much, Much Bigger Than You (and the Government) Think." *Atlantic*, July 2013. http://www.theatlantic.com/business/archive/2013/07/the-data-economy-is-much-much-bigger-than-you-and-the-government-think/278113/.
McLure, Merinda et al. "Data Curation: A Study of Researcher Practices and Needs." *portal: Libraries and the Academy* 14, no. 2 (2014).
Mohr, Alicia Hofelich, et al. "Surveying Academic Researchers to Identify Disciplinary-Specific Needs for Research Data Management Services." 2015.
Nosek, B. A. et al. "Promoting an Open Research Culture." *Science* 348, no. 6242 (2015).
Rotella, Perry. "Is Data the New Oil?" *Forbes*, April 2, 2012. http://www.forbes.com/sites/perryrotella/2012/04/02/is-data-the-new-oil/.
Si, Li, et al. "Investigation and Analysis of Research Data Services in University Libraries." *Electronic Library* 33, no. 3 (2015).
Stoffle, Carla J., Robert Renaud, and Jerilyn R. Veldof. "Choosing Our Futures." *College & Research Libraries* 76, no. 3 (2015).
University of Minnesota Board of Regents. "Open Access to Scholarly Articles." 2015, http://policy.umn.edu/research/scholarlyarticles.
———. "Research Data Management: Archiving, Ownership, Retention, Security, Storage, and Transfer." 2015. https://policy.umn.edu/research/researchdata.
University of Minnesota Libraries. "Data Repository for University of Minnesota (DRUM)." http://z.umn.edu/drum.
Vassilakaki, Evgenia, and Valentini Moniarou-Papaconstantinou. "A Systematic Literature Review Informing Library and Information Professionals' Emerging Roles." *New Library World* 116, nos. 1–2 (2015).
Wallis, Jillian C., Elizabeth Rolando, and Christine L. Borgman, "If We Share Data, Will Anyone Use Them? Data Sharing and Reuse in the Long Tail of Science and Technology," *PLoS ONE* 8, no. 7 (2013).
Weller, Travis, and Amalia Monroe-Glick. "Understanding Methodological and Disciplinary Differences in the Data Practices of Academic Researchers." *Library Hi Tech* 32, no. 3 (2014).

Chapter 10

Contextualizing Visualization in Library Services

Marci D. Brandenburg, University of Michigan Taubman Health Sciences Library, and Justin Joque, University of Michigan Library

While the present book is focused on data management, visualization and other data-related activities can be the most effective when combined with careful thinking about data management, discovery, exploration, and analysis. Data visualization can play an important role in the life cycles of various types of data, as it both requires that data be well managed and provides efficient means to understand the data one has, further informing its management, collection, and analysis. Moreover, data visualization provides a means to communicate research results and data to diverse audiences.

As libraries expand their data offerings and collection of research data, providing data visualization services presents an opportunity to enhance and further develop these services. In addition to being closely related to data management and analysis, data visualization services provide an opportunity for libraries to aid patrons in utilizing and exploring collections of data. Data visualization services can allow researchers and students access to and understanding of the datasets that libraries are now collecting. Librarians can play an important role by offering instruction and consultations, along with being valuable collaborators for patrons exploring their own research data. Moreover, it is not always necessary to have a librarian devoted exclusively to data visualization. While one of us is a visualization librarian, the other is a health sciences librarian who has provided visualization services and instruction for a number of years. Through visualization, we can help patrons understand and utilize data, whether private or publicly available.

Data visualization includes a rich spectrum of activities ranging from simple bar charts to immersive 3D environments displaying terabytes of data. Lev Manovich offers a broad definition of data visualization, stating that its goal "is to discover the structure of a (typically large) dataset. This structure is not known a priori; a visualization is successful if it reveals this structure."[1] Likewise, Edward Tufte states that graphics, as meaning visual displays of data, "reveal data."[2] Data visualization is thus a technique for making visible some of the deep structures that organize datasets and the underlying reality they express. Manovich further stresses that this definition connects diverse data visualization tools from ink to computers: "while availability of computers led to the development of new visualization techniques (scatter plot matrix, treemaps, etc.), the basic visual language of infovis remained the same as it was in the 19th century—points, lines, rectangles and other graphic primitives."[3] In this direction, we understand visualization as the process of mapping data to a visual space so that one can better understand the structure, distribution, and composition of different types of data in diverse media.

A number of writers, including Manovich, make a distinction between information visualization and scientific visualization, distinguishing between arbitrary spatial coordinates in the former (for example, income and unemployment rates on a scatter plot) and the given spatial layout of an object in the latter (for example, an MRI of a brain or a coastline on a map).[4] Regardless, in both cases one still often uses color, scale, and other spatial markers to communicate the various aspects of the data even if it has a fixed spatial form; thus, in our work, and for the purposes of this chapter, we understand data visualization to encompass all of these various activities aimed at understanding data and the world by mapping and presenting it so that it can be visually comprehended.

Throughout this chapter, we will explore the history of visualization, outline important principles, and discuss the role that libraries can play in leading the way in research visualization services.

Visualization in Context

Data visualization and scientific discovery, especially in medical research, have a rich and complicated history that offers a unique perspective on the role that data visualization can play in research. While there is not space here to document this history fully, and this work is already represented in a variety of places,[5] a little bit of this historical context can help situate the role data visualization can play today. Despite a long history of map making and displaying geographic information in visual form, statistical graphs (such as bar charts, scatterplots, and line charts) and data visualization are much more recent phenomena. The first known map dates back to 3800 BCE, but it was not until the mid-seventeenth century that graphical space was used to display statistical rather than geographic information.[6]

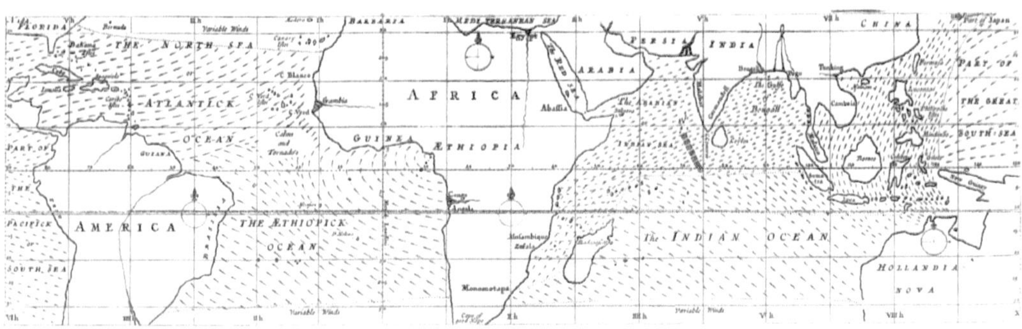

Figure 10.1. Edmond Halley's 1686 map of global trade winds. Edmund Halley, "An Historical Account of the Trade Winds, and Monsoons, Observable in the Seas between and Near the Tropicks, with an Attempt to Assign the Phisical Cause of the Said Winds," Philosophical Transactions 16, nos. 179–91 (1686): 153–68.

During the seventeenth century, a number of visualizations were created that displayed data on geographic maps, such as Edmond Halley's 1686 map of trade winds (see figure 10.1), as well as more abstract displays of data, such as Michael Florent van Langren's 1644 graph of estimates of the difference in longitude between Toledo and Rome (see figure 10.2).[7] Thus, over five thousand years elapsed from the time of the first known maps to the abstraction of these technologies and methods to describe statistical information.

Since these beginnings in the seventeenth century, visualization has been used both in scientific pursuits directly and in communicating the results to larger audiences. Two centuries after Halley and van Langren's pioneering work, John Snow's cholera map provides an exemplary use of data visualization to understand a health emergency. In the midst of an 1854 outbreak of cholera in central London,

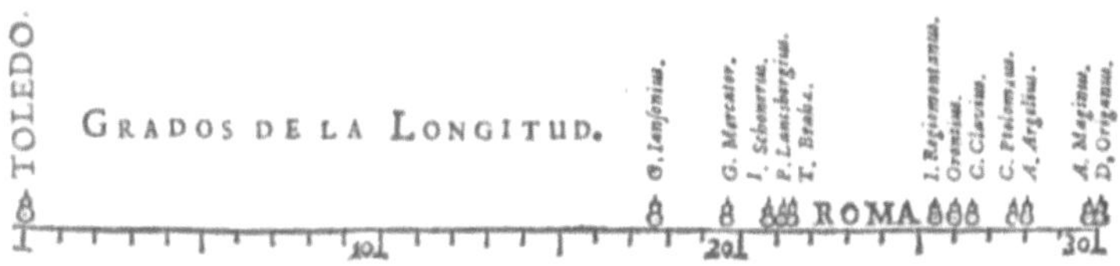

Figure 10.2. Florent van Langren's 1644 graph of longitude difference between Toledo and Rome. Michael Florent van Langren, 1644, from: Michael Friendly, "Milestones in the History of Data Visualization: A Case Study in Statistical Historiography," in *Classification—the Ubiquitous Challenge*, ed. Claus Weihs and Wolfgang Gaul (Berlin: Springer, 2005), 37.

Snow collected data on cholera deaths and plotted the deaths on a map that also showed the location of water wells. On the resultant map, it was very clear that the deaths clustered around a single well, which played a key role in the outbreak. With this information, Snow was able to get the well pump's handle removed, disabling it. The map and the insights that can be seen from it suggest how effective visually displaying information can be in understanding complex phenomena. Tufte, in recounting this story, makes an important observation, noting, "The link between the pump and the disease might have been revealed by computation and analysis without graphics, with good luck and hard work. But, here at least, graphical analysis testifies about the data far more efficiently than calculation."[8] At least in this instance, and given the computational tools and techniques available to Snow, the visualization was able to demonstrate a potential association much more effectively than calculating a statistical relationship.

The relationship between statistical methods and visualization is of incredible import for thinking about the role of visualization in research. While visualization offers unique insights into data and its structure, one can often arrive at some of the same insights through calculation. This distinction—and with it a certain tension—between the insights offered through visualization and calculation of statistics dates back to the earliest statistical graphics. As Beniger and Robyn note, many early applied scientists were proponents of tabular data, despite the instrumentation of the time often directly producing visualizations: "Between 1660 and 1800, scores of different mechanical recorders were invented that produced moving line graphs of various natural time series: temperature, barometric readings, wind speed and direction, tidal movements, etc. Such automatic graphs were considered useless for analysis and were routinely translated into tabular logs."[9] This complex relationship between visualization and calculation continues to affect present research and should, at the very least, be kept in mind when developing and providing visualization services.

Humans are incredibly adept at recognizing patterns, which means that we are able to find relationships that sometimes do not show up in certain calculations, but also that we often believe we see patterns where we are merely looking at noise or random variation. Anscombe's quartet exemplifies the first case, identifying important information visually that may escape calculation. The quartet consists of four sets of data that all share the same summary statistics, so each dataset has the same mean, regression coefficient, and so on. However, when graphed, they show very distinct structural characteristics, such as a straight line versus a curved line, that suggest other modes of analysis.[10] As in the case of Snow's cholera map, it would have been difficult to know what to calculate for in this scenario, yet he was able to see something important via the visualization. In regard to the second case, examples abound of significance being attached to chance events from the sometimes-believable predictive power of astrology to claims that cold spells disprove global warming or relationships between vaccines and autism. In sum, one must be careful in placing too much emphasis on observed visual patterns, but at the same time these visual patterns can inform research in ways that calculation alone cannot.

Visualization Principles

Given the interdisciplinary nature of visualization, and the wide range of visualization types, it is important to have a familiarity of visualization principles. Color, shape, and size are all characteristics that can be changed to alter one's perception of an image. For example, the use of colors may lead to discovering patterns that otherwise were not recognized,[11] and the human eye is generally drawn to larger shapes before smaller shapes. In addition, proximity can be important, for we detect clusters of objects that are spaced close together.[12] For example, network visualization can be used to understand a group of interacting genes, where each gene would be represented by a circle, known as a node, and the interaction between two genes would be represented by a line, known as an edge, connecting the two representative circles. When looking at a network visualization of interacting genes, a cluster showing that one gene interacts with many other genes might lead a researcher to focus additional research on that specific gene. Pattern detection can help researchers better understand and represent their data, so many visualization tools allow for the manipulation of visualizations to take advantage of these principles. To best help a researcher create a data visualization, an understanding of these visualization principles is imperative.

Design principles should also be considered when creating or using visualization tools. Librarians bridge the gap between the people who create a software tool and the user. Before we can recommend specific visualization resources and techniques, we must have a solid understanding of good versus bad visualization and the criteria necessary for evaluating visualization software. Heuristics are often used when evaluating visualization software. Heuristics relate to "exploratory problem-solving techniques that utilize self-educating techniques (as the evaluation of feedback) to improve performance."[13] Understanding visualization best practices and tool evaluation criteria is important for librarians to best help their researchers. Librarians can conduct usability studies to compare various features of tools from a user's perspective to determine where they perform well and where they need improvement. This knowledge provides librarians guidance for recommending the best tools to users based on their needs.

There are numerous tools for creating and manipulating data visualizations, ranging from scripting languages (programming languages that allow for writing specialized programs that work in specific environments and execute specific tasks) to network visualization tools (software that transforms raw data into shapes that represent items and connecting lines that represent a relationship between two items) to combination packages (programs that create a variety of different visualization types). Having knowledge of a range of visualization tools can enhance the visualization services offered by a library. It is not necessary to be an expert on all tools, but instead to have an understanding of several tools' overall functionality in order to recommend the appropriate tool based on a researcher's needs. We recommend learning about both freely available and commercial tool alternatives, since funds may or may not be a prohibitive factor for using a specific tool.

Visualization in the Library

While it took over five thousand years to develop data visualization out of technologies for map making, visualization has advanced rapidly since these beginnings, especially in the last decades as the size and complexity of digital data and our ability to process it has grown. Data visualization has become a complex field in its own right, including techniques from simple bar charts to interactive 3D environments for exploring terabytes of data. The broad spectrum of activities and skillsets that now fall under the term data visualization, along with the aforementioned complexities in the relationship between visualization and calculation, requires that libraries and librarians think carefully about their constituents' needs when developing and providing data visualization services. Often researchers and students require assistance with the entire spectrum of visualization, from aesthetic choices to selecting graphs to working with software to developing systems and methods for working with large datasets.

The authors of this chapter are both librarians at the University of Michigan (U-M), founded in 1817, and located in Ann Arbor, Michigan. It consists of nineteen schools and colleges, and in 2014 it had over forty-three thousand students, over six thousand eight hundred faculty, and more than fourteen thousand staff.[14] U-M has an expansive library system that consists of over forty libraries and departments, including Taubman Health Sciences Library, which collaborates closely with U-M's Medical School, School of Nursing, School of Dentistry, College of Pharmacy, School of Public Health, and the U-M Health System;[15] Stephen S. Clark Library for maps, government information, and spatial and numeric data;[16] Digital Media Commons, which includes audio and video recording, virtual reality, 3D printing, and maker spaces;[17] and the Shapiro Science Library, which collaborates with researchers in fields such as astronomy, geological sciences, biology, chemistry, and natural resources.[18] U-M Library's mission is to "support, enhance, and collaborate in the instructional, research, and service activities of the faculty, students, and staff, and contribute to the common good by collecting, organizing, preserving, communicating, and sharing the record of human knowledge."[19] As we look for innovative ways to work with our community, the library has expanded its services to incorporate data and visualization.

Faculty, students, and staff are all engaged in visualization activities. Researchers, whether faculty or staff, often use visualization techniques to explore and represent their data. Many students learn about visualization techniques as part of their studies and often use visualization in class projects. As a result, visualization services can target all members of an academic community.

Services

Traditionally, a library is not the first place that comes to mind when someone needs help visualizing data. With the exponential increase in the amount of data being collected, and the movement toward libraries offering data services, the next logical step is for libraries to offer visualization services.

When initially embarking on the journey of offering visualization services, we recommend creating a working group of librarians to assess institutional needs and determine an appropriate role for the library within the visualization domain. Given that the term "visualization" encompasses a broad range of disciplines and categories, librarians should collaborate with each other to determine the existing knowledge base and skills that can be leveraged to best serve the community. Providing visualization services should be a communal activity where librarians across disciplines look to each other for help in answering questions and learning about resources. Education and promotion of services are extremely important for providing successful visualization activities.

Like with many library services, it is important for visualization librarians to be well-versed in conducting reference interviews. A data visualization request begins like any other reference question or consultation in that the first step is to get more information about the researcher's needs and desires. It is important to ask questions to determine whether or not visualization is the most appropriate and best way to represent the researcher's data. This requires gaining context and background on the dataset and asking questions such as: What is the purpose of the visual representation of data? What personnel are available and what skills do you have for generating the data visualization? Are you looking for additional data to combine with your existing data? The more information that librarians can get initially, the more efficiently they will be able to help.

Libraries can offer an assortment of visualization services, specific to the skills and experiences of their librarians. The U-M Library provides a variety of services around visualization activities, including in-depth consultations, instruction sessions, a referral service, partnering, and help finding and manipulating data. Employees throughout the library work together, and with researchers, to ensure that their visualization needs are met with the best resources available to them, including people, software, and hardware.

Instruction

Providing detailed step-by-step instructions for using resources, such as PubMed, is a typical activity for librarians. As a result, and given the value of data visualization, it is a natural transition for librarians to provide instruction on data visualization techniques and tools. Important topics to consider covering in training include data management practices to ease the transformation of raw data into a visual representation, the difference between a good and bad visualization, and how to use specific visualization-generating tools.

Seminar-style workshops are an appropriate format for teaching the first two concepts, and we offer these to researchers and librarians at U-M. For example, in April 2015, we, along with the Manager of the UM3D Lab, which is part of the Library's Digital Media Commons and offers tools and expertise for computer modeling and visualization, offered a one-hour "Introduction to Visualization" workshop. This workshop was aimed at librarians and covered the visualization landscape, several design concepts, interpretation of a visualization, and who to contact within the library for visualization help. We believe that all subject librarians and informationists should have basic knowledge of visualization techniques and tools in order to direct researchers appropriately.

The teaching of specific tools is often better handled in a hands-on workshop format. Many of these tools are complex, and we have found users prefer to actively walk through the steps, helping them learn when and where to click in order to visualize and manipulate data. Researchers first want to know how to get their data from an Excel spreadsheet or text file into the chosen software program. Then they want to know how to manipulate the data to create a desired visual representation and/or perform data analysis. Depending on the complexity of the tool, a series of hands-on workshops can be best, with each having a different focus.

The U-M Library has been offering hands-on instruction on visualization tools, such as Cytoscape, an open-source network visualization tool,[20] for over six years and attendance continues to be high. Based on user feedback and in order to reach a wider audience, these sessions have evolved over the years to include different content and presentation media.[21] Other visualization tools on which we provide instruction are R,[22] a statistical and graphics package; MetScape,[23] a Cytoscape app used for visualizing relationships between compounds and genes; and ConceptGen,[24] an enrichment and concept mapping tool. Teaching these sessions presents an opportunity to further our own knowledge of the tools, combined with meeting user needs, as often questions are asked that lead us to learn something new about a resource. To provide instruction on visualization resources, it is not necessary to understand everything about a specific discipline; the goal is to teach how to use the tool. This also provides an opportunity for collaboration, as sessions can be co-taught by one person who is experienced in using the tool and a second person who has discipline-specific knowledge related to the training dataset. This collaboration model is one that we use quite frequently at U-M when teaching on visualization resources.

In the academic environment, there are opportunities for teaching visualization concepts and tools within the curriculum. For example, for the last five years, one of the authors, along with a research specialist in a nephrology lab, co-taught a ninety-minute hands-on lab session, titled "Network analysis for systems biology," for the graduate-level bioinformatics course "Foundations in Bioinformatics and Systems Biology." Although the majority of this session focused on one open-source network visualization tool, Cytoscape, at least one other visualization tool, ConceptGen, was shown each of the last three years, and additional resources, such as LRpath,[25] a tool for gene set enrichment testing, were mentioned. Whereas the previous example represents a case of teaching one session within a semester-long class, we also offer more expansive visualization instruction within the curriculum. For example, the other author, along with a faculty member in the humanities, co-teaches a mini-course, "Mapping Moby-Dick," which requires students to think visually in new ways. The author helped design the course and taught it with the faculty member, as a supplement to his responsibilities in the library. Although this specific example comes from the humanities, it shows how librarians can work collaboratively with faculty to teach visualization concepts, which is true not only within the humanities, but also in all of the health sciences. Seeking out opportunities to integrate visualization instruction in the curriculum is a great way to solidify the library's role and expertise in this area.

Although in-person workshops provide great learning opportunities for users, we do not limit ourselves to these standard instruction-related activities. In addition to onsite seminars and hands-on workshops, we have offered webinars to reach a wider audience. In addition, we are involved in working with the creators of certain visualization software tools to develop video tutorials and write user manuals. Many tools lack good user documentation because this is not a strength or priority of the developers who write the software. However, good documentation is a requirement for a tool to gain widespread usage. This is an area where we can use our strengths as librarians to develop documentation in a way that is most useful for the user. Librarians may want to consider looking into what visualization tools and software are being created at their institution or organization, and then collaborate with the creators to develop the documentation. This partnership can turn into a long-term collaboration as tools get regularly updated and new ones are created, all needing up-to-date documentation.

Consultations

After learning about visualization techniques and tools, researchers will attempt to apply this information to their own datasets. At this point, many researchers contact us for consultations, where we can look more in-depth at using specialized tools with specific research data. Researchers run experiments, collect data, and perform data analysis, but they are often at a loss as to what to do next with the large amounts of data they have generated. As discussed in this chapter, visualization can lead to improved interpretation and an increased understanding of data. Once librarians become knowledgeable of visualization concepts, techniques, and some of the tools, they can offer consultations with researchers to help them through this stage of the research life cycle. Ideally, a researcher participates in an initial consultation with a librarian before beginning the data collection stage, but realistically, this is rarely the case. Regardless of the stage in the process, librarians can work with researchers to get the data in the correct format, evaluate visualization tools to determine the most appropriate one for the desired result, and provide instruction for using the tool. This instruction may be provided directly by the librarian or may involve guidance to useful web-based tutorials and existing documentation. Depending on the researcher's needs, this process could include one consultation or result in a series of consultations throughout the research life cycle.

At U-M, we often receive consultation requests from researchers who are interested in visualizing data. Consultations are requested for two main reasons: (1) a researcher is working on a publication or presentation and wants to represent the data visually, or (2) a researcher has a large amount of data and wants to make sense of it. The first type of consultation request often results in one or two meetings, and requires knowledge of visualization categories, principles, and tools. Our role is to help determine the best type of visualization (for example, bar chart, pie graph, network graph, overlaid map, etc.) and the best tools for creating it. The second type of consultation request can be a longer-term, collaborative relationship that involves meeting at various stages throughout the research process. As the researcher begins to make sense of the data, needs may change, leading to an iterative process. We help researchers choose an appropriate tool, get the data into that tool, and understand how to use the tool to appropriately manipulate the data. However, we do not interpret the data visualization results, as this requires detailed knowledge about the data and study.

Visualization consultations provide a unique opportunity to stress the importance of good data management practices. Exceptional data management skills can ease the process of transforming raw data into a visually pleasing and informative data visualization. The use of column headings within a data file can ensure that the correct variables are appropriately mapped and used in the visual representation. In addition, sometimes it is necessary to visualize only a portion of a dataset. To ensure the correct data are being incorporated into the visualization, it is important to use a clearly defined file naming convention. We usually start a consultation by discussing the dataset to determine the best method of visualization. Often, the researcher provides a portion, if not all, of the data to us, so that we can sit down together and try several visualization options. At this point, we also discuss data formatting and management.

As we get deeper into the consultation, where we are visualizing the data, it is not uncommon for the researcher to discover new patterns about the data. Researchers are often extremely grateful for these consultations, as they walk away with a better understanding of their data and how to visualize and manipulate it in a way that furthers their research mission. The credit we receive for our help varies from an in-person thank you to a publication acknowledgment to potential co-authorship, depending on the researcher, the project, and the extent of our help.

Referral Service

Connecting researchers with available services is an important role of librarians. To implement a visualization referral service, librarians must be familiar with the visualization landscape within their institution or organization. This requires knowing the correct people to contact and the location of desired technology. For example, the U-M Library's Digital Media Commons has a UM3D Lab that provides the community access to a variety of hardware, software, and people to help visualize data in three dimensions.[26] If researchers approach us with the desire to visualize their data in 3D, we refer them to the UM3D Lab. Another example is referring a researcher with extremely intense computational needs to the U-M Advanced Research Computing unit, which provides the necessary infrastructure for high-performance computing.[27] Knowing when to refer someone and to whom can be challenging, especially in larger institutions.

To facilitate the implementation of a referral service, we have created a U-M Library data visualization web page that summarizes services we provide, along with appropriate contact information.[28] Both researchers and librarians can go to this web page to determine whom to contact, based on a specific need. In addition, we created a group e-mail address that includes library employees who are involved with visualization activities, spanning the Taubman Health Sciences Library, the Digital Media Commons, and the Clark Library. This group e-mail list was recently created, so we have only received a couple of requests so far, but when a request is sent to this e-mail address, we appropriately triage the inquiry so that it is handled by the most knowledgeable person based on availability and desired outcome. As mentioned earlier in this chapter, we also offered an "Introduction to Visualization" workshop, targeting librarians, in an effort to increase awareness about visualization methods, techniques, and the role of the library. The goal of this workshop was to educate librarians, thereby enhancing their ability to provide referrals. Referring researchers appropriately instills confidence in the library and its librarians, which can lead to valuable collaborations and partnerships.

Partnering

Visualization is a term that encompasses a wide breadth of categories. As a result, we try to partner with people both within and outside of the library in order to offer the best services possible. As previously mentioned, the U-M Library system consists of many libraries and units, such as the Clark Library, the Digital Media Commons, and the Taubman Health Sciences Library. In order to provide the best visualization services possible, partnering is necessary across the various U-M libraries and units.

A Visualization Working Group was established within the U-M Library to stimulate the implementation and growth of visualization services offered by the library. Members of this group span the various libraries and units within the larger U-M Library system, encouraging collaboration. It quickly became clear that offering visualization services is not a one-person job, but instead, is best done as a collaborative group. The larger Working Group has created several subgroups, focusing on internal communication, education, and funding. The internal communication subgroup ensures seamless communication within the library about visualization needs and services, including new hardware, software, and student availability. The education subgroup works to educate the U-M community, including the library, about visualization concepts and services. The funding subgroup searches for grant and other funding opportunities related to visualization. The subgroups include additional library stakeholders outside the Working Group and meet regularly to maintain momentum.

Not only does the offering of visualization services provide an opportunity for partnering within the library, but it also provides a terrific opportunity for partnering outside of the library. Working with researchers to visualize data often leads to repeated and long-term partnerships. In addition, library personnel can offer certain skills that work well with resources and personnel outside of the library. As mentioned earlier, long-term collaborations can form as a result of curriculum-based instruction, consultations, and the creation of instructional resources on visualization tools developed in-house. As a result, partnering with others, both within and outside of the library, leads to the most beneficial outcomes in terms of time, cost, and deliverables.

Finding and Manipulating Data

Besides developing a visualization framework and linking it with other data-related activities, the libraries also aid researchers and students in finding data. At the U-M libraries, many of our data services have grown out of the Clark Library, which focuses on both government and geographic information. The Clark librarians often help researchers across fields find, manipulate, and utilize various types of data. Librarians evaluate and purchase subscriptions to databases that include everything from social science data to remote sensing data to datasets of chemical structures. We are also in the process of developing infrastructure, such as a research data repository, to preserve datasets produced by researchers. Especially in the social sciences—with the abundance of freely available government data—but also in other disciplines, we assist in the discovery and use of datasets that exist outside our collections (such as census, soil, hydrography, transportation data, etc.).

In our visualization collaborations, we often find that researchers require assistance in locating either appropriate data for their visualization work or additional context for publicly available data that they use in their research. Librarians also help researchers utilize this data with different software. Data regularly have to be reformatted, aggregated, or otherwise manipulated to work with different systems from mapping software to network analysis software. By helping to find appropriate datasets and manipulating or cleaning the data in order to be useable in common visualization software, it is often possible to assist patrons who might not have been able to work with visualization otherwise. Moreover, as researchers and students learn new visualization tools and techniques, having a sample dataset that works well can be an unforeseen and challenging step before even beginning to develop a familiarity with the software or method. Providing access and help with datasets can be of immense benefit in helping patrons learn data visualization. As libraries grow their collections, both of commercially purchased data and archived research data, we can leverage these collections, and our abilities to navigate these complex collections, in providing visualization services.

Discussion

As data visualization increases in popularity and becomes more essential with the advent of big data, librarians have an opportunity to solidify themselves as important collaborators in the visualization field. The U-M Library has successfully implemented visualization services, although we continue to improve upon them and work to implement new services. Before offering services, librarians need to become educated about visualization principles, tools, and more. Suggestions would be to attend seminars, workshops, and webinars on visualization tools and concepts, along with potentially taking courses, such as those provided by Coursera or other online courses. However, it is also important to take the time for hands-on exploration of tools and to learn from coworkers and collaborators. One of the best ways to learn a visualization tool can often be to complete a project using the tool.

It is extremely important for librarians to do their own research on visualization topics and tools in order to learn new skills and technology. Exploration and discovery is one of the best ways to educate oneself on new techniques and technology. We set aside time to do our own data visualization and research, which inform our recommendations to researchers.

Once services are developed, it is necessary to educate the community and promote the services. Since the library is not the first place people think of for visualization help, this can be a challenge. A good place to start is by educating other librarians about visualization concepts, along with informing them of offered services, so that they can refer researchers appropriately. Next, it is necessary to promote the services outside the library. Offering workshops, presenting at discipline-specific seminars and meetings, and providing promotional handouts are all proposed methods for increasing awareness. Data visualization is complex, but libraries are good resources for offering a variety of data services, and librarians already have many of the skills that are required for successfully providing these services.

Conclusion

The types of services offered by libraries have evolved over the years, but the ultimate goal of working with users to meet their needs has not changed. Based on existing skills and a willingness to explore new areas, libraries and librarians are capable of offering valuable visualization services. Although this is relatively new territory for many libraries, we believe that offering these types of services will be beneficial to both libraries and their communities. The U-M Library already offers several visualization services, yet we continually work to determine user needs in order to offer additional data visualization services. We believe that it is only a matter of time before libraries become a commonly recognized institution for visualization services, partnerships, and instruction.

Pearls

- Data visualization is an actively developing field that has a complex relation to research.
- In order for libraries and librarians to provide visualization services, they must actively be involved in their research and teaching communities.
- Libraries are an ideal home for many visualization services, including instruction, consultations, referrals, partnering, and finding and manipulating data.
- Visualization services can complement and multiply the impact of other data services, such as data collections and data management support.
- Visualization services should be a collaborative effort that includes librarians with a variety of skills and knowledge.
- Visualization is complex; knowledge about principles, techniques, and tools are all required for offering comprehensive visualization services.

Notes

1. Lev Manovich, "What Is Visualisation?," *Visual Studies* 26, no. 1 (2011): 38.
2. Edward Tufte, *The Visual Display of Quantitative Information Second Edition* (Cheshire, CT: Graphics Press, 2001), 13.
3. Manovich, "What Is Visualisation?," 38.

4. Manovich, "What Is Visualisation?," 41.
5. See, for example: Michael Friendly, "Milestones in the History of Data Visualization: A Case Study in Statistical Historiography," in *Classification—the Ubiquitous Challenge*, eds. Claus Weihs and Wolfgang Gaul (Berlin: Springer, 2005), 34–52.
6. James Beniger and Dorothy Robyn, "Quantitative Graphics in Statistics: A Brief History," *American Statistician* 32, no. 1 (1978): 1–2. Tufte, *Visual Display of Quantitative Information*, 20–22.
7. Beniger and Robyn, "Quantitative Graphics in Statistics," 2; Friendly, "Milestones," 36–37.
8. Tufte, *Visual Display of Quantitative Information*, 24.
9. Beniger and Robyn, "Quantitative Graphics in Statistics," 2.
10. Frank Anscombe, "Graphs in Statistical Analysis," *American Statistician* 27, no. 1 (1973): 17–21.
11. Colin Ware, *Visual Thinking for Design* (Burlington, MA: Morgan Kaufmann, 2008), 81.
12. Ware, *Visual Thinking for Design*, 56.
13. *Webster's Third New International Dictionary, Unabridged*, s.v. "heuristic" (Springfield, MA: Merriam-Webster), accessed March 27, 2015, http://unabridged.merriam-webster.com.
14. *Michigan Almanac*, 5th ed. (Ann Arbor: University of Michigan Office of Budget and Planning, 2015), 6, http://obp.umich.edu/wp-content/uploads/almanac/Almanac_Ch1_Jan2015.pdf.
15. "University of Michigan Taubman Health Sciences Library," accessed February 7, 2016, http://www.lib.umich.edu/taubman-health-sciences-library.
16. "University of Michigan Clark Library," accessed February 7, 2016, http://www.lib.umich.edu/clark-library.
17. "University of Michigan Digital Media Commons," accessed February 7, 2016, http://www.lib.umich.edu/digital-media-commons.
18. "University of Michigan Shapiro Science Library," accessed February 7, 2016. http://www.lib.umich.edu/shapiro-science-library.
19. "About the Library," University of Michigan Library, accessed June 25, 2015, http://www.lib.umich.edu/about-library.
20. Paul Shannon, et al., "Cytoscape: A Software Environment for Integrated Models of Biomolecular Interaction Networks." *Genome Research* 13 (2003): 2498–504.
21. Marci D. Brandenburg and Jean Song, "Broadening Instructional Scope with Network Visualization," *Journal of the Medical Library Association* 100, no. 4 (2012): 313–16.
22. R Development Core Team, *R: A Language and Environment for Statistical Computing* (Vienna: R Foundation for Statistical Computing, 2008).
23. Alla Karnovsky et al., "Metscape 2 Bioinformatics Tool for the Analysis and Visualization of Metabolomics and Gene Expression Data," *Bioinformatics* 28, no. 3 (2012): 373–80.
24. Maureen Sartor et al., "ConceptGen: A Gene Set Enrichment and Gene Set Relation Mapping Tool," *Bioinformatics* 26, no. 4 (2010): 456–63.
25. Jung H. Kim et al., "LRpath Analysis Reveals Common Pathways Dysregulated via DNA Methylation across Cancer Types," *BMC Genomics* 13, no 526 (2012).
26. "University of Michigan 3D Lab," accessed February 7, 2016, http://um3d.dc.umich.edu/.
27. "University of Michigan Advanced Research Computing," accessed February 7, 2016, http://arc.umich.edu/.
28. "University of Michigan Library Data Visualization," accessed February 7, 2016, http://www.lib.umich.edu/data-visualization.

Bibliography

Anscombe, Frank. "Graphs in Statistical Analysis." *American Statistician* 27, no. 1 (1973): 17–21.

Beniger, James, and Dorothy Robyn. "Quantitative Graphics in Statistics: A Brief History." *The American Statistician* 32, no. 1 (1978): 1–11.

Brandenburg, Marci D., and Jean Song. "Broadening Instructional Scope with Network Visualization." *Journal of the Medical Library Association* 100, no. 4 (2012): 313–16.
Friendly, Michael. "Milestones in the History of Data Visualization: A Case Study in Statistical Historiography." In *Classification—the Ubiquitous Challenge*, edited by Claus Weihs and Wolfgang Gaul, 34–52. Berlin: Springer, 2005.
Halley, Edmond. "An Historical Account of the Trade Winds, and Monsoons, Observable in the Seas between and Near the Tropicks, with an Attempt to Assign the Phisical Cause of the Said Winds." *Philosophical Transactions* 16, nos. 179–191 (1686): 153–68.
Karnovsky, Alla, Terry Weymouth, Tim Hull, V. Glenn Tarcea, Giovanni Scardoni, Carlo Laudanna, Maureen A. Sartor, et al. "Metscape 2 Bioinformatics Tool for the Analysis and Visualization of Metabolomics and Gene Expression Data." *Bioinformatics* 28, no. 3 (2012): 373–80.
Kim, Jung H., Alla Karnovsky, Vasudeva Mahavisno, Terry Weymouth, Manjusha Pande, Dana C. Dolinoy, Laura S. Rozek, and Maureen A. Sartor. "LRpath Analysis Reveals Common Pathways Dysregulated via DNA Methylation across Cancer Types." *BMC Genomics* 13 (2012): 526.
Manovich, Lev. "What Is Visualisation?" *Visual Studies* 26, no. 1 (2011): 36–49.
Sartor, Maureen A., Vasudeva Mahavisno, Venkateshwar G. Keshamouni, James Cavalcoli, Zachary Wright, Alla Karnovsky, Rork Kuick, et al. "ConceptGen: A Gene Set Enrichment and Gene Set Relation Mapping Tool." *Bioinformatics* 26, no. 4 (2010): 456–63.
Shannon, Paul, Andrew Markiel, Owen Ozier, Nitin S. Baliga, Jonathan T. Wang, Daniel Ramage, Nada Amin, Benno Schwikowski, and Trey Ideker. "Cytoscape: A Software Environment for Integrated Models of Biomolecular Interaction Networks." *Genome Research* 13, no. 11 (2003): 2498–504.
Tufte, Edward. *The Visual Display of Quantitative Information*. Cheshire, CT: Graphics Press, 2001.
Ware, Colin. *Visual Thinking for Design*. Burlington, MA: Morgan Kaufmann, 2008.

Part III

Data Management in Practice

In 2015, the National Institutes of Health (NIH) awarded grant funding to researchers at nearly two thousand five hundred different institutions, from large universities like Johns Hopkins University and the University of California, San Francisco, which received over twelve hundred grants each, to small liberal arts colleges like St. Mary's College, from academic medical centers to hospitals to corporations.[1] If you work in a biomedical or academic library of any type, there is most likely research going on at your institution. As the previous chapters have demonstrated, a wide variety of opportunities exist for developing library services in support of data management. Part III of this collection explores considerations for developing a successful service for supporting the research being conducted at your institution, whether you're a solo librarian at a small hospital library or a member of a large team in an academic medical center—or anywhere in between.

As with planning any new service, it can be useful to start the process by thinking strategically about the institution's needs and the library's capacity to support those needs. In a 2010 survey of their member institutions about data support services, the Association of Research Libraries found that more than a third of respondents had conducted or were planning to conduct a needs assessment to inform the development of their data support programs.[2] A needs assessment may be a formal research project, gathering and analyzing quantitative data from library users, but could also take the form of casual conversations with researchers at your institution about their data practices and needs. In addition, it can be useful to identify services already being offered at the institution by other units, such as the information technology department or Office of Sponsored Research (or equivalent), to avoid duplication of effort.

Offering new services can involve a substantial commitment of time, effort, and, potentially, funding. It is essential to ensure that any planned data management support services are both sustainable (they can feasibly be continued on a long-term basis) and scalable (small pilot projects can potentially be expanded to provide services to other users or groups). Staffing of such services should be carefully considered. Librarians do not necessarily need to be data specialists to succeed in providing data services, and many successful programs are conducted by librarians for whom providing data support is not their only job or even their primary focus, such as subject specialist or liaison librarians. However, for libraries planning to offer substantial, long-term services, hiring a librarian (or even a team of librarians) who will specialize in data management may be essential.

Even with careful planning, it should be recognized that not every service will be a success. Developing a new program often involves experimenting with a variety of services that may or may not end up working out in the long run. Librarians exploring new ways of supporting data management at their institutions should consider the process iterative, and management of the library should be supportive of such experimentation. In addition, the needs of research communities, even at a single institution, can substantially evolve over time as new technologies emerge and new policies regarding data management and sharing come into effect. A successful data services program is often a moving target, not a final destination. Assessment and evaluation of services play an important role in this process of experimentation and iterative development, and can help with improving or adjusting services and making determinations about whether services should be continued.

Libraries of all types and sizes can have a role in providing support for data management at their institution. Though smaller libraries may be hesitant to take on the challenge of providing such new services, Bonnie L. Fong, Minglu Wang, and Ann Vreeland Watkins demonstrate in chapter 11 that data services programs can be highly successful in small- and medium-size libraries. In fact, librarians at smaller institutions that do not have as much research infrastructure and support as their larger peers may find their services are especially helpful, and that the library can provide support for data management needs that are currently unmet.

Many data services programs focus their attention on researchers and graduate students, but as Yasmeen Shorish and Carolyn Schubert discuss in chapter 12, undergraduate students are also increasingly likely to be actively engaged in research. In fact, the undergraduate level may be the ideal time at which to provide data management training, reaching students at an early stage in their educational process and giving them essential skills and knowledge that will benefit them throughout the rest of their academic career. Librarians who work with undergraduates often have unique opportunities to be embedded in classes and can be actively engaged in helping to develop instruction.

While librarians at academic institutions often have such chances to be integrated into instruction to students, opportunities to reach active researchers may not be as common. Researchers don't necessarily think of the library as a place to look for help with data management, so launching a data services program often involves being proactive and approaching researchers, rather than waiting for them to come to the library. In chapter 13, Alisa Surkis and Kevin Read describe their approach to providing data services as "entrepreneurial." Their experience also provides a useful example of iterative development of services. As Surkis and Read found, not every service or class will be successful, and librarians who develop data services must be able to think critically about why new approaches do (or don't) work and adjust their efforts accordingly.

In addition to adjusting efforts to the institution, it's also often necessary to adjust efforts to specific individuals or groups. Data practices are not necessarily homogenous across all disciplines, even within the biomedical research community. The approach to instruction that Caitlin Bakker describes in chapter 14 involves working closely with research groups to help them devise workflows and data practices in the context of their unique lab setting. Such an approach may be labor intensive, but it is essential to recognize that different groups may have widely different needs.

While data management is often discussed in the context of academic or research settings, hospital librarians also have opportunities to provide support for data management at their institutions. As Jeannine Cyr Gluck points out in chapter 15, clinicians often conduct research in addition to clinical care and may not have the benefit of research support services that are typically available in academic medical centers. In such settings, libraries can play an essential role in providing support for and training in data management that would not otherwise be available. Gluck provides useful guidance for hospital librarians who wish to gain expertise in data management but who may find it difficult to get the time or resources for in-depth training. Her experience demonstrates that there are many opportunities, often free, for librarians of all backgrounds to prepare to dive into providing data services.

As the authors in this section demonstrate, librarians who are interested in providing data services should not feel limited by the size or type of library. Opportunities exist for providing data management support across a wide variety of institutions. Indeed, anywhere research is conducted, researchers at some level will likely need some type of support in meeting new data management requirements and effectively working with their data. In addition, librarians who work with students have an important chance to help train the next generation of researchers.

Notes

1. National Institutes of Health, "NIH Awards by Location and Organization," https://report.nih.gov/award/index.cfm?ot=&fy=2015&state=&ic=&fm=&orgid=&distr=&rfa=&om=n&pid=.
2. Catherine Soehner, Catherine Steeves, and Jennifer Ward, *E-Science and Data Support Services: A Study of ARL Member Institutions* (Washington, DC: Association of Research Libraries, 2010).

Bibliography

National Institutes of Health. "NIH Awards by Location and Organization." https://report.nih.gov/award/index.cfm?ot=&fy=2015&state=&ic=&fm=&orgid=&distr=&rfa=&om=n&pid=.

Soehner, Catherine, Catherine Steeves, and Jennifer Ward. *E-Science and Data Support Services: A Study of ARL Member Institutions*. Washington, DC: Association of Research Libraries, 2010.

Chapter 11

Data Services at a Medium-Size Academic Library

Minglu Wang, Bonnie L. Fong, and Ann Vreeland Watkins, John Cotton Dana Library,
Rutgers University-Newark

As computing capacity and digital technology applications coalesced to transform scientific research in the early 1990s, investigators began to create immense amounts of data and conduct analyses to find patterns that might lead to a significant discovery. Concerns about data management, curation, and preservation emerged very quickly. Much of the data creation was expensive and supported by federal grant funding. Fiscal responsibility dictated that the data be openly accessible, shared with other researchers, and preserved for future use by scholars. Federal agencies, such as the National Institutes of Health (NIH)[1] and National Science Foundation (NSF),[2] have since added data management plans as part of grant applications. When large research universities responded to the data deluge and compliance measures with new federal agency requirements, they initially invested in greater storage capacity for data and then realized a more comprehensive program was necessary. Librarians, recognizing that data services are an extension of their traditional areas of expertise in information description, organization, preservation, and instruction, sought opportunities to get involved in more stages of the research data life cycle.[3]

Research data support can vary widely due to a range of factors, including human, financial, and technological resources that are available at an institution. While librarians may view finding datasets for researchers as part of their reference responsibilities, data computing services is one aspect of data services that is seldom seen as an opportunity for librarians to help researchers with the challenges of research data management. A survey of science librarians affiliated with the Association of Research Libraries (ARL) revealed that they were uncertain about their roles in data services and the skills that would be required.[4] In their white paper, *Academic Libraries and Research Data Services*, written for the Association of College & Research Libraries (ACRL), Tenopir and her coauthors reported that, based on a 2012 survey of 223 academic libraries in the United States and Canada, many were not yet involved in providing data services, although they were preparing themselves to do so in the future. Libraries at larger research universities receiving national research funding were the exception.[5]

Literature on the development of data services programs has focused primarily on initiatives at large public and private research university libraries for which data curation infrastructure and data management services are standard components or project goals.[6] In a majority of case studies, libraries offer services based on the development and use of a data repository. Akers et al.[7] analyzed programs at eight university libraries for the timing of data service development and determined there are usually five key steps in the development of a new library-sponsored data service and infrastructure: starting with traditional data acquisition, reference, or data analysis services and an institutional repository for scholarly publications, followed by a researcher needs assessment, data management services, and an institutional repository with data curation capabilities. Raboin, Reznik-Zellen, and Salo[8] described in depth the development and delivery of research data management services at their respective institutions and noted the differences. While the services at University of Massachusetts–Amherst and Tufts University are delivered with limited repository facilities and the University of Wisconsin–Madison library offers services that are not based on a repository, the authors noted commonalities such as university support, building new services within current or modified staffing patterns, and remaining proactive to researchers' changing needs.

With such a predominance of reports from large research libraries, librarians supporting smaller campuses and those institutions with masters and baccalaureate programs only might have reservations about grasping the opportunity to offer data services. However, there is growing interest in doing so. Partlo et al. shared strategies for data services at liberal arts colleges during a workshop at the 2015 IASSIST conference.[9] Shorish wrote encouragingly about her experience at James Madison University, a smaller institution where she coordinated a data management support plan for faculty that included collaborations across campuses and across institutions (see chapter 12 for additional discussion of the program at James Madison University).[10]

On the medium-size Rutgers University–Newark campus, the John Cotton Dana Library has been successful in developing a suite of data services to serve both faculty and student researchers. This is possible due to the knowledge and skills of our data services librarian, her close collaborations with subject specialist librarians, partnerships with campus units (such as the Research Office and Computing Services), and utilization of the expertise of external groups (such as vendors and disciplinary organizations).

Setting

Rutgers University–Newark (RU-N) is one of four campuses that make up Rutgers, the State University of New Jersey. Prior to the integration of the University of Medicine and Dentistry of New Jersey (UMDNJ) into Rutgers in July 2013, Rutgers had been one of the nation's few public research universities without a medical school. Now Rutgers has medical schools in Newark and New Brunswick, extensive allied health programs based in Newark, and a merged School of Nursing offering undergraduate and graduate programs in both locations. The current School of Nursing has twice as many students and faculty as the former UMDNJ School of Nursing or the Rutgers College of Nursing.

RU-N has an incredibly diverse student body and has, in fact, been deemed the most diverse national university in the United States every year since 1997 (*U.S. News & World Reports*).[11] Students are predominantly local residents, reflecting the city's population of immigrants and minorities. Many are the first in their family to attend college. There are approximately seven thousand four hundred undergraduate and three thousand nine hundred graduate students enrolled in one of five professional schools (business, criminal justice, law, nursing, and public administration) or the undergraduate or graduate programs in the arts and sciences at RU-N.

The campus's Carnegie Classification is Research University (high research activity). The faculty, numbering 585, are fully engaged in research in addition to their teaching responsibilities. A large number support their research through grant funding from the NSF, NIH (including the National Institute of Neurological Disorders and Stroke, the National Institute of Mental Health, the National Institute of Allergy and Infectious Diseases, the National Institute on Drug Abuse, and the National Eye Institute), the Health Resources and Services Administration, the Department of Defense, and the Department of Labor. Over the past five years, total faculty grant awards have averaged $30 million a year.

The John Cotton Dana Library is centrally located on campus. It is one of twenty-five libraries and centers within the Rutgers University Libraries (RUL), a system that spans all four Rutgers campuses. Print and online library resources are shared throughout the system. At the Dana Library, researchers have access to over three hundred online indexes or databases, a book collection numbering seven hundred thousand items, a repository of federal and state government documents, and a media collection of six thousand items. The library facility houses a computer lab with ninety desktop computers; two computer classrooms seating fifteen and thirty students, respectively; and two collaborative multimedia rooms with advanced software. Eight subject specialist librarians provide information support for students, faculty, and staff in all disciplines, with the exception of law and criminal justice, for which there are separate libraries on campus.

There is a nice sense of community among the librarians and library staff on the four Rutgers campuses. Going beyond infrastructure building, everyone is willing to share their skills and knowledge with each other and provide instruction or consultations for colleagues or researchers on another campus. To prepare librarians and library staff to support researchers' data curation needs, the associate university librarian for digital library systems and the data librarian in New Brunswick organized and presented a course in 2011–2012 titled, "Data Management Training to Support Faculty Research Needs." All who were involved in the course have continued to meet regularly as the RUresearch Team, where they participate in continuing education programs, hear updates on the RUL research data management program, and share how they are progressing with data services on their campus.[12] The inclusion of health sciences librarians following the UMDNJ integration has helped strengthen knowledge of acceptable data management practices in the medical and health sciences field.

At the Dana Library, there are three librarians on the RUresearch Team—the data services librarian, life sciences librarian, and physical sciences librarian. The science librarians recognized the growing importance of data management in their field, so they built their knowledge of research data support in order to better collaborate with the data services librarian on outreach to researchers, as well as instruction and consultation services. This partnership has become one of the key factors in the continual development of a more comprehensive suite of data services on the RU-N campus.

Dana Library's data services librarian was hired in 2009 through a two-year grant because the faculty in the campus's social science research centers had expressed a need for assistance with managing large amounts of data. It was later discovered that the faculty's actual data management needs were a Web-based database setup, maintenance, and website data visualization—all of which fall outside of the library's scope and capacity of services. Still, value was seen in expanding data services on campus, so after the grant ended, the data services librarian's position was changed to a regular faculty line. Based on analysis of a log the data services librarian created about her individual consultations with students and faculty, she reflected on the data needs of researchers on campus and developed a framework for new services.[13]

Description of Services

Medium-size academic libraries have the capability to expand traditional reference and instruction services to develop a relevant data services program. By working with partners from within the library and across the campus, librarians can maximize support for researchers throughout the research data life cycle. Through leveraging diverse skills and knowledge from multiple sources, researchers benefit from a much fuller suite of data-related services.

Following a review of many research data life cycle models[14] within the context of our researchers' data management practices, we found the Carnegie Mellon University Libraries' (CMUL) model[15] to be most suitable for visualizing our understanding of the process and development of appropriate services (see figure 11.1). The CMUL data life cycle model begins with research project design and planning, at which point a good data management strategy should be set. At the next stages of data collection and analysis, it is expected researchers will adhere to this strategy, implementing best practices in their field of research. During the final stages of the life cycle, when researchers are considering data repository options and may have interest in data curation support for the purposes of sharing and archiving their data, librarian involvement is critical.

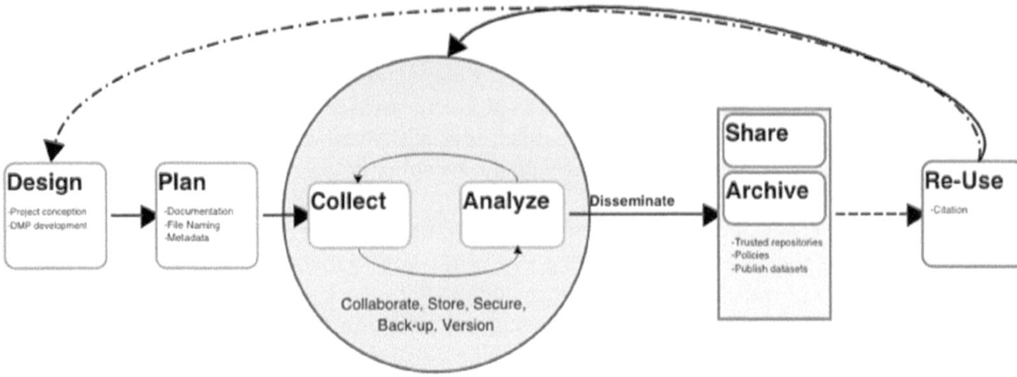

Figure 11.1. Carnegie Mellon University Libraries (CMUL) Data Life Cycle Model. "Data Management 101," Carnegie Mellon University Libraries, accessed July 14, 2015, http://library.cmu.edu/datapub/dms/data/101.

Research data services at most institutions have been developed with a focus on data management best practices training, data management plan consultation, and data curation; however, based on working with faculty and graduate students on the RU-N campus these past few years, we have identified additional data service training, consultation, and assistance opportunities for each stage of the research data life cycle. The overlaid boxes in figure 11.2 illustrate our services in greater detail, as they relate to the CMUL data life cycle model.

Partnerships are necessary to provide the Dana Library's suite of data services shown in figure 11.2. The data services librarian might be involved in almost all aspects, although may also require close collaboration between her and subject specialist librarians. On the RU-N campus, we participate in the RUL-wide data infrastructure (for example, the institutional data repository) and services development, as this contributes to our library offerings. We also actively reach out to other service departments on campus and work with them to round out our research data support for faculty and students.

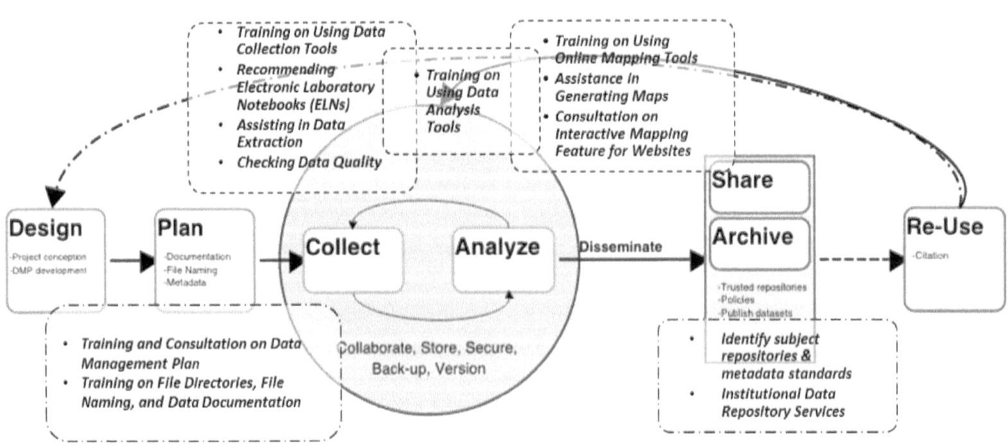

Figure 11.2. Our Data Services Programs Overlaid on CMUL Data Life Cycle Model.

Research Design and Plan

The research data life cycle is typically seen as a continuous loop; however, it is recommended that researchers have a clear plan about how to manage their data before beginning research. These days, many funding agencies ask for a data management plan (DMP) at the grant proposal stage. Writing a DMP should go hand-in-hand with planning for a research project. Thinking carefully about how data is handled throughout the entire process—from where and how data will be collected, to how it will be analyzed and presented, to how it will be stored, preserved, and accessed in the future—ensures valuable data will not be lost, but will instead be findable and understandable. Similarly, it is important to consider early on how to set up file directories, name files, and provide sufficient data documentation. At the Dana Library, we provide consultation services and training through seminars or workshops to address the usual components of DMPs as well as best practices for file directory setup, file naming conventions, and documentation.

TRAINING AND CONSULTATION ON DATA MANAGEMENT PLANS

Researchers across the disciplines are finding that more and more funding agencies—public and private—require DMPs with grant proposal applications. The agencies want to see that the researchers they support will manage their data in an accountable manner. With their expertise in organizing information in multiple formats in an easily accessible fashion, librarians have applied their more traditional information management skills to data management. They now train researchers on how to develop DMPs for their various projects. On the RU-N campus, we provide DMP workshops for faculty and graduate students in collaboration with the Research Office. With the Research Office promoting the workshops, researchers seeking grants may pay closer attention to the announcement.

Individual consultations about creating DMPs are available to both faculty and student researchers. On the RU-N campus, requests have come from the Department of Earth and Environmental Science (DEES), Psychology Department, and School of Criminal Justice. The data services librarian usually works closely with one of the science librarians, depending on the discipline under discussion. They review a draft of the researcher's DMP, compare it against the relevant grant agency's specific requirements or available templates, research suitable metadata standards, and identify possible disciplinary data repositories. Feedback is provided fairly quickly so that researchers may make revisions in time for their grant proposal deadlines. Faculty and graduate students have been very pleased with such assistance. In the case of DEES, one faculty member invited the physical sciences librarian and the data services librarian to serve as the data manager and a data management team member, respectively, of his proposed project.

TRAINING ON FILE DIRECTORIES, FILE NAMING, AND DATA DOCUMENTATION

Before they begin to collect data, researchers must carefully consider how they will set up their file directories and how they will consistently and descriptively name their files. Such organization ensures ease in finding data and getting a quick sense of where a researcher may be in her or his study. Faculty advisors appreciate how highly useful it is to know at a glance how far their students are in their research. Well-organized and clearly labeled files are also necessary when research projects involve internal or external collaborators.

Data documentation is a crucial strategy that ensures collected data can be accurately used in later stages of research and data can be understood and reused by other researchers completing relevant studies. Therefore, it is very important to decide at the design and planning stage what to document and the structure, standards, and terminology to be applied throughout the project. Some disciplines already have developed data file templates and normalized terminology and measurements to assist with data interoperability in their field. Researchers are encouraged to create a data dictionary for their data collection. During this process, they are asked to consider whether variables are in the correct analysis level (for example, continuous numbers vs. a few aggregated categories); whether variables are recorded in appropriate formats (such as text vs. integers vs. decimals); whether meaningful variable names are used; what the descriptions of each variable are; what values are documented in the codebook; and how to ensure more accurate data entry that adheres to the codebook.

We regularly teach data organization and documentation best practices during basic data management seminars and workshops. However, a data needs assessment of DEES graduate students and some of their faculty advisors revealed that they considered learning proper file directory creation to be high in importance, so the physical sciences librarian taught it during the department's annual retreat for the students.[16] Since researchers have different needs, they are encouraged to contact either their subject specialist librarian or the data services librarian for an individual consultation. One faculty member in the School of Nursing took advantage of this option and later sent her research assistants to the data services librarian for training before they began data entry for the faculty member's research projects.

Data Collection

Depending on their projects, researchers may extract data from existing sources or collect new data. Librarians' expertise can be valuable in both cases. In addition to helping researchers find the data that they need, librarians can assist researchers with extracting the data in the correct format that fits the requirement of their data analysis and presentation tools. For researchers collecting their own data, librarians who stay up to date on new data collection tools can advise and train them on the most appropriate one(s) for their research. If time allows, librarians may also perform a data quality check at this early stage of the research data life cycle.

TRAINING ON USING DATA COLLECTION TOOLS

Many electronic data collection tools exist today. They range from those that may be free (such as Google Forms, REDCap, and SurveyMonkey) to those that are proprietary (such as Qualtrics). Researchers who have relied on paper questionnaires may appreciate learning about online tools that have a number of advantages, such as greater legibility, time savings, and the elimination of errors that sometimes result from migration of data from paper questionnaires to electronic files.

Continuously learning about new data-related tools results in the librarians having more knowledge and more confidence when recommending tools to researchers. If Rutgers subscribes to a data collection tool (such as Qualtrics), we take the initiative to learn how to use it and then begin to provide support through workshops and individual consultations. If we think a free data collection tool (such as Google Forms) might be useful for our researchers, we offer hands-on workshops about it. We also try to keep our eyes and ears open for other tools that may help the faculty and students on campus improve their data collection practices and make efforts to familiarize ourselves with them. This was the case with REDCap, which is widely used in health sciences research. When we learned that it was installed at our neighboring health sciences campus just blocks away, we contacted the technician who administers the system and scheduled a training workshop. Upon hearing that the IT Department could provide limited support for REDCap, we noted that this might be an area for potential outreach to help researchers who use it.

RECOMMENDING ELECTRONIC LABORATORY NOTEBOOKS (ELNS)

Given that data services are still relatively new in academic libraries, our philosophy has been to keep an open mind about where this may lead. We were a little surprised when a new faculty member in the

Department of Biological Sciences contacted us for assistance in identifying an appropriate electronic lab notebook (ELN) for his research. He had attended our presentation about the data portal of the University Libraries' institutional repository during his department meeting and hoped we might be able to provide some advice for him on what he perceived as a closely related topic. He had asked around campus and found that the science faculty still preferred the traditional laboratory notebook, so he expanded his field of query and reached out to us. Following a consultation session with the researcher, the authors conducted a comprehensive investigation into ELN options appropriate for biology, including reaching out to science librarian colleagues via listserv posts; sending similar inquiries to Rutgers' Office for Research Information Technology, Division of Life Sciences, and Discovery Informatics Institute; and contacting ELN software companies and the Broad Institute at Harvard University. Findings were summarized and shared with the researcher to help him make a more informed decision. Following his inquiry, we have paid particular attention to the progress of ELNs as they are growing increasingly important in scientific research and can be quite useful for data management.

ASSISTING IN DATA EXTRACTION

Researchers interested in using existing data must first be able to find and access that data. They might seek assistance from their subject specialist librarian or data librarian. Once the data has been located, however, it must be carefully extracted. Data may be available in a variety of formats and cover different data collection date ranges. The level of detail in the metadata may also differ. Therefore, it is vital that researchers extract enough metadata to help them fully understand the context of the original research. The metadata is also important for proper reuse and helps with accuracy when merging multiple datasets; for example, geographic identification numbers can be used to match up spatial data obtained from other datasets. Formats make a difference, too, because some allow for direct transfer into statistical software programs (such as Stata or SPSS), making data extraction quite efficient. In a rapidly changing digital world, researchers may not necessarily be able to keep up with all the new tools and features data providers offer, so librarians may see this as another opportunity to assist them with the data collection part of the research data life cycle.

CHECKING DATA QUALITY

As careful as researchers may be when collecting data, it is important to double-check the quality of the data collected. Having someone who is not on the project team check the data may be more effective because the researchers themselves may be too immersed in the data and not notice some errors. At RU-N, the data services librarian has used technical strategies to help faculty members in the School of Nursing and the School of Social Work conduct data quality checks. She runs frequency tables to check the patterns of values entered for all variables in datasets. This reveals outliers as well as abnormal or missing values that researchers may pursue to ensure the data's accuracy. The data services librarian shares this strategy with the researchers, providing detailed documentation on the process so that the researchers (and their research assistants) know how to conduct similar quality checks on their own in the future.

Data Analysis

Researchers may use a variety of tools during the data analysis part of the research data life cycle. Some are free or open-source, whereas others are proprietary; however, either type can be quite sophisticated. These tools may be general enough to serve multiple disciplines or they may be specific to a field of study. At the Dana Library, we provide consultation services and workshops for both qualitative and quantitative data analysis tools. Although numerous tools exist, we focus on those for which Rutgers has a subscription, as well as freely available tools in high demand by faculty and students on campus.

TRAINING ON USING DATA ANALYSIS TOOLS

When she first arrived at the Dana Library, the data services librarian surveyed the graduate students on campus about their interest in training for data analysis software tools. Their very positive response resulted in a series of data analysis tool workshops that have been offered at the beginning of each semester since 2010.[17] Initially, the workshops were limited to statistical software (including SPSS, Stata, and R). When Rutgers University purchased site licenses for the qualitative data analysis tool NVivo and the survey software tool Qualtrics, these tools were added to the growing list of graduate student workshops.

Data analysis tool workshops are among the most popular on the RU-N campus. Each semester, over one hundred graduate students from the different schools and departments register for them. A contributing factor may be the encouragement given by faculty from multiple disciplines including public administration, neuroscience, global affairs, psychology, and business to their students to attend the workshops. Some students learn statistical software to complete their dissertations while others need it for homework assignments.

Workshops about data analysis tools are introductory in nature, generally consisting of a demonstration followed by hands-on exercises that reinforce student learning. In addition to a technical demonstration of the various tools, data analysis best practices are discussed during workshops. For example, the data services librarian teaches attendees how to document their research procedures using annotating program codes that make their analyses replicable—something that is increasingly becoming the norm for current and future scholarly communication. A guide with links to online learning opportunities, user group resources, and screencasts of workshop videos complements and supplements the workshop sessions, allowing anyone who is interested to easily review content from the workshops and find additional information.[18]

Once researchers have collected data for their specific project, they may wish to schedule an individual consultation with a librarian to discuss analysis. In fact, a number of workshop participants have done just that and continue to seek such help on an ongoing basis. Consultations typically focus on technical issues related to data analysis. Both faculty and student researchers in the sciences and social sciences can rely on the data services librarian to help them with troubleshooting or quick data analysis programming in a timely manner.

Data Presentation

With the development of mapping technology, researchers now have the option of presenting their data in a manner that is more sophisticated than basic tables and graphs. Libraries are starting to subscribe to online mapping tools that can generate maps without requiring advanced geographical skills, although users new to the tools still appreciate and benefit from some guidance at the very beginning. Although there is no geographic information system (GIS) specialist at the Dana Library, our data services librarian learned the basic functions of Esri GIS and Tableau software and has become especially familiar with mapping census data. In fact, she has further refined her skills in these areas when she consults on research projects involving these tools. One possible area for future collaborative data services might be developing interactive maps appropriate for websites aimed at the public.

TRAINING ON USING ONLINE MAPPING TOOLS

On the RU-N campus, students and faculty have access to three mapping tools—ArcGIS, Social Explorer, and PolicyMap. ArcGIS is installed on all machines in computer labs on campus. Students and faculty can purchase a license through the University's Computing Services Department. Social Explorer and PolicyMap are RUL subscriptions. As impressive as ArcGIS may be, it has a steep learning curve, so few researchers use it. Social Explorer and PolicyMap, on the other hand, are much easier to use. Researchers can generate maps to visualize their numerical data and tell interesting stories. When the data services librarian began to offer Census Data Mapping workshops, she taught attendees how to accomplish the same tasks using each of the three mapping tools and pointed out the different features available from each tool. At the end of the workshop, students appeared well informed, confident, and excited about using the mapping tools and further exploring the tools' advanced techniques.

ASSISTANCE IN GENERATING MAPS

Mapping as a form of data visualization is still relatively new, so researchers may not be very familiar with the tools involved. They may need help understanding which visualizations are most suitable for different types of data. Although technical staff may be able to handle the technical aspects of using mapping tools, librarians understand the nature of research and may also possess subject knowledge that can be more beneficial for researchers seeking assistance with their data visualization. After all, recognizing which data to gather and how to gather it for mapping is the most important part of this process. On the RU-N campus, the data services librarian has been helping faculty members generate maps for their research projects. She learned basic mapping skills while interning at another academic library and then learned ArcGIS through Esri's online course. She learned Tableau on the job, just as the researcher was doing. Still, the librarian was able to acquire suitable spatial data and transform them into the correct format for use in Tableau, solving technical problems for the researcher in a timely manner so project deadlines were met without compromising the quality of the maps used in her reports.

CONSULTATION ON INTERACTIVE MAP FEATURE FOR WEBSITES

For a variety of reasons, researchers may want to place an interactive map on their website. The online dissemination of research products might fulfill grant funding agency requirements that expect a public outreach component such as an informative website. It may also be a way for researchers to increase the visibility and impact of their work beyond the traditional publication venues of books and journal articles. As a result of the close relationships that developed between the data services librarian and the researchers she worked with in other areas of data services, she was approached about developing interactive map features for project websites geared toward the public. Limited in technical expertise and restricted by time constraints, the data services librarian was only able to provide consultation advice on possible solutions. However, this seems to be an opportunity for additional data services in the future.

Share and Archive Data

Following the completion of a research project, researchers are usually heavily focused on publishing the results of their studies in journals or books. The sharing or archiving of their research data may be just an afterthought. However, as grant funding agencies begin to require data sharing, researchers' interest in sharing and archiving data will likely increase. Similarly, as publishers start mandating data sharing—at times suggesting specific repositories for deposits—researchers may appreciate the library's help with this final stage of the research data life cycle. Data services librarians and subject specialist librarians should leverage their respective areas of expertise and collaborate to identify suitable disciplinary data repositories and metadata standards for researchers on their campus. At the Dana Library, we also take note of developments concerning our institutional repository because researchers without an appropriate disciplinary repository might choose the institutional repository to deposit their data.

IDENTIFY DISCIPLINARY DATA REPOSITORIES & METADATA STANDARDS

Although many disciplines are paying closer attention to data sharing and data archiving, some are further along than others in developing data repositories and metadata standards to support this activity. As the NIH requires data sharing for certain of their grantees, they also helpfully provide a list of sixty-five NIH-supported data sharing repositories on their website.[19] In the biosciences, many publishers work with the Dryad Digital Repository in an effort to integrate the article and data submission process, making it more streamlined.[20] In neuroscience, the Neuroscience Information Framework[21] has the capability for researchers to register resources stored in local databases. Then the Framework connects them as part of an aggregate through vocabulary terms and ontologies. Resources become easily accessible through searching. The Framework also features a community effort to develop the taxonomy system for the field to improve communication about research and data through standardized terminology. Supported by the NSF's EarthCube grant, the earth sciences community is creating a complex integrated system to make the variety of research data in that discipline interoperable and, thus, easier to discover and reuse (EarthCube 2015).[22] Researchers in the social sciences have ICPSR (Inter-University Consortium for Political and Social Research), which maintains a data archive and provides learning opportunities for those interested in furthering their education about data. At the Dana Library, we make recommendations for potential disciplinary data repositories and metadata standards or controlled vocabulary for researchers preparing their data for archiving. We also direct researchers to existing file templates and anything else that is relevant and useful to them in the data sharing and archiving stage.

INSTITUTIONAL DATA REPOSITORY SERVICES

When there are no existing disciplinary data repositories that are a good match for a researcher's data, an institutional repository may be the best option. If a researcher has identified and deposited data into a disciplinary repository, he or she should consider a duplicate deposit into his or her institutional repository. While disciplinary repositories can help make researchers' data more easily discovered by others in their field, depositing valuable research data in two repositories provides extra assurance that it will not become lost; rather, it ensures long-term preservation and enables broader access to the data beyond a specific discipline. At Rutgers, repository deposits are nonexclusive, meaning researchers are free to deposit their data elsewhere as well. Therefore, when we make recommendations for repositories, we make sure we also mention our institutional repository.

RUL has been working on developing the institutional data repository for several years now. The data librarian and research data manager on the larger Rutgers campus in New Brunswick handle infrastructure development and lead RUresearch, a research data support team composed of subject specialist librarians, metadata librarians, and library technicians from across all four Rutgers campuses. The authors have been active members of this data support team since its beginning. It is this extended support network, where members of the data team each have their own areas of expertise, that is most valuable.

Discussion

In medium-size libraries, limited human, technological, and financial resources may prevent librarians from being able to provide in-depth and complete support throughout the entire research data life cycle; however, it is certainly possible to meet many of researchers' data management needs through most of the life cycle. The expertise that librarians already have in managing information and organizing accessible library collections can easily be transferred and applied to the areas of managing, sharing, and archiving research data. New skills such as those necessary for data collection, data analysis, and data presentation can be learned by librarians, or librarians might refer researchers to existing experts—whether local or afar. Researchers generally do not expect a medium-size library to be able to completely address any and all of their data needs or questions.

At the Dana Library, our work with researchers provides us with an opportunity to both share our own expertise concerning handling research data and to learn more about the varying needs of researchers. As we work together with researchers to try and answer a question they may have—such as identifying an appropriate ELN or metadata standards for a specific field—we expand on our own knowledge. This helps us to be more informed and better prepared to answer similar questions from other researchers in the future. When we know a topic is of interest to our researchers, we make a note to stay aware of any news or trends in that area, continuously building our knowledge and expertise.

Opportunities to learn abound—and many are available free of charge. Grants have funded a number of in-person training sessions, such as the EarthCube Summer Institute for Technology Exploration. Many colleges and universities post guides and tutorials online about how to deal with research data. Vendors typically offer free webinars. E-mail listservs can be a venue to ask and help answer research data questions. Colleagues are often willing to teach sessions or provide one-on-one assistance. We learn from each other and rely on each other to more fully support the data needs of our researchers.

Utilizing the expertise of others is essential for medium-size libraries. In cases where the data needs of researchers may be met by others on or off campus, librarians can serve as facilitators, helping to arrange a meeting or training opportunity between the groups. On the RU-N campus, we have set up meetings between researchers and the Computing Services unit to discuss storage and backup options. We also arrange for NVivo webinars and host viewings in our library for those who prefer a more social learning environment. As we promote others' services, we hope they do the same for us.

Faculty and students see value in learning data-related skills throughout the research data life cycle although their attendance at optional workshops and webinars is not always high. At the Dana Library, we have found that targeting specific groups during mandatory attendance activities such as department meetings, seminar series, or retreats is best for guaranteeing an audience. In instances where students must learn a specific data analysis software to complete a course assignment, registration and attendance for that workshop is also high.

When offering workshops, we take into consideration the large number of commuters and full-time workers among our student population. We offer workshops later in the afternoons to accommodate their schedules and those of evening students. Still, too often, students who register are unable to attend workshops due to scheduling conflicts. Librarians offering workshops may create online guides with workshop slides or other materials for students unable to attend. In some cases, screencast videos of workshops may be made available.

Generally, the more closely librarians meet the research data needs of faculty and students, the more useful it will be for them, and therefore, the more successful the interaction. This requires working closely with faculty and student researchers to identify their needs—for which Data Profile forms can be quite helpful—and then clearly addressing them. One successful DMP consultation leads to another, whether for the same researcher or for a colleague. In some cases, successful DMP consultations have also resulted in library instruction requests.

Efforts to improve the promotion of how the library can help throughout the research data life cycle have not been especially successful. At the Dana Library, it has been mostly a bottom-up approach. Word-of-mouth can only do so much. Although we have collaborated with the Research Office to offer DMP workshops for faculty, they do not yet actively refer researchers to us during the grant-writing process. The vice chancellor for research and collaborations has also recently tried to help increase awareness of our offerings by sending out a campus-wide e-mail describing them, although it has not resulted in a noticeable increase in requests. Perhaps a top-down approach with more intense promotion earlier on—when DMP requirements were still quite new—might have been more effective.

By now, most faculty researchers have figured out what they need to do and do not require as much help. Their students, however, may still benefit from what we have to offer. Partnering with deans and department chairs to introduce research data skills to their students is something we are considering for the future.

At the Dana Library, data information literacy is something we see as involving both data librarians and subject specialist librarians. As each of the librarians contributes her or his own set of knowledge and skills—whether it is data or subject expertise—the lesson becomes more complete. This is the same philosophy we take when assisting researchers with their data needs. A solid partnership between data librarians and subject specialist librarians who complement each other is vital to successful data services.

Conclusion

Library data services do not need to be limited to building data curation infrastructure, consulting on data management plans, and providing data management training. Having a holistic vision of the data life cycle and awareness of researchers' varied needs at each stage of research can stimulate librarians' continuous learning and service innovation. A similar philosophy might be applied to develop other academic services where we need to change our traditional role as information gatekeepers to be research facilitators or partners.

While librarians at medium-size libraries may face some limitations, they can provide service by leveraging the expertise of campus partners and facilitating connections with external parties to help ensure faculty and student researchers are served as best as possible. Interactions with researchers provides librarians with the chance to learn more about their needs, and if time allows, librarians can take advantage of learning opportunities—many of which are free—to increase their knowledge and skills in order to address those same needs.

Seminars and workshops geared toward a general audience may be useful in providing an overview of a topic, although specifics are best addressed in a more targeted session such as a department event or individual consultation. On the RU-N campus, researchers are encouraged to make individual appointments with the data services librarian. Subject specialist librarians also make it a habit to refer users to the data services librarian as appropriate. In these cases, if the subject specialist librarian has been trained in data management, she or he will often sit in on the meeting and, when helpful, use her or his subject area expertise to serve as a communication bridge between the researcher and the data services librarian.

Researchers may not necessarily think of the library as being helpful with research data management or other parts of the research data life cycle, so it is important to actively promote this service. To ensure that word spreads, librarians might consider reaching out to multiple audiences on campus—from student and faculty researchers to campus administrators (such as provost, deans, and department chairs) to related campus units (such as Research Office, Computing Services, and Graduate School). There is a demand for data-related expertise and researchers need to know that librarians are ready and able to fill this role.

Pearls

- Librarians at medium-size libraries can develop and deliver viable data services to support researchers throughout the research data life cycle. Start small with a basic DMP service or workshops on one or two data collection or analysis tools and see where they take you.
- As librarians work with researchers, both groups continuously learn from each other about the complexities of data management and resulting best practices.

- As researchers delve deeper into eScience, they increasingly need data support. By providing research data services, academic libraries become more relevant to the faculty and students in their institutions.
- Build your relevance in data-driven research by carefully assessing faculty and students' needs and then develop services to meet those needs.
- Data librarians and subject librarians should leverage their respective knowledge and skills and work closely together to provide data services to researchers.
- Consider making referrals when appropriate (for example, to librarian colleagues, campus partners, or external parties).
- If there are any gaps in data-related skills on campus that would be appropriate for librarians to fill, learn them.
- Be sure to promote the library's data services to student and faculty researchers, campus administrators, and any other related or relevant campus units.
- Include graduate students in your data services offerings. They are frequently dealing with data either in the conduct of their own research or for their professor's research with very little preparation in research data management.
- Forge partnerships with campus departments with interests in research data management, such as the Research or Grants Office and Computing Services or IT.

Recommended Reading and Resources

Books

- Corti, Louise, Veerle van den Eynden, Libby Bishop, and Matthew Woollard. 2014. *Managing and Sharing Research Data: A Guide to Good Practice*. Los Angeles: Sage.
- Fearon, David Jr., Betsy Gunia, Sherry Lake, Barbara E. Pralle, and Andrew L. Sallans. 2013. *SPEC Kit 334: Research Data Management Services (July 2013)*. Washington DC: Association of Research Libraries.
- Pryor, Graham, Sarah Jones, and Angus Whyte. 2014. *Delivering Research Data Management Services: Fundamentals of Good Practice*. London: Facet Publishing.
- Ray, Joyce M., ed. 2014. *Research Data Management: Practical Strategies for Information Professionals*. Charleston Insights in Library, Archival, and Information Sciences. West Lafayette, IN: Purdue University Press.

Data Management Best Practices

- ICPSR (Inter-University Consortium for Political and Social Research). "Guide to Social Science Data Preparation and Archiving." http://www.icpsr.umich.edu/files/ICPSR/access/dataprep.pdf.
- DataONE (Data Observation Network for Earth). "Data Management Best Practices." https://www.dataone.org/all-best-practices?page=1.
- UK Data Archive. "Managing and Sharing Data: A Best Practice Guide for Researchers." http://www.data-archive.ac.uk/media/2894/managingsharing.pdf.

Online Training Modules

- University of Minnesota Libraries. "Data Management Course Module for Graduate Students." https://sites.google.com/a/umn.edu/data-management-course_structures/.
- University of Edinburgh. "Research Data Management Training for PhD Students." http://datalib.edina.ac.uk/mantra/.

- Northumbria University. "Research Data Management Training for Health Studies." https://www.northumbria.ac.uk/sd/academic/ee/work/research/clis/dlar/datum/health/materials/?view=Standard.
- UK Data Archive. "Create and Manage Data Training Resources Developed." http://www.data-archive.ac.uk/create-manage/training-resources.

Notes

1. "Final NIH Statement on Sharing Research Data," National Institutes of Health, last modified February 26, 2003, http://grants.nih.gov/grants/guide/notice-files/NOT-OD-03-032.html.
2. "Dissemination and Sharing of Research Results," National Science Foundation, accessed July 14, 2015, http://www.nsf.gov/bfa/dias/policy/dmp.jsp.
3. See Geoffrey Little, "Managing the Data Deluge," *Journal of Academic Librarianship* 38 (2012): 263-64, doi:10.1016/j.acalib.2012.07.005; Tony Hey, Stewart Tansley, and Kristin Tolle, eds., *The Fourth Paradigm: Data-Intensive Scientific Discovery* (Redmond, Washington: Microsoft Research, 2009), accessed July 14, 2015, http://research.microsoft.com/en-us/collaboration/fourthparadigm/; Gordon Bell, Tony Hey, and Alex Szalay, "Beyond the Data Deluge," *Science* 323 (March 6, 2009): 1297–98, doi:10.1126/science.1170411; Committee on Science, Engineering, and Public Policy (U.S.) and Committee on Ensuring the Utility and Integrity of Research Data in a Digital Age, *Ensuring the Integrity, Accessibility, and Stewardship of Research Data in the Digital Age* (Washington, DC: National Academies Press, 2009).
4. Karen Antell, Jody Bales Foote, Jaymie Turner, and Brian Shults, "Dealing with Data: Science Librarians' Participation in Data Management at Association of Research Libraries Institutions," *College & Research Libraries* 75 (2014): 557–74, doi:10.5860/crl.75.4.557.
5. Carol Tenopir, Robert J. Sandusky, Suzie Allard, and Ben Birch, "Research Data Management Services in Academic Research Libraries and Perceptions of Librarians," *Library & Information Science Research* 36 (2014): 84–90, doi:10.1016/j.lisr.2013.11.003.
6. See Brian Westra, "Developing Data Management Services for Researchers at the University of Oregon," in *Research Data Management: Practical Strategies for Information Professionals*, ed. Joyce M. Ray (West Lafayette, IN: Purdue University, 2014), 375–91; D. Scott Brandt, "Purdue University Research Repository: Collaborations in Data Management," in *Research Data Management: Practical Strategies for Information Professionals*, ed. Joyce M. Ray (West Lafayette, IN: Purdue University Press, 2014), 325–45; Gail Steinhart, "An Institutional Perspective on Data Curation Services: A View from Cornell University," in *Research Data Management: Practical Strategies for Information Professionals*, ed. Joyce M. Ray (West Lafayette, IN: Purdue University Press, 2014), 303–24; Regina Raboin, Rebecca C. Reznik-Zellen, and Dorothea Salo, "Forging New Service Paths: Institutional Approaches to Providing Research Data Management Services," *Journal of eScience Librarianship* 1 (2012): article 2, doi:10.7191/jeslib.2012.1021; Katherine G. Akers, F. C. Sferdean, Natsuko H. Nicholls, and Jennifer A. Green, "Building Support for Research Data Management: Biographies of Eight Research Universities," *International Journal of Digital Curation* 9 (2014): 171–91, doi:10.2218/ijdc.v9i2.327.327.
7. Akers et al., "Building Support for Research Data Management."
8. Raboin, Reznik-Zellen, and Salo, "Forging New Service Paths," 329.
9. Kristin Partlo, Danya Leebaw, Paula Lackie, Peter Rogers, Diana Symons, and Aaron Albertson, "Where Everybody Knows Your Name: Building Credible and Sustainable Data Services in a Liberal Arts College" (presented at the IASSIST Annual Conference, Minneapolis, MN, June 2–5, 2015), http://iassist2015.pop.umn.edu/program/workshops#w2.
10. Yasmeen Shorish, "Data Curation Is for Everyone! The Case for Master's and Baccalaureate Institutional Engagement with Data Curation," *Journal of Web Librarianship* 6 (2012): 263–73, doi:10.1080/19322909.2012.729394.

11. "College Ranking List: Campus Ethnic Diversity," *U.S. News & World Reports*, accessed July 14, 2015, http://colleges.usnews.rankingsandreviews.com/best-colleges/rankings/national-universities/campus-ethnic-diversity.
12. Ryan Womack, "Data Management Training to Support Faculty Research Needs: Lessons Learned" (presented at the IASSIST Annual Conference, Washington, DC, June 7, 2012), doi:10.7282/T3DB83H8.
13. Minglu Wang, "Supporting the Research Process through Expanded Library Data Services," *Program: Electronic Library & Information Systems* 47 (2013): 282–303, doi: 10.1108/PROG-04-2012-0010.
14. Jake R. Carlson, "The Use of Life Cycle Models in Developing and Supporting Data Services," in *Research Data Management: Practical Strategies for Information Professionals*, ed. Joyce M. Ray (West Lafayette, IN: Purdue University Press, 2014), 63–86.
15. "Data Management 101," Carnegie Mellon University Libraries, accessed July 14, 2015, http://library.cmu.edu/datapub/dms/data/101.
16. Bonnie Fong and Minglu Wang, "Required Data Management Training for Graduate Students in an Earth and Environmental Sciences Department," *Journal of eScience Librarianship* 4 (2015): article 3, doi:10.7191/jeslib.2015.1067.
17. Wang, "Supporting the Research Process."
18. "Dana Library's Data Support: Stata," last modified February 3, 2016, http://libguides.rutgers.edu/danadata/Stata.
19. "NIH Data Sharing Repositories," U.S. National Library of Medicine, accessed July 14, 2015, http://www.nlm.nih.gov/NIHbmic/nih_data_sharing_repositories.html.
20. "Frequently Asked Questions," Dryad, accessed July 14, 2015, http://datadryad.org/pages/faq.
21. "NIF Data Sharing," Neuroscience Information Framework, accessed July 14, 2015, http://www.neuinfo.org/datasharing/index.shtm.
22. "About EarthCube," EarthCube, accessed July 14, 2015, http://earthcube.org/info/about.

Bibliography

Akers, Katherine G., F. C. Sferdean, Natsuko H. Nicholls, and Jennifer A. Green. "Building Support for Research Data Management: Biographies of Eight Research Universities." *International Journal of Digital Curation* 9 (2014): 171–91, doi:10.2218/ijdc.v9i2.327.327.

Antell, Karen, Jody Bales Foote, Jaymie Turner, and Brian Shults. "Dealing with Data: Science Librarians' Participation in Data Management at Association of Research Libraries Institutions." *College & Research Libraries* 75 (2014): 557–74, doi:10.5860/crl.75.4.557.

Bell, Gordon, Tony Hey, and Alex Szalay, "Beyond the Data Deluge." *Science* 323 (March 6, 2009): 1297–98, doi:10.1126/science.1170411.

Brandt, D. Scott. "Purdue University Research Repository: Collaborations in Data Management." In *Research Data Management: Practical Strategies for Information Professionals*, edited by Joyce M. Ray, 325–45. West Lafayette, IN: Purdue University Press, 2014.

Carlson, Jake R. "The Use of Life Cycle Models in Developing and Supporting Data Services," in *Research Data Management: Practical Strategies for Information Professionals*, ed. Joyce M. Ray (West Lafayette, Indiana: Purdue University Press, 2014), 63–86.

Carnegie Mellon University Libraries, "Data Management 101," accessed July 14, 2015, http://library.cmu.edu/datapub/dms/data/101.

Committee on Science, Engineering, and Public Policy (U.S.) and Committee on Ensuring the Utility and Integrity of Research Data in a Digital Age. *Ensuring the Integrity, Accessibility, and Stewardship of Research Data in the Digital Age*. Washington, DC: National Academies Press, 2009.

Dryad. "Frequently Asked Questions." Accessed July 14, 2015. http://datadryad.org/pages/faq.

EarthCube. "About EarthCube." Accessed July 14, 2015. http://earthcube.org/info/about.

Fong, Bonnie, and Minglu Wang. "Required Data Management Training for Graduate Students in an Earth and Environmental Sciences Department." *Journal of eScience Librarianship* 4 (2015): article 3, doi:10.7191/jeslib.2015.1067.

Hey, Tony, Stewart Tansley, and Kristin Tolle, eds. *The Fourth Paradigm: Data-Intensive Scientific Discovery*. Redmond, Washington: Microsoft Research, 2009. Accessed July 14, 2015. http://research.microsoft .com/en-us/collaboration/fourthparadigm.

Little, Geoffrey. "Managing the Data Deluge." *Journal of Academic Librarianship* 38 (2012): 263–64, doi:10.1016/j.acalib.2012.07.005.

National Institutes of Health. "Final NIH Statement on Sharing Research Data." Last modified February 26, 2003. http://grants.nih.gov/grants/guide/notice-files/NOT-OD-03-032.html.

National Science Foundation. "Dissemination and Sharing of Research Results." Accessed July 14, 2015. http://www.nsf.gov/bfa/dias/policy/dmp.jsp.

Neuroscience Information Framework. "NIF Data Sharing." Accessed July 14, 2015. http://www.neuinfo .org/datasharing/index.shtm.

Partlo, Kristin, Danya Leebaw, Paula Lackie, Peter Rogers, Diana Symons, and Aaron Albertson. "Where Everybody Knows Your Name: Building Credible and Sustainable Data Services in a Liberal Arts College." Presented at the IASSIST Annual Conference, Minneapolis, MN, June 2–5, 2015. http:// iassist2015.pop.umn.edu/program/workshops#w2.

Raboin, Regina, Rebecca C. Reznik-Zellen, and Dorothea Salo. "Forging New Service Paths: Institutional Approaches to Providing Research Data Management Services." *Journal of eScience Librarianship* 1 (2012): article 2, doi:10.7191/jeslib.2012.1021.

Shorish, Yasmeen. "Data Curation Is for Everyone! The Case for Master's and Baccalaureate Institutional Engagement with Data Curation." *Journal of Web Librarianship* 6 (2012): 263–73, doi:10.1080/1932 2909.2012.729394.

Steinhart, Gail. "An Institutional Perspective on Data Curation Services: A View from Cornell University." In *Research Data Management: Practical Strategies for Information Professionals*, edited by Joyce M. Ray, 303–24. West Lafayette, IN: Purdue University Press, 2014.

Tenopir, Carol, Robert J. Sandusky, Suzie Allard, and Ben Birch. "Research Data Management Services in Academic Research Libraries and Perceptions of Librarians." *Library & Information Science Research* 36 (2014): 84–90, doi:10.1016/j.lisr.2013.11.003.

U.S. National Library of Medicine. "NIH Data Sharing Repositories." Accessed July 14, 2015. http:// www.nlm.nih.gov/NIHbmic/nih_data_sharing_repositories.html.

U.S. News & World Report. "College Ranking List: Campus Ethnic Diversity." Accessed July 14, 2015. http://colleges.usnews.rankingsandreviews.com/best-colleges/rankings/national-universities/ campus-ethnic-diversity.

Wang, Minglu. "Dana Library's Data Support: Stata." Last modified February 3, 2016. http://libguides .rutgers.edu/danadata/Stata.

———. "Supporting the Research Process through Expanded Library Data Services." *Program: Electronic Library & Information Systems* 47 (2013): 282–303, doi: 10.1108/PROG-04-2012-0010.

Westra, Brian. "Developing Data Management Services for Researchers at the University of Oregon." In *Research Data Management: Practical Strategies for Information Professionals*, edited by Joyce M. Ray, 375–91. West Lafayette, IN: Purdue University, 2014.

Womack, Ryan, "Data Management Training to Support Faculty Research Needs: Lessons Learned." Presented at the IASSIST Annual Conference, Washington DC, June 7, 2012, doi:10.7282/ T3DB83H8.

Chapter 12

Data Information Literacy

ENGAGING WITH THE UNDERGRADUATE HEALTH SCIENCES POPULATION

Yasmeen Shorish and Carolyn Schubert, Rose Library, James Madison University

Data management has been recognized as important for faculty and graduate students, yet developing the foundational content and necessary skills should begin in undergraduate curriculum. A significant body of research regarding data management knowledge, attitudes, and behaviors provides opportunities for translation back into the undergraduate experience. To help identify strategies and areas in the health curriculum that are relevant to data management for undergraduates, this chapter will explore three areas of engagement: liaison librarians, the undergraduate research experience, and the research process as it relates to the Institutional Review Board. By integrating data information literacy into these areas, librarians can help prepare undergraduate populations interested in health-related fields to engage with data in their careers and graduate studies.

Background

Since the formation of the Council on Undergraduate Research (CUR) in 1978, undergraduate research has grown into a recognized area of importance in higher education and continues to shape higher education curriculum, research, and funding.[1] The Boyer Commission in 1998 called for significant reforms in undergraduate education, such as focusing on research-based learning and creating capstones for a culmination of learning.[2] Research in this area has identified key areas of benefit associated with undergraduate research, such as the development of critical thinking skills, increasing student engagement and retention, receiving mentorship, and promoting innovation.[3] Further research into the outcomes of undergraduate research has found self-reported improvements in domain knowledge, research skills, and higher educational satisfaction.[4] As a result of these findings and growth in undergraduate research endeavors, CUR has grown to seven hundred institutional members and over ten thousand individual members.[5]

In addition to calls for educational reform, grant funding from major government institutions has aided the advancement of undergraduate research centers. The National Science Foundation (NSF) developed a Research in Undergraduate Institutions (RUI) program in 1983 and further refined opportunities with programs such as Facilitating Research at Primarily Undergraduate Institutions.[6] In

1985, the National Institutes of Health (NIH) also started an allocation of funds for undergraduate training and research under the Academic Research Enhancement Award (AREA) Program.[7] In the ten years from 2002 to 2012, the NSF funded $488 million under the RUI program and the NIH funded $481 million under the AREA program, which helped to actualize some of these educational reform suggestions and establish undergraduate research programs more broadly around the United States.[8] For example, Western Michigan University received funding in 2015 to support undergraduate student research on recreational designer drugs.[9] These programs, alongside other research trends, have been strong motivators for undergraduate research experiences at primarily undergraduate institutions.

James Madison University (JMU) represents a large and growing population of such undergraduate research programs. JMU is a comprehensive, undergraduate-focused institution with some graduate programs. Approximately 9.7 percent of all universities match this profile.[10] Large, comprehensive institutions capture large student numbers, accounting for 16.9 percent of all college enrollment—the largest percentage of all classifications, according to the Carnegie Classification of Institutions of Higher Education.[11] In 2014, JMU had a total student population of 20,855, of which 19,144 (about 89 percent) were undergraduates.[12] JMU secured over $18.7 million in external funding in 2013–2014.[13] According to the Office of Research Integrity, the number of protocols seeking Institutional Review Board approval increased 17 percent in 2013–2014 and 27 percent in 2014–2015, suggesting that the research community is active and engaged across the campus population.[14] Eighty percent of JMU's undergraduates participate in research, an internship, and/or a practicum, and the university's strategic plan calls for an integrative capstone experience for all majors by 2016–17, which for many programs may be a research experience.[15]

As a participant in these larger trends of supporting and developing undergraduate research, JMU provides a good case to study data information literacy skills of undergraduates and the implications for library involvement. JMU accepts approximately 215 incoming freshmen into the Honors Program, with most identifying as biology, nursing, health sciences, psychology or interdisciplinary liberal studies majors.[16] Forty-three of these incoming Honors students also identify as a preprofessional health emphasis. To further these research activities, JMU holds MADRUSH, the annual undergraduate research conference, and supports the *James Madison Undergraduate Research Journal* for student publications across the campus. In addition to these campus-wide events, individual colleges and departments regularly host undergraduate research posters and presentations, such as Pi Mu Professional Day, an annual event highlighting research and continuing education in nursing.

Given the growth in a variety of health care positions, allied health programs at JMU comprise a significant component of undergraduate research occurring on campus. JMU offers a variety of allied health and nursing programs, as well as a dedicated preprofessional health track. The College of Health and Behavioral Studies contains a diverse array of departments, including communication sciences and disorders, health sciences, kinesiology, nursing, psychology, and social work. Moreover, the Department of Health Sciences itself contains undergraduate programs such as athletic training, dietetics, general health studies, and graduate programs for dietetics, occupational therapy, and physician assistant. Undergraduate students account for approximately 90 percent of the student enrollment in the college, which is reflective of overall JMU student composition. Overall, the College of Health and Behavioral Studies accounts for 17 percent of all student enrollment at JMU.[17] The Pre-Professional Health (PPH) program is a dedicated preparation program for students who wish to attend professional programs in medicine, dentistry, optometry, pharmacy, physical therapy, veterinary medicine, occupational therapy, physician assistant, and forensic studies.[18] Students in the PPH program come from all majors across the campus, but are most heavily represented in biology, chemistry, health sciences, kinesiology, and psychology. In 2014, there were 2,733 students associated with the PPH program, with over 50 percent of those students declaring a Pre-Med or Pre-Physician Assistant concentration.[19]

Across these programs, there is a wide range of applied learning activities. Some programs may offer students an opportunity to join a faculty member's lab, working alongside graduate students on grant-funded research. A number of programs offer clinical experiences, while others use a traditional written research project as the research activity for the program. Libraries have naturally supported these undergraduate research activities through traditional and emerging services. Hensley, Shreeves, and Davis-Kahl documented these types of library services in their survey and analysis of 281 academic libraries.[20] In that study, they found that many of the ways that libraries support undergraduate research are expansions or modifications of existing services. Some libraries have introduced services that leverage a data librarian/specialist position to provide qualitative and quantitative data manipulation support. This service model is present in a variety of academic libraries, including University of California, Berkeley's Data Lab, Barnard College Library's Empirical Reasoning Lab, and the Research Data Department at Purdue University Libraries.

An area of need across these programs is a consistent approach to using and creating data as a scholarly product. Understanding how to manage the data that one produces, while also recognizing how to find and use data effectively and ethically, is an activity that is seldom formally taught.[21] While the ability to collect, process, manage, evaluate, and use data has been defined as science data literacy,[22] this—and other related literacies (statistical, data, and information)—often implies a consumer role for the researcher. However, increasingly researchers engage in collaborative or large-scale projects that require some level of data sharing. These actions of a data producer require training in data information literacy. Data information literacy (DIL) is a relatively new term in librarianship and has not achieved the same penetration in the profession as information literacy. Carlson et al. define DIL as merging "the concepts of researcher-as-producer and researcher-as-consumer."[23]

The members of the Data Information Literacy Project, an Institute of Museum and Library Services (IMLS) grant-funded initiative, investigated the DIL needs of researchers and developed a curriculum to address those needs.[24] They created twelve competencies associated with DIL. The competencies include cultures of practice, data management and organization, data curation and reuse, ethics and attribution, data conversion and interoperability, data preservation, data processing and analysis, data quality and documentation, data visualization and representation, databases and data formats, and discovery and acquisition of data.[25] It is possible that not all of the related activities will be relevant to the undergraduate health science or PPH populations, but a basic awareness of the concepts is important to help form a foundation for the students to build upon as they continue their studies or start careers.

Some DIL competencies, such as data management and organization, data curation and reuse, data preservation, discovery and acquisition of data, and ethics and attribution easily fall within the purview of librarian expertise. Others, such as cultures of practice, data conversion and interoperability, data processing and analysis, data quality and documentation, data visualization and representation, and databases and data formats may be most effectively taught within the discipline. However, it is important to note that this is a very fluid landscape. Some libraries may have the expertise and resourcing to provide data analysis training and some disciplines may have a well-defined data discovery practice in place. As data take on a more prominent role as a primary source of information, and good data management becomes more important to the reuse of data, the ways in which researchers and librarians engage with the competencies will evolve with the research environment.

Case 1: Engagement With Liaison Librarians

At JMU, PPH students represent nearly every major on campus. Utilizing the department liaison librarian model, the library can act as a resource for good data management practices for researchers in any field. This could occur during reference consultations, or through course development with departmental faculty. While not every liaison needs to be an expert in data management, creating a shared, foundational level of knowledge of DIL can help every liaison triage data management requests. Moreover, framing data management and DIL as aspects of scholarly communication can help reduce the anxiety that some liaisons may feel when confronted with data questions. Data can be treated as another information medium, with some unique characteristics, but otherwise philosophically identical to any other information source.

Within JMU Libraries, a shared foundation for DIL is still being built. In 2011, a new science librarian joined the faculty and began to work with her departmental faculty to meet NSF data management plan (DMP) requirements. This work identified areas for further engagement with entities across campus, including the Office of Research and Scholarship, Central Information Technology (IT), and the Office for Sponsored Programs. Stakeholders from those offices met with the science librarian and library dean to discuss strategies to effectively serve faculty, but the conversations were mostly limited to the science disciplines.

The science librarian's heavy engagement with DIL resulted in interest from faculty across campus, as faculty collaborated on interdepartmental projects and shared experiences with one another. After one year, it became clear that additional methods of engagement beyond one liaison were necessary. One way that the library increased impact across campus was through the adoption of the DMPTool. As one of the first universities in Virginia to become a partner institution, JMU has been able to provide DMP support across a range of funders irrespective of discipline. A subject guide on data was another immediate solution to provide a single reference point to users. This passive learning object provides resources and references to anyone with a data management question.[26] Looking for ways to build more active engagement, JMU became an organizing member of the Virginia Data Management Boot Camp, a collaborative event across universities in Virginia that offers two-and-a-half days of programming on data management prior to the start of the spring semester.[27] Any student, faculty, or staff member from the JMU community and environs can attend the event at no cost to build his or her skills.

JMU began participating in 2013 with initially small attendance numbers—mostly administrators, some instructional faculty, and only one other librarian. However, it was clearly an area of growth, as the 2014 boot camp exceeded the small registration capacity and resulted in a waiting list. Additional seating was secured to accommodate as many registrants as possible. That year, the majority of attendees were instructional faculty from across the campus, with smaller numbers of graduate students, staff, and a handful of liaison librarians. Given the variety of roles involved in data management services, the Libraries and Educational Technology's Scholarly Communication Steering Committee coordinated a professional development workshop on key issues such as open access, research impact, and research data management.

This workshop framed data and DIL as analogous to the research support activities that libraries currently provide. Instruction in information seeking, the evaluation of sources, and the ethical use of information are considered part of the bedrock of librarianship. The workshop queried participants about the ways that they provide these and other services, then illustrated the ways that these behaviors occur with respect to data. Just as one directs a student to the most appropriate database or journal for a particular research need, the same activity occurs when that student's research need includes data as a source. The cognitive leap that must occur for subject librarians is when the research support must be given to the researcher as a content (or data) creator. This is an area of growth further identified in Hensley, Shreeves, and Davis-Kahl's survey findings.[28]

The boot camp and the workshop represent "in-reach" or "up scaling" activities within the library organization, which are critical to build foundational knowledge and hone the skills that liaisons need to engage with students and faculty. Framing DIL within the familiar framework of information literacy and scholarly communication can help demystify the content. Librarians can pair with faculty in their liaison departments to integrate DIL competencies into assignments in much the way that information literacy instruction currently takes place. With this knowledge, liaisons in any department can better partner with faculty to address areas of need, and the organization reduces the risk of sequestering all information about data management within one person.

As important as educating all liaisons about the relevance of DIL to their departments is using the connections of these liaisons to help form a picture of cross-campus data scenarios and concerns. Liaisons working with their departments in an ad hoc or siloed manner will not help the institution anticipate needs with respect to data, nor will it help devise efficient workflows. Liaisons must have a way to communicate the data patterns that they see across campus with one another. This should, ideally, be communicated to administration to help inform the strategic direction of library support, and to ensure that the liaisons are using all appropriate resources to serve their communities.

Case 2: The Undergraduate Research Experience

In 2012, CUR adopted three strategic pillars to guide the organization's actions in connecting undergraduate research with existing higher education policies. These pillars include "broadening participation in undergraduate research, embedding undergraduate research into the curriculum, and assessing the impacts of undergraduate research."[29] At JMU, many departments strive to find ways to further embed the research experience into their curriculum. These investigations present opportunities for liaison librarians to work with their departments and identify points in the curriculum for information literacy and DIL instruction.

As mentioned previously, the majority of PPH students at JMU come from STEM-H majors where they may have the opportunity to work with faculty on a research project via for-credit independent study courses. One key difference between undergraduate students and graduate students working in faculty labs is in the required training that they may receive. Often, graduate students must complete a Responsible Conduct of Research (RCR) course through the Graduate School or the Office of Research as part of their research assistantship. For undergraduate students, no such unifying, non-major specific research course exists. Each department may offer a general research methods course, or each faculty researcher may have standard lab procedures, but the content can vary. At JMU, liaison librarians who are engaged with DIL and data management concerns have tried to find gateway research courses to reach students who are engaged with research. Due to inconsistency across departmental curricula, this can be a challenging undertaking.

The Science Librarian has found that the most effective, but least efficient, way to reach students engaged in research is directly through the research laboratory faculty member. Her liaison departments of biology, chemistry, and physics do not offer a research course that is translatable across majors, or that all students engaged in research labs must take. Similarly, the Health Sciences & Nursing Librarian has observed siloed research methods courses across the health programs that also range in content and research expectations. Given the overlap in populations, many of the students in those departments who are accepted into a research lab are PPH students. As a result of this decentralization, individual consultations with faculty researchers have been the best way to introduce DIL concepts to a research group.

Since joining the faculty, the science librarian proactively approached her departments to advocate for DIL instruction throughout courses and lab groups. As a result of these efforts, faculty contact her when they recognize that a research project may encounter difficult data scenarios. Before meeting with a research group, the faculty researcher and the librarian meet to discuss the research question, anticipated data collection, instrumentation use, and duration of active research. Essentially, a data-specific reference interview takes place between the researcher and librarian and they create a streamlined Data Curation Profile.[30] In this discussion, the librarian and faculty researcher determine what the outcomes for the lab group should be, and the librarian builds her instruction around these outcomes as they relate to the DIL competencies.

A successful example of this in the biology department occurred with a research group focused on an ecological research question. In this research group, faculty are most appropriate to cover the areas of community of practice and data processing and analysis. The librarian gave instruction in the competencies data management and organization, data curation and reuse, data preservation, and ethics and attribution. This research group planned to collect original data in the field, transfer it between instruments, normalize it, analyze it, and derive secondary data from the analysis for further study. The librarian drew the research life cycle on the whiteboard, with notes for each area that required documentation and procedures, which helped the group visualize what needed to happen prior to data collection and what actions were needed as research progressed.

The students remarked that they could see how easy it would be to inconsistently document the data and how difficult this would make the data analysis later in the year. The group discussed agreeing on a standard operating procedure, which would detail naming conventions and define the standard workflow for data transfer from the instruments. As one student talked about the work required to get data into Excel from the instrument download, it became clear that she hadn't adequately documented the process for other group members. The ensuing discussion provided the research group with exactly the type of "real world" example that connected with them on an individual level and they enthusiastically remarked on the relevance of good documentation. Upon follow-up, the faculty research indicated improvement in documentation practices and a desire to introduce this training even earlier in the process. Nonetheless, a single data management instruction session has limitations. While faculty reinforced the concepts discussed in the session, the students' ability to scaffold and incorporate this new information into their knowledge base may be limited. Incorporating a semester-long strategy similar to the approach of Mooney, Collie, Nicholson, and Sosulski, which involved an embedded library data team with a social work undergraduate research group, could allow for further integration and deeper understanding of data management competencies.[31]

For non-laboratory settings, undergraduate allied health and nursing programs provide other opportunities to engage DIL through coursework and clinical practice. On a broad level, the Council of Education in Public Health specifies that "the basic concepts, methods and tools of public health data collection, use and analysis" are some of the required domains in undergraduate public health curriculum.[32] Statistics or biostatistics courses are common program requirements in the early years of a program, serving as a foundation for basic statistical concepts and a general introduction to statistical software. At JMU, many allied health programs require a research methods course that addresses data use and understanding of existing data. In junior- or senior-level research methods courses, foundational concepts of quantitative versus qualitative data and study design comparisons, which relate to the DIL competencies of cultures of practice and databases and data formats, commonly occur as students navigate the literature, learn about the levels of evidence, and refine queries to find best practices. Traditional library instruction on search development, search refining by study design, and study design evaluation is often connected to this level of data consumption.

Some courses push students a step beyond the data consumption role to begin to learn how to be a data creator. In their research methods coursework, many JMU health sciences students develop a study, complete the Institutional Review Board (IRB) process, and conduct a study over the course of a semester. The opportunity for students to conduct a study introduces them to the challenges of instrumentation, data collection, and data analysis. In addition to the competencies gained as a data consumer, these active roles engage undergraduates in the application of other DIL competencies, such as data management and organization, data processing and analysis, and ethics and attribution. For these advanced needs, the health sciences and nursing librarian teaches students about resources that evaluate instruments, such as the Health and Psychosocial Instruments (HAPI), and that offer full-text instruments for educational use, such as PsycTESTs. Similar to the science librarian, the health sciences and nursing librarian's consultations with students and discussion with faculty are the primary modes of engaging these advanced DIL competencies. These librarians continue to grow their knowledge of the cultures of practice competency through collaborations with research offices across campus.

Outside of formalized research courses, similar DIL skills are forming in clinical settings and in informatics education. The American Association of Colleges of Nursing identifies "information management and application of patient care technology" as one of the essential criteria for baccalaureate nursing curriculum.[33] At the most basic level, undergraduate students learn discovery and acquisition of data through health assessment didactic education and patient simulation experiences. They learn to connect their data to other objective test data and subjective patient histories. They practice these skills by completing patient records during their clinical education experiences and receiving feedback from their instructors, helping them develop a stronger sense of data quality and documentation needed in practice. For example, nursing students need "to use and [understand] standardized terminologies," which complement the concept of metadata and data description;[34] examples of these standardized terminologies include the International Statistical Classification of Diseases and Related Health Problems (ICD-10) used for reimbursement and comparative worldwide statistics and the North American Nursing Diagnosis Association (NANDA) for nursing diagnoses. Ethics and attribution are repeatedly addressed, as students must understand the ethical responsibilities of patient data under HIPAA. In this case, these DIL competencies together inform the nursing culture of practice and focus on working with existing data infrastructures, making it best taught by the nursing faculty.

The data curation and reuse competency creates a natural space for health librarians to meet these undergraduate students and faculty. Nursing informatics, an increasingly common component in the nursing curriculum, bridges didactic and clinical nursing skills and incorporates the use of information technology to "promote the health of people, families, and communities worldwide."[35] Electronic health record (EHR) adoption is opening opportunities to advance nursing students' DIL skills; larger governmental policies, like the HITECH Act, are also incentivizing EHR adoption in order to improve health care quality and efficiency.[36] These programs aim to gather data on individual patients in electronic formats, which allows for easier reuse and further analysis of trends and outcomes across the health care system. As librarians are acutely familiar with the ability to not just create information structures, but also access them and reuse the information in diverse ways, informatics is a natural fit to engage the DIL competencies.

In a unique campus opportunity, the health sciences and nursing librarian developed an interprofessional health informatics course for undergraduates to start this broader conversation about data, information technology, and improving patient care.[37] Activities include discussion of structured versus unstructured data formats and hands-on activities with electronic health records. Reuse of data from the Center for Medicare and Medicaid Services, such as in Hospital Compare, also provides opportunities to review quality and efficiency of care. In the nursing program itself, the librarian has helped develop nursing informatics and has provided information about the HITECH Act and its meaningful use criteria. These senior-level students had already begun the development of some DIL skills, such as discovery and data acquisition, and were now applying their understanding to a larger systems perspective. The course centered on developing a quality improvement project that required students to consider a data measure to assess the project's outcome. While the projects were only proposed and not actually deployed, the experience does mirror the emerging expectations of nurses to develop or critically contribute to projects.

DIL competencies are still in an early stage of understanding and integration, particularly in the undergraduate environment. Faculty collaborations and strategic course connections are critical first steps. Curriculum revisions and accreditation standards can help to translate the DIL competencies to other disciplinary realms and gain greater acceptance. Beyond the individual department or librarian, broader campus engagement with research offices and regulatory bodies provide additional avenues for engaging and building undergraduate DIL competence.

Case 3: Involvement with the Institutional Review Board

Given the growing engagement of undergraduates with research activities, campus regulatory bodies like the Institutional Review Board (IRB) are increasing their contact with undergraduates. The IRB is responsible for overseeing the ethical treatment of human subjects involved in research studies; each institution has its own local IRB to help ensure proper regulation and meet the federal requirements.

In particular, the IRB's role in reviewing research design, methods, and data security creates an ideal opportunity for librarians to understand the data management behaviors and educational needs of faculty and student researchers. Furthermore, collaborating with the IRB can create moments for individual consultations between librarians and researchers and can confer an association of librarians with the overall research life cycle, not just the literature.

Because of research participants' rights to confidentiality, data management concerns—particularly those related to data security and privacy—are naturally within the IRB's purview. As research moves from collecting data in physical formats, such as with paper and pencil, to more electronic data formats, knowledge and awareness of electronic data management becomes increasingly important. With data management education just beginning to enter the graduate curriculum,[38] there is still a need among faculty for guidance or training in these new and evolving platforms. Therefore, librarians have the opportunity to draw from their expertise in data management and DIL to shape the conversation within the values of IRB.

Over the last few decades, medical librarians have collaborated with IRBs and researchers completing IRB-reviewed research, ranging from conducting literature reviews to providing feedback from the non-expert point of view. As questions circulated in 2001 after the death of Ellen Roche, a research participant in a Johns Hopkins University study on asthma, librarians have been called on to help support researchers and mitigate participant risk.[39] Librarians have provided support through literature reviews that thoroughly examine the literature for any preexisting information on contraindications in an effort to minimize participant risk.[40] Medical librarians at the University of Maryland have also helped researchers develop appropriate language for informed consent documents.[41] In 2004, they started providing workshops about patient literacy and the consent process. Recognizing the liability related to a lack of informed patient or research participant consent, the librarians developed a consent review service in 2011. Elsewhere, librarians are merging their expert literature-searching skills and nonscientist perspective to serve as full IRB board members.[42] Despite these various options, few medical librarians serve in these roles; a 2010 survey of academic health science libraries in the United States and Canada, found that only 16.9 percent of respondents served on IRBs or the Institutional Animal Care and Use Committee (IACUC).[43] As Internet research methods and tools become increasingly popular, IRBs must develop data security guides for researchers, opening the door to data management conversations and more librarian involvement.

Starting in 2013, the health sciences and nursing librarian became a full board member for the JMU IRB, filling a position previously established by the communication sciences and disorders librarian. As previously discussed, engaged learning through research is a key component to the educational experience at JMU, so the IRB reviews protocols for faculty, graduate students, and undergraduate students. Graduate and undergraduate students have faculty advisors for each project. In 2014–2015, faculty IRB protocols accounted for 51.6 percent of submitted proposals, graduate student protocols accounted for 20.9 percent, and undergraduate student protocols accounted for 27.5 percent.[44] For convenience, future references to IRB researchers will refer to all of these populations under the general umbrella of "researcher."

From her experiences on the IRB, the health sciences and nursing librarian noticed that researchers were struggling with data security across different phases of the research life cycle. While most faculty successfully offered security for signed consent forms, typically in a locked filing cabinet within a locked lab or locked office, digital security was less clear. In some cases, researcher protocols were not in alignment with campus data security policy. Data security requires conversations about data across the research life cycle, not just at the final storage location. Data security is a concern during data collection and analysis, as well as data retention, sharing, or destruction after the end of a project. Working with the science librarian, Campus IT, the director of Research Integrity, and the DMPTool, the librarians developed a framework to help researchers understand how to address these elements when developing a research protocol.

Data Collection Stage

The IRB expects researchers to understand how they acquire data and the implications of these methods and associated technologies. Surveys are a popular research methodology due to easy e-mail or social media distribution to a large group. Depending on the information requested, varying degrees of security are important to consider. To have a truly anonymous survey, researchers must be aware of the IP address recording that occurs in some Web-based survey software. Sensitive questions containing identifiable information also face a potentially greater risk, as many survey packages are hosted on cloud-based systems. Therefore, the researcher must understand the security of the software or consider the use of pseudonyms to minimize individual risk. For example, SurveyMonkey is a common tool with different membership levels that offer different levels of security.[45] The top Platinum level is HIPAA compliant, but the Gold, Select, and Basic are not. While other common survey programs utilized by academic institutions, such as Qualtrics and REDCap, can be made HIPAA compliant, undergraduate students are not always given access to these tools and instead rely on freely available resources like Google Forms, which may not guarantee data privacy for the survey results.[46]

Other common research methods deployed by undergraduates include direct participant interaction through interviews, focus groups, and observation. The ubiquity of technology and low cost of digital storage makes the recording participants easier than ever before. Cell phones and mobile devices have audio, video, and photographic capabilities. However, understanding the backend functionality of these data collection methods and intermediate storage of the data is important. Auto-configuration of resources like Apple's iCloud put data captured through mobile devices at risk of unsecure transmission, even if unintended by researchers. These mobile devices are easily stolen or lost, meaning that data transfer to a more secure device or encryption of these mobile devices is important to avoid accidental disclosure. Security of these devices while traveling between research sites and data storage sites must also be considered. Typically, researchers use mobile devices to capture data, but then migrate the data to a more secure platform like a personal computer or department server. Ensuring proper data conversion and interoperability are important considerations for migrating. As undergraduates begin to rely heavily on their personal devices to conduct research and as technologies change, it is becoming increasingly difficult for the IRB to create a predetermined, prescriptive list of requirements for data gathered through these devices. Instead, triaging the data needs must address the unique realities of each project team, its resources, and its capabilities

Data Retention, Sharing, and Destruction Stage

Just as mobile devices have eased the creation of data, the decreasing cost of storage has allowed researchers to consider data retention for longer periods of time with little apparent cost. Researchers may want to use items like Google Drive and Dropbox as data storage locations due to flexibility; these options are especially attractive to undergraduates who are less likely to have access to campus computing resources or server space. However, interpretation of each company's Terms of Service or Use Agreement does not guarantee that data will remain private, so IRBs often discourage these platforms for any potentially sensitive information. For example, Google's Terms of Service, as of April 2014, states that:

> When you upload, submit, store, send or receive content to or through our Services, you give Google (and those we work with) a worldwide license to use, host, store, reproduce, modify, create derivative works (such as those resulting from translations, adaptations or other changes we make so that your content works better with our Services), communicate, publish, publicly perform, publicly display and distribute such content.[47]

Researchers must weigh the terms of service and the potential associated risks therein with the use and convenience of the product. Larger institutional policies around data storage can also influence acceptable storage and retention options.

Sharing sensitive data in the digital age has proven to be a challenge, as access to more information or other datasets can increase the possibility of re-identification. While personally identifiable information, such as names, social security numbers, or other unique identifiers are secured or removed, discussion about reverse identification (or identification of anonymized data through unique characteristics or attributes, possibly when triangulated with other secondary data sources) has become more critical. A 2006 example of reverse identification occurred with AOL's release of search keywords. After replacing unique number strings for user names, AOL released a text file of search terms from over six hundred fifty-seven thousand users for researchers to analyze.[48] However, the ability to track each user individually and match patterns of keywords over time enabled reporters from the *New York Times* to reidentify individual users. In other studies, anonymous DNA information could be used, in conjunction with public information available online, to reidentify participants.[49] As these examples illustrate, researchers need to determine how much data should be shared and identify the risks of reidentification.

Certain disciplines have established a standard retention period; for example, psychology has a professional expectation of storing research data for a minimum of five years.[50] Other disciplines have not provided specific guidance. For faculty, greater IRB emphasis is on the timeline and methods for data destruction. The culture of practice policies for data retention, like psychology, are not always useful since the student may graduate before the retention period has ended and is not likely to return to campus a few years later to complete the data destruction. Moreover, the destruction of digital data is different from the physical shredding of paper data. Electronic files require more than simply putting them in the virtual trash; instead, electronic deletion software may be necessary to fully remove all traces of the files and avoid any accidental access. Researchers who wish to retain data indefinitely will have to address how they will migrate data into future formats and avoid obsolescence, a skill that aligns with the DIL competency of data conversion and interoperability.

With respect to these concerns, consultations and recommendations from the health sciences and nursing librarian, as an IRB member, have helped guide researchers on safe data management practices. At JMU, the Libraries & Educational Technologies unit works closely with campus IT to address campus-wide computing needs, providing the librarians with a greater understanding of IT use on campus than the average faculty member or student. As librarians often interact with students in the middle of their projects, over a variety of courses, and for a number of years, they have a sense of the technological capabilities of these students, perhaps more so than the average staff member in the Office of Research Integrity. Lastly, librarians are able to network with colleagues at other institutions who are leading DIL and data management conversations.

Conclusion

Data information literacy, with its characteristics of data documentation, preservation, and sharing, requires engagement with a wide array of information skills. To that end, DIL should be treated as any of the other literacy competencies and incorporated into the workflow of outreach librarians, with the acknowledgment that this may require input from other library units, such as metadata and scholarly communication.[51] Pre-professional health students and students engaged in research experiences would benefit from DIL instruction for a myriad of reasons, including a competitive edge in the marketplace or graduate programs. As knowledge of data security, data sharing, and critical data analysis become more valued as scholarly currency, exposure at the undergraduate level will help produce a more informed citizenry.

Pearls

- Work with liaison librarians to gain understanding of student research activities and disciplinary expectations.
- Identify programmatic places in the curriculum to engage data information literacy concepts.
- Create partnerships across campus with other research offices
- Distribute RDM knowledge—no silos!
- Recognize data as a scholarly product.
- Data information literacy is a facet of scholarly communication.

Recommended Reading and Resources

- ACRL Scholarly Communication Toolkit: http://acrl.ala.org/scholcomm/ A consistently updated resource covering the breadth of scholarly communication concerns, including data management.
- Clearinghouse of data information literacy sources from the e-Science portal for New England Librarians: http://esciencelibrary.umassmed.edu/DIL_Course_Materials
- Data Management videos from the University of Wisconsin Data Services on YouTube: https://www.youtube.com/channel/UC9MT-uDcJJgSXQWC9JvlfeQ
- Johnston, L., and Jeffryes, J. "Steal This Idea: A Library Instructors' Guide to educating students in data management skills." *College & Research Libraries News* 75, no. 8 (2014): 431–34. http://crln.acrl.org/content/75/8/431.full. While written with the graduate student in mind, lessons can be adapted for the undergraduate audience.
- Medeiros, Norm, and Richard Ball. "Project TIER: Protocol 2.0 DEMO." *Open Science Framework*. February 25, 2015. osf.io/he87a. Collaborative effort between a librarian and economic faculty to teach undergraduate students data management as a basic part of research in order to help assign responsibility and accountability to the findings. This is an exceptional example of delivering DIL instruction within a discipline's curriculum.

Notes

1. Mitchell Malachowski, et al., "Realizing Student, Faculty, and Institutional Outcomes at Scale: Institutionalizing Undergraduate Research, Scholarship, and Creative Activity within Systems and Consortia," *New Directions for Higher Education* 2015, no. 169 (2015): 3-13, doi: 10.1002/he.20118.
2. Boyer Commission on Educating Undergraduates in the Research University. *Reinventing Undergraduate Education: A Blueprint for America's Research Universities* (Stony Brook, NY: Boyer Commission on Educating Undergraduates in the Research University, 1998), http://eric.ed.gov/?id=ED424840.
3. David Lopatto. *Science in Solution: The Impact of Undergraduate Research on Student Learning* (Tucson, AZ: Research Corporation for Science Advancement, 2009); Shouping Hu, et al., *Reinventing Undergraduate Education: Engaging College Students in Research and Creative Activities* (Hoboken, NJ: Wiley, 2008); CarolAnne Kardash, "Evaluation of an Undergraduate Research Experience: Perceptions of Undergraduate Interns and Their Faculty Mentors," *Journal of Educational Psychology* 92, no. 1 (2000): 191–201, doi: 10.1037/0022-0663.92.1.191; George Kuh, et al., *Student Success in College: Creating Conditions That Matter* (San Francisco, CA: Wiley, 2010).
4. John Aubrey Douglas and Chun-Mei Zhao, "Undergraduate Research Engagement at Major US Research Universities," Center for Studies in Higher Education, November 2013, http://files.eric.ed.gov/fulltext/ED545187.pdf
5. Malachowski, et al., "Realizing Student, Faculty, and Institutional Outcomes at Scale."
6. "Facilitating Research at Primarily Undergraduate Institutions," National Science Foundation, accessed June 17, 2015, http://www.nsf.gov/funding/pgm_summ.jsp?pims_id=5518

7. Department of Health and Human Services, "Academic Research Enhancement Award (Parent R15)," accessed on June 17, 2015, http://grants.nih.gov/grants/guide/pa-files/PA-13-313.html.
8. Robert D. Slocum and Jacob D. Scholl, "NSF Support of Research at Primarily Undergraduate Institutions (PUIs)," *CUR Quarterly* 34, no. 1 (2013): 31–40, accessed June 17, 2015, http://www.cur.org/assets/1/23/Fall2013_v34.1_slocum.scholl.pdf.
9. Mark Scherwin, "Prof Wins $416,385 NIH Grant to Involve Students in Research," Western Michigan University, accessed September 11, 2015. http://wmich.edu/news/2015/06/24634.
10. Carnegie Classification of Institutions of Higher Education, "Distribution of Institutions and Enrollments by Classification Category," 2010, accessed June 17, 2015, http://carnegieclassifications.iu.edu/summary/ugrad_prog.php.
11. Ibid.
12. James Madison University, "Factsheet," accessed June 17, 2015, http://www.jmu.edu/_images/news/2014/JMU_Factsheet_03-2015.pdf.
13. Office of Sponsored Programs, "Annual Report Fiscal Year 2014, July 1, 2013–June 30, 2014," accessed June 17, 2015, http://www.jmu.edu/sponsoredprograms/newsletters-and-reports/annual-fy14.pdf.
14. Carrie Tillman, e-mail message to author, May 14, 2015.
15. Office of the President, "James Madison University Strategic Plan 2014–2020: The Madison Plan," accessed on June 17, 2015, http://browndigital.bpc.com/publication/?i=223226.
16. Sharon Babcock, e-mail message to author, May 21, 2015.
17. Office of Institutional Research, "Statistical Summary 2014," accessed June 17, 2015, http://www.jmu.edu/instresrch/statsum/2014_15/T3-11_2014.pdf.
18. University Studies, "Pre-Professional Health Programs," James Madison University, 2013, accessed June 17, 2015, http://www.jmu.edu/advising/preprofessional/health.shtml
19. Babcock, e-mail message to author, May 21, 2015.
20. Merinda Kaye Hensley, Sarah L. Shreeves, and Stephanie Davis-Kahl, "A Survey of Library Support for Formal Undergraduate Research Programs," *College & Research Libraries*, 75, no. 4 (2014): 422-41. doi:10.5860/crl.75.4.422.
21. Jake Carlson, et al., "An Exploration of the Data Information Literacy Competencies," in *Data Information Literacy: Librarians, Data, and the Education of a New Generation of Researchers* (West Lafayette, IN: Purdue University Press, 2015), 53.
22. Jian Qin and John D'Ignazio, "Lessons Learned from a Two-Year Experience in Science Data Literacy Education," Purdue University, 2010, http://docs.lib.purdue.edu/iatul2010/conf/day2/5.
23. Jacob Carlson, et al., "Determining Data Information Literacy Needs: A Study of Students and Research Faculty." *Portal: Libraries & the Academy* 11, no. 2 (2011): 634, http://muse.jhu.edu/journals/portal_libraries_and_the_academy/v011/11.2.carlson.html.
24. Purdue University, University of Minnesota, University of Oregon and Cornell University, "Data Information Literacy," accessed April 14, 2015, http://wiki.lib.purdue.edu/display/ste/Home.
25. Carlson, et al., "An Exploration of the Data Information Literacy Competencies," 55–68.
26. Yasmeen Shorish, "Data Management," accessed February 8, 2016, http://guides.lib.jmu.edu/data.
27. "VA Data Management Boot Camp," accessed February 8, 2016, http://guides.lib.odu.edu/VADMBC.
28. Hensley, et al., "A Survey of Library Support for Formal Undergraduate Research Programs," 422–41.
29. Malachowski, et al. "Realizing Student, Faculty, and Institutional Outcomes at Scale: Institutionalizing Undergraduate Research, Scholarship, and Creative Activity within Systems and Consortia," 8.
30. "Data Curation Profiles," accessed February 8, 2016, http://datacurationprofiles.org/.

31. Hailey Mooney, et al., "Collaborative Approaches to Undergraduate Research Training: Information Literacy and Data Management," *Advances in Social Work* 15, no. 2 (2014): 368–89, accessed June 17, 2015, https://journals.iupui.edu/index.php/advancesinsocialwork/article/viewFile/15089/18390.
32. Council on Education for Public Health, "Accreditation Criteria: Standalone Baccalaureate Programs," 6, accessed June 13, 2015, http://ceph.org/assets/SBP-Criteria.pdf.
33. American Association of Colleges of Nursing, "The Essentials of Baccalaureate Education for Professional Nursing Practice," 1, accessed June 13, 2015, http://www.aacn.nche.edu/education-resources/BaccEssentials08.pdf.
34. Ibid, 18.
35. American Medical Informatics Association, "Nursing Informatics," accessed June 13, 2015, https://www.amia.org/programs/working-groups/nursing-informatics
36. HealthIT.gov. "Health IT Legislation," accessed June 13, 2015, http://healthit.gov/policy-researchers-implementers/health-it-legislation.
37. Carolyn Schubert, "What Is Biomedical Informatics? An Overview and a Case Study," in *Curriculum-Based Library Instruction: From Cultivating Faculty Relationships to Assessment*, ed. Amy Blevins and Megan Inman (Lanham, MD: Rowman & Littlefield, 2014), 177–86.
38. Amanda Whitmire, "Implementing a Graduate-Level Research Data Management Course: Approach, Outcomes and Lessons Learned," *Journal of Librarianship and Scholarly Communication*, 3, no. 2 (2015): eP1246, doi: 10.7710/2162-3309.1246; Christine Borgman. "Courses," accessed June 19, 2015, http://christineborgman.info/courses/; Jennifer Muilenburg, Mahria Lebow, and Joanne Rich, "Lessons Learned from a Research Data Management Pilot Course at an Academic Library," *Journal of eScience Librarianship* 3, no. 1 (2014): 67–73, doi:10.7191/jeslib.2014.1058.
39. Eva Perkins, "Johns Hopkins' Tragedy: Could Librarians Have Prevented a Death?" accessed on May 14, 2015, http://newsbreaks.infotoday.com/nbreader.asp?ArticleID=17534.
40. Jessica Adamick, "Librarian Involvement in Research Ethics: An Entry Point into the World of Sponsored Research," *Issues in Science and Technology Librarianship* 65 (2011): 11–21, doi: 10.5062/F44Q7RW0.
41. Paula Raimondo, et al.. "Health literacy and Consent Forms: Librarians Support Research on Human Subjects." *Journal of the Medical Library Association* 102, no. 1 (2014): 5–8. doi: 10.3163/1536-5050.102.1.003.
42. Rachel Resnick, "IRB and You, the Hospital Librarian," *National Network: Newsletter of the Hospital Libraries Section of the Medical Library Association* 26 (2001): 5, 8, accessed May 7, 2015, https://www.academia.edu/841736/IRB_and_You_the_Hospital_Librarian.
43. Fern Cheek and Pamela S. Bradigan, "Academic Health Sciences Library Research Support," *Journal of the Medical Library Association*, 98, no. 2 (2010): 167–71, doi: 10.3163/1536-5050.98.2.011.
44. Carrie Tillman, e-mail message to author, May 14, 2015.
45. SurveyMonkey, "Plans and Pricing," accessed June 17, 2015, https://www.surveymonkey.com/pricing/?ut_source=header.
46. Qualtrics, "Security Statement," accessed on September 11, 2015, http://www.qualtrics.com/security-statement/; REDCap. "Software," accessed on September 11, 2015, http://project-redcap.org/software.php.
47. Google, "Terms of Service," accessed June 13, 2015, https://www.google.com/intl/en/policies/terms/.
48. Michael Barbaro and Tom Zeller, "A Face Is Exposed for AOL Searcher No. 4417749," *New York Times*, August 9, 2006, accessed June 13, 2015, http://query.nytimes.com/gst/abstract.html?res=9E0CE3DD1F3FF93AA3575BC0A9609C8B63.
49. Melissa Gymrek, et al., "Identifying Personal Genomes by Surname Inference," *Science* 339, no. 6117(2013):321-324, doi: 10.1126/science.1229566.

50. Deborah Smith, "Five principles for research ethics," *Monitor on Psychology*, accessed June 13, 2015, http://www.apa.org/monitor/jan03/principles.aspx.
51. Association of College and Research Libraries, Working Group on Intersections of Scholarly Communication and Information Literacy, *Intersections of Scholarly Communication and Information Literacy: Creating Strategic Collaborations for a Changing Academic Environment* (Chicago, IL: Association of College and Research Libraries, 2013), accessed February 8, 2016, http://www.ala.org/acrl/sites/ala.org.acrl/files/content/publications/whitepapers/Intersections.pdf.

Bibliography

Adamick, Jessica. "Librarian Involvement in Research Ethics: An Entry Point into the World of Sponsored Research." *Issues in Science and Technology Librarianship* 65 (2011): 11–21. doi: 10.5062/F44Q7RW0.

American Association of Colleges of Nursing. "The Essentials of Baccalaureate Education for Professional Nursing Practice." Accessed June 13, 2015. http://www.aacn.nche.edu/education-resources/BaccEssentials08.pdf.

American Medical Informatics Association. "Nursing Informatics." Accessed June 13, 2015. https://www.amia.org/programs/working-groups/nursing-informatics.

Association of College and Research Libraries. Working Group on Intersections of Scholarly Communication and Information Literacy. *Intersections of Scholarly Communication and Information Literacy: Creating Strategic Collaborations for a Changing Academic Environment*. Chicago, IL: Association of College and Research Libraries, 2013. Accessed February 8, 2016. http://www.ala.org/acrl/sites/ala.org.acrl/files/content/publications/whitepapers/Intersections.pdf.

Barbaro, Michael, and Tom Zeller. "A Face Is Exposed for AOL Searcher No. 4417749." *New York Times*, August 9, 2006. Accessed June 13, 2015. http://query.nytimes.com/gst/abstract.html?res=9E0CE3DD1F3FF93AA3575BC0A9609C8B63.

Borgman, Christine. "Courses." Accessed June 19, 2015. http://christineborgman.info/courses/

Boyer Commission on Educating Undergraduates in the Research University. *Reinventing Undergraduate Education: A Blueprint for America's Research Universities*. Stony Brook, NY: Boyer Commission on Educating Undergraduates in the Research University, 1998. http://eric.ed.gov/?id=ED424840.

Carlson, Jacob, Michael Fosmire, C. C. Miller, and Megan Sapp Nelson. "Determining Data Information Literacy Needs: A Study of Students and Research Faculty." *Portal: Libraries & the Academy* 11, no. 2 (2011): 629–57. http://muse.jhu.edu/journals/portal_libraries_and_the_academy/v011/11.2.carlson.html.

Carlson, Jake, Jon Jeffryes, Lisa R. Johnston, Mason Nichols, Brian Westra, and Sarah J. Wright. "An Exploration of the Data Information Literacy Competencies." In *Data Information Literacy: Librarians, Data, and the Education of a New Generation of Researchers*, ed. Jake Carlson and Lisa R. Johnston. West Lafayette, IN: Purdue University Press, 2015.

Carnegie Classification of Institutions of Higher Education. "Distribution of Institutions and Enrollments by Classification Category." Accessed June 17, 2015. http://carnegieclassifications.iu.edu/summary/ugrad_prog.php.

———. "Distribution of Institutions and Enrollments by Classification Category." Accessed June 17, 2015. http://carnegieclassifications.iu.edu/summary/basic.php.

Cheek, Fern M., and Pamela S. Bradigan. "Academic Health Sciences Library Research Support." *Journal of the Medical Library Association* 98, no. 2 (2010): 167–71. doi: 10.3163/1536-5050.98.2.011.

Council on Education for Public Health. "Accreditation Criteria: Standalone Baccalaureate Programs." Accessed June 13, 2015. http://ceph.org/assets/SBP-Criteria.pdf.

Department of Health and Human Services. "Academic Research Enhancement Award (Parent R15)." Accessed on June 17. http://grants.nih.gov/grants/guide/pa-files/PA-13-313.html.

Douglas, John Aubrey, and Chun-Mei Zhao. "Undergraduate Research Engagement at Major US Research Universities." Center for Studies in Higher Education, November 2013. http://files.eric.ed.gov/fulltext/ED545187.pdf.

Google. "Terms of Service." Accessed June 13, 2015. https://www.google.com/intl/en/policies/terms/.

Gymrek, Melissa, Amy L. McGuire, David Golan, Eran Halperin, and Yaniv Erlich. "Identifying Personal Genomes by Surname Inference." *Science* 339, no. 6117 (2013): 321–24. doi: 10.1126/science.1229566.

HealthIT.gov. "Health IT Legislation." Accessed June 13, 2015. http://healthit.gov/policy-researchers-implementers/health-it-legislation

Hensley, Merinda Kaye, Sarah L. Shreeves, and Stephanie Davis-Kahl. "A Survey of Library Support for Formal Undergraduate Research Programs." *College & Research Libraries*. 75: 422–41. doi:10.5860/crl.75.4.422.

Hu, Shouping, Kathyrine L. Scheuch, Robert A. Schwartz, Joy G. Gayles, and Shaoqing Li. *Reinventing Undergraduate Education: Engaging College Students in Research and Creative Activities*. Hoboken, NJ: Wiley, 2008.

James Madison University. "Factsheet." Accessed June 17, 2015. http://www.jmu.edu/_images/news/2014/JMU_Factsheet_03-2015.pdf.

Kardash, CarolAnne M. "Evaluation of an Undergraduate Research Experience: Perceptions of Undergraduate Interns and Their Faculty Mentors." *Journal of Educational Psychology* 92, no. 1 (2000): 191–201. doi: 10.1037/0022-0663.92.1.191.

Kuh, George D., Jillian Kinzie, John Schuh, and Elizabeth Whitt. *Student Success in College: Creating Conditions that Matter*. San Francisco, CA: Wiley, 2010.

Lopatto, David. *Science in Solution: The Impact of Undergraduate Research on Student Learning*. Tucson, AZ: Research Corporation for Science Advancement, 2009

Malachowski, Mitchell, Jeffrey M. Osborn, Kerry K. Karukstis, and Elizabeth L. Ambos. "Realizing Student, Faculty, and Institutional Outcomes at Scale: Institutionalizing Undergraduate Research, Scholarship, and Creative Activity within Systems and Consortia." *New Directions for Higher Education* 2015, no. 169 (2015): 3–13. doi: 10.1002/he.20118.

Mooney, Hailey, W. Aaron Collie, Shawn W. Nicholson, and Marya R. Sosulski. "Collaborative Approaches to Undergraduate Research Training: Information Literacy and Data Management." *Advances in Social Work* 15, no. 2 (2014): 368–89. Accessed June 17, 2015. https://journals.iupui.edu/index.php/advancesinsocialwork/article/viewFile/15089/18390.

Muilenburg, Jennifer, Mahria Lebow, and Joanne Rich. "Lessons Learned from a Research Data Management Pilot Course at an Academic Library." *Journal of eScience Librarianship* 3, no. 1 (2014): 67–73. doi:10.7191/jeslib.2014.1058.

National Science Foundation. "Facilitating Research at Primarily Undergraduate Institutions." Accessed June 17, 2015. http://www.nsf.gov/funding/pgm_summ.jsp?pims_id=5518.

Office of Institutional Research. "Statistical Summary 2014." Accessed June 17, 2015. http://www.jmu.edu/instresrch/statsum/2014_15/T3-11_2014.pdf.

Office of Sponsored Programs. "Annual Report Fiscal Year 2014, July 1, 2013–June 30, 2014." Accessed on June 17, 2015, http://www.jmu.edu/sponsoredprograms/newsletters-and-reports/annual-fy14.pdf

Office of the President. "James Madison University Strategic Plan 2014–2020: The Madison Plan." Accessed on June 17, 2015. http://browndigital.bpc.com/publication/?i=223226.

Perkins, Eva. "Johns Hopkins' Tragedy: Could Librarians Have Prevented a Death?" Accessed May 14, 2015. http://newsbreaks.infotoday.com/nbreader.asp?ArticleID=17534.

Purdue University, University of Minnesota, University of Oregon, and Cornell University. "Data 308 Information Literacy." Accessed April 14, 2014, http://wiki.lib.purdue.edu/display/ste/Home.

Purdue University Libraries, University of Michigan, Institute of Museum and Library Services, and D2C2 Distributed Data Curation Center. "Data Curation Profiles." Accessed February 8, 2016. http://datacurationprofiles.org/.

Qin, Jian, and John D'Ignazio. "Lessons Learned from a Two-Year Experience in Science Data Literacy Education." Purdue University, 2010. http://docs.lib.purdue.edu/iatul2010/conf/day2/5.

Qualtrics. "Security Statement." Accessed on September 11, 2015. http://www.qualtrics.com/security-statement/

Raimondo, Paula G., Ryan L. Harris, Michele Nance, and Everly D. Brown. "Health Literacy and Consent Forms: Librarians Support Research on Human Subjects." *Journal of the Medical Library Association* 102, no. 1 (2014): 5–8. doi: 10.3163/1536-5050.102.1.003.

REDCap. "Software." Accessed on September 11, 2015. http://project-redcap.org/software.php.

Resnick, Rachel. "IRB and You, the Hospital Librarian." *National Network: Newsletter of the Hospital Libraries Section of the Medical Library Association*. 26 (2001): 5, 8. Accessed May 7, 2015. https://www.academia.edu/841736/IRB_and_You_the_Hospital_Librarian.

Scherwin, Mark. "Prof Wins $416,385 NIH Grant to Involve Students in Research." Western Michigan University. Accessed September 11, 2015. http://wmich.edu/news/2015/06/24634.

Schubert, Carolyn. "What Is Biomedical Informatics? An Overview and a Case Study." In *Curriculum-Based Library Instruction: From Cultivating Faculty Relationships to Assessment*, ed. Amy Blevins and Megan Inman, 177–86. Lanham, MD: Rowman & Littlefield, 2014.

Shorish, Yasmeen. "Data Management." Accessed February 8, 2016. http://guides.lib.jmu.edu/data.

Slocum, Robert D., and Jacob D. Scholl. "NSF Support of Research at Primarily Undergraduate Institutions (PUIs)." *CUR Quarterly* 34, no. 1: 31–40. Accessed June 17, 2015. http://www.cur.org/assets/1/23/Fall2013_v34.1_slocum.scholl.pdf.

Smith, Deborah. "Five Principles for Research Ethics." *Monitor on Psychology*. Accessed June 13, 2015. http://www.apa.org/monitor/jan03/principles.aspx.

SurveyMonkey. "Plans and Pricing." Accessed June 17, 2015. https://www.surveymonkey.com/pricing/?ut_source=header.

University Studies. "Pre-Professional Health Programs." James Madison University, 2013. Accessed June 17, 2015. http://www.jmu.edu/advising/preprofessional/health.shtml

"VA Data Management Boot Camp." Accessed February 8, 2016. http://guides.lib.odu.edu/VADMBC.

Whitmire, Amanda. L. "Implementing a Graduate-Level Research Data Management Course: Approach, Outcomes and Lessons Learned." *Journal of Librarianship and Scholarly Communication* 3, no. 2 (2015): eP1246. doi: 10.7710/2162-3309.1246.

Chapter 13

Building Data Management Services at an Academic Medical Center

AN ENTREPRENEURIAL APPROACH

Alisa Surkis and Kevin Read, New York University Health Sciences Library

The New York University Health Sciences Library (NYUHSL) offers data management services that include a data catalog, a lab organization tool, data management education, and individualized lab support. The core of our approach has been to develop services in direct response to needs expressed by researchers. We have put ourselves in a position to find these opportunities by building strong ties with the research community through liaison work, performing a series of data interviews, and using broad outreach strategies to identify informationist supplement opportunities. We have then taken the external landscape around data management and sharing into account when strategizing how to develop these services. This entrepreneurial approach, which we consider a key to our success, will be described in detail in this chapter.

NYUHSL's participation in the Association for Research Libraries (ARL) E-Science Institute in 2011[1] was the first step toward the development of our data management services. NYUHSL librarians joined librarians from across NYU in this effort to assess the institutional environment's readiness for "E-Science" services, defined by ARL as services in support of computational research, including support for data curation and production. Members of the team interviewed stakeholders from across NYU—researchers, administrators, and information technology professionals—to assess what was currently being offered and to gauge opinions on the role of the library in this undertaking. The final exercise was to perform a SWOT (Strengths, Weaknesses, Opportunities, and Threats) analysis of the institution.

The interviews and the SWOT analysis provided several important pieces of information. First, most stakeholders did not recognize a role for the library as a provider of services in the E-Science arena, particularly in the area of data management. Second, not many services were being offered by anyone in this area. Finally, we saw that there was no coordination of the services that were available. It was clear to us that a great deal of opportunity existed, but major hurdles needed to be overcome, particularly around perceptions of the library.

Since that environmental scan in 2011, NYUHSL has established itself as a significant provider of data services within the NYU School of Medicine. The set of services we offer has begun to coalesce into a coherent whole, but this happened organically over time; we did not come out of our ARL E-Science Institute participation with a plan for a suite of services. We were wary of planning services based on our own agenda or on funding agency and publisher requirements, rather than in response to the direct needs of the researchers as seen by the researchers. To bastardize an idiom, we knew that as much as we could lead a researcher to a data policy, we couldn't make that researcher drink of its requirements—at least not until they either were forced to or saw the direct benefit to their work.

Setting

The NYU Health Sciences Library is positioned within an academic medical center that has a strong emphasis on data governance. NYU, in partnership with the New York City Health and Hospitals Corporation (HHC), has a Clinical and Translational Science Institute (CTSI) that has been a key player in building centralized data services at the institution. This focus on data aligns with the vision of our library director, Neil Rambo, who has brought a strong interest in developing data related services to the library. Also of note, since Hurricane Sandy in October 2012, we have not had a physical library or books, which has forced us out into our user community more, and has helped our user community to recognize that library services go beyond the physical space.

Who We Are

A number of people from the library have coalesced around data services over the past four years, forming an ad hoc data services team. The authors of this chapter are core members of this team. Alisa Surkis is the translational science librarian and has been at NYUHSL since 2011. She received an MS in physics and a PhD in neuroscience and then worked for more than ten years writing software to collect and analyze research data and model the visual system for vision science researchers. Kevin Read is the knowledge management librarian and originally came to the library as a National Library of Medicine associate fellow in 2013, a position where he gained experience working on large-scale projects with researchers within the NIH and exploring federal data management and sharing initiatives.

The core team has recently expanded to include a second knowledge management librarian, Fred LaPolla, to meet the growing demand for data services by both providing support for ongoing projects and seeking out new opportunities to expand service areas. In addition, the team works closely with the library's systems group, collaborating regularly with the Web services librarian, Catherine Larson, and a developer, Ian Lamb, both of whom have been vital to our role in developing and supporting the tools that we will outline in this chapter. A number of other librarians have contributed to these efforts over the years to build our data management services, most notably Karen Hanson, formerly our knowledge systems librarian, who was instrumental in initial efforts to build data management services. Together our team provides a diverse, yet complementary approach to providing data services within our academic medical center, encompassing research experience, technical expertise, archival training, and experience with NIH initiatives.

Education (2012–present)

Teaching to Researchers

THE START OF IT ALL: POSTDOC CLASS

Our first step in establishing data services was to offer an introductory data management class for postdoctoral scholars (postdocs). There were two reasons that we chose this as an entry point into data services. First, Alisa had experience as a basic science researcher and programmer, and Karen Hanson had extensive programming and database experience and had worked with digital archives.

These complementary skill sets brought together knowledge of the research process, an archival background, and hands-on experience in working with data, all of which allowed us to build an effective course around data management best practices. The second reason we chose this approach was that we could partner with the Postdoctoral Office, with which we had worked on other projects, to provide the course under their auspices. They offered a lab management series and saw our content as a good fit. Because of this partnership, we did not have to rely on researchers' acceptance of the library in a data management role, a key barrier identified as part of the ARL E-Science institute.

While data management best practices taken from trusted resources[2] formed the core of the class, a number of elements were added to the course as ways to more effectively engage the students. One was a "carrots and sticks" motivational section where we discussed the current landscape around data management and sharing, including evolving funder and publisher requirements, stories of poor data management leading to dire consequences like retraction, successes of data sharing, and emerging ways for researchers to get credit for sharing their data. Another element that we added to the class was a short, humorous video demonstrating some of the issues that arise in data management and sharing, "Data Sharing and Management Snafu in 3 Short Acts."[3]

As we neared the time of our data management debut, we realized that the lab management series for postdocs, of which our class was supposed to be a part, had never actually materialized. We decided to open the class up to the entire medical center, and ended up with almost thirty attendees from a range of research types and research roles. Despite the wide range of attendees, the class was very well received, as evidenced by the positive course evaluations, with all attendees indicating they either definitely or probably would use the material learned in the course, and two-thirds indicating an interest in future, more detailed classes.

A success that grew beyond the scope of the class was the Data Snafu video we made. We put the video up on YouTube, sent the link around to a few key people, and it took off. It has been viewed over forty-one thousand times and incorporated into research guides, educational materials, and conference keynote talks. Because the video was able to hit so many key points in under five minutes, it established that we understood the issues around data management and served as an effective calling card both within and outside of our institution.

In the aftermath of Hurricane Sandy and the loss of our library, we weren't able to teach the class again until 2014. Outreach for the class was done exclusively by the Postdoctoral Office for this class. By this time, Kevin had joined the library and was able to add his perspective to the class, bringing in new federal requirements and highlighting initiatives that were under development at the NIH, like the Big Data to Knowledge (BD2K) initiative.

Another change was a move away from some of the more library-centric material we had presented in 2012 in favor of researcher-friendly terminology (for example, replacing the term "metadata" with "data description and documentation"). We took the opportunity to update the postdocs on recent changes in publisher requirements around data sharing. Not long before the class, *PLOS* had released its new requirements,[4] becoming the first journal to require researchers to demonstrate proof of data sharing in the form of a unique identifier like a DOI. Using *PLOS* as an example, we stressed that the attitude of scholarly publishers toward data sharing was changing, and encouraged postdocs to manage their data so that they would be in a position to easily comply with the requirements of *PLOS* and other scientific journals as they moved toward similar requirements.

While the 2014 class again received very positive evaluations, turnout was poor. Thirty postdocs registered for the class, but only thirteen attended. We discussed the turnout with the course coordinator, who had had similar issues with other courses offered around that time, but other than the possibility that there were just too many competing courses and seminars at that time, we were unable to explain the poor showing.

We returned to the material again for the 2015 class and made further adjustments. We did not make many changes to the core material, but once again tried to update our "carrots and sticks" to include recent events in the world of data management. For example, we provided more focus on the topic of experiment reproducibility, a popular issue in the news and scholarly community at that time. The NIH's Genomic Data Sharing Policy[5] and new Data Management Requirements[6] had also been released only a few weeks before our class, so we took the opportunity to outline these. With each passing year, we found that there were more convincing carrots and sticks for our presentation.

In 2015, we also expanded our discussion of data sharing. We presented a variety of discipline-specific data repositories from the NIH Data Sharing Repositories website, and provided examples of online research sharing communities like the Collaborative Research for Computational Neuroscience (CRCNS) website to demonstrate that data sharing could lead to increased collaboration within specific communities. We presented alternative options for data sharing including large-scale general data repositories like Figshare, data publications such as *Scientific Data* and *GigaScience*, and data repository registries like the Registry of Research Data Repositories (re3data).

While the course was again well received, the turnout was even worse than the previous year, with thirty-three people registered for the class, and only six attending. While we learned that there had been confusion over the location, the poor attendance for these classes was a concern. However, one extremely positive outcome was that, upon learning of this poor attendance, the associate dean for biomedical sciences and the director of the Sackler Institute of Graduate Biomedical Sciences asked the library to submit a proposal for a twelve-week required graduate course focusing on data management.

HOW TO GET THEM IN THE DOOR: HAPPY HOUR

Only a few months after the disappointing turnout for our 2015 data management class for postdocs, we learned what was needed to get people to care about data management: a happy hour. Our most recent class on data management was presented to the Skirball Institute of Biomolecular Medicine. This class was organized in collaboration with Kevin, who serves as liaison librarian for Skirball, and the director and assistant director of the department. It was decided that the class would be presented before the regular Skirball happy hour social event. The directive from the heads of the department and the incentive of a happy hour afterward led to a high turnout, with over sixty postdocs, graduate students, and faculty members in attendance. This was a stark contrast to the attendance at the class for the postdocs, a community with which we did not have a strong connection.

The course followed a nearly identical format to our postdoc course taught a few months prior, but we focused more on fostering discussion with the audience. Where possible, we directed questions to the audience, asking them to share their opinions on and struggles with collecting, documenting, managing, and storing their data. Much of the discussion from the audience focused on issues around storage and the lack of trust in the medical center's IT department. Other points the audience raised included struggles to comply with new data management and sharing requirements from the NIH and publishers and difficulties in finding a standardized way to document their experiments and keep track of all the data collected within a single lab. The class also provided us with an opportunity to promote our data management services, such as the Lab Organization Tool. The Skirball Institute directors conveyed to us both that they felt that the class was an important contribution and passed along the positive feedback they had received from others in the class; we felt this was an important step toward connecting with the basic science community.

Teaching to Librarians

THE BEGINNING

As the scope of our library's data management services grew, we recognized that there were relatively few academic medical libraries providing data management services, despite evident interest in this area. In those few libraries, the librarians providing these services often had a significant biomedical research background, usually a PhD. In nonmedical academic libraries, librarians often have a master's degree or PhD in the subject for which they provide liaison services, so they are very familiar with the language and practice of research in that area. This is rarely the case in medical libraries, putting medical librarians at a disadvantage in talking to researchers about their data. With a data team consisting of librarians both with and without a biomedical research background, we straddled this divide and thus felt that we were well positioned to bridge this gap for other librarians. We therefore proposed two continuing education classes on data management at the annual Medical Library Association meeting in 2014, consisting of a two-hour introductory lecture class, and a two-hour workshop consisting of lecture, hands-on exercises, and group work.

THE FIRST ROUND: THE STORY OF DATA

We intended for these classes to provide not just an understanding of data management concepts, but also context to help librarians gain comfort with the process, culture, and language of researchers. The first class included an introduction to data management concepts, not dissimilar to other available introductory materials. Where our material differed from other data management education materials was in the context we provided about data and how researchers interact with that data.

The class included a section on the "story of data"—ways in which raw data, processed data, and analyzed data could be generated and how the different types of data might relate to each other. Another section of the class provided an explanation of the differences between bench and clinical researchers, including differences in culture, team roles, workflow, and data management issues. This distinction is critical to help librarians understand that different researcher communities talk about data differently and have very different data management issues. In the second class, the lecture portion focused more on practical advice for how to initiate data management services and included a number of hands-on exercises, such as finding errors in data collection forms and answering data management reference questions, as well as group work designed to help each attendee develop at least one action item related to starting data management services at their institution. Overall, the classes were very well received, and we were fortunate to have the MLA CE committee extend an invitation to us to teach them again in Austin, Texas, in 2015.

THE SECOND ROUND: A HANDS-ON APPROACH

The MLA CE in Austin, Texas, again consisted of two classes of two hours each. The first class had received uniformly positive reviews the previous year and we felt the material was quite strong, so we made only minor updates on the previous year's materials. Reviews for the second class, while positive overall, had been less favorable than those for the first. We decided a complete redesign was needed if we were to achieve our goal of having the attendees leave the class with the skills and comfort level to begin providing data management services at their own institutions. We kept the group exercise at the end of the class, cut back considerably on the lecture portion, and spent most of the two hours working through a hands-on exercise based on a clinical research case study on smoking cessation.

The exercise began with the attendees reading an article[7] to learn about the researcher's data types and data collection methods. We asked attendees to think about the data interview questions they would ask the researcher based on a list of "researcher" problems that we compiled based on our previous conversations with researchers about their data issues. Next, attendees looked at example data collection forms and identified and fixed errors, such as variables that were poorly defined or for which units were not specified. Similarly, they examined a spreadsheet of data that we had constructed and identified data quality issues, such as inconsistent use of null values or confusing variable names. Next they created a section of a data dictionary, identified a solution to poor file-naming conventions, and found potential venues through which the researchers could share their data.

Both classes were well received, with the revamped second class receiving more favorable reviews than the previous year. We received valuable feedback that the classes should be combined into one four-hour class. Without the context from the first class, librarians were less prepared to address the issues in the exercises compared to those librarians that did. This problem will be rectified next year as we have been invited to teach again at the MLA Conference in Toronto, Canada, this time in a four-hour continuous format.

NLM Informationist Supplements (2012–present)

Informationist Supplements: Round 1 (2012)

In 2012, the National Library of Medicine established a funding mechanism to facilitate the establishment of data management and other nontraditional services by libraries, the Informationist Administrative Supplements. NYUHSL leadership used this funding mechanism as an opportunity to reach out broadly to all researchers at our institution who met the criteria for the supplements.[8] The outreach served to both solicit potential collaborators and inform researchers of the types of services that the library offered. The library reached out to a total of forty-four researchers, received interested responses from nine, and ultimately submitted two applications, both of which were funded, and one of which involved providing data management support.

The data management supplement was for the grant on Clinical Management of Cochlear Implant Patients with Contralateral Hearing Aids awarded to principal investigator (PI) Dr. Mario Svirsky. This support consisted of building a custom database and data entry tool for the research team. This would replace their existing approach of using a Microsoft Access database, written in an old version of the software and supplemented by spreadsheets where new data were no longer supported by the original data model. This project provided the library with valuable hands-on experience in working with a research team on their data and understanding their research process and data management practices. However, in delving into the researchers' data, problems emerged that neither the PI nor the library had anticipated, resulting in the need to devote effort that far exceeded the amount allotted by the grant. The mounting needs of this project provided a valuable cautionary tale for the library in considering the scalability of a service and the potential pitfalls that might be unseen at the time of initial commitment. The project did serve as a positive example of the library providing assistance to a researcher with serious data management issues.

Informationist Supplements: Round 2 (2014)

Library leadership again engaged in broad outreach when the second round of informationist supplements was announced in 2014 and identified two projects for which to submit applications. The first was a clinical study, Multicultural Community Dementia Screening, with PI Dr. James Galvin. The second was a basic science study, Synaptic Basis of Perceptual Learning in Primary Auditory Cortex, with PI Dr. Robert Froemke. Both applications were funded, but shortly thereafter informationist project members from each grant left the library. The authors of this chapter joined the remaining original team members for each project. The new project teams brought different skill sets and approaches, and in light of this, we reexamined the supplement aims. The new teams met with the researchers to discuss their core data management needs and to determine whether the library could still address the researchers' issues, without necessarily taking the paths that had originally been outlined.

MULTICULTURAL COMMUNITY DEMENTIA SCREENING

Dr. Galvin's project involved collecting results from dementia screenings of study participants. Multiple study personnel collected data using paper forms, and a data analyst entered the data into a statistical package. The study data were then combined with screening data from Dr. Galvin's other studies for analysis. The variable names were idiosyncratic and followed no standards. The combined dataset used for analysis was constructed manually within the statistical package.

The original aims of the informationist supplement for Dr. Galvin's project were to establish a data model and data dictionary to facilitate searching, sharing, and expansion over time; to build a web-based input tool for data capture at point of collection; and to develop a web-based approach for sharing anonymized datasets to foster further research. After the personnel change, the new team met with Dr. Galvin and members of his research team to reexamine the issues in his research process, rather than rely on secondhand knowledge of what had led the initial team to that particular set of aims.

The first aim involved building a data model and a data dictionary. In approaching the data dictionary, we saw that the variable names did not conform to any standard and were often quite cryptic, which hindered data sharing. This aim was therefore expanded to map the variable names to more intuitive names, using the Clinical Data Acquisition Standards Harmonization (CDASH) standard from Clinical Data Interchange Standards Consortium (CDISC), when possible, to facilitate interoperability with other clinical research. We also dropped the data model from the project; the new team did not have data modeling expertise and, since building a database was not explicitly included in the specific aims, the data model would have provided no immediate benefit.

The second aim of building a Web-based input tool addressed a clearly critical need. Collecting data on paper and then manually entering hundreds of variables for hundreds of participants is time consuming and increases the likelihood of data errors. The library recommended building electronic data collection forms using REDCap, a HIPAA-compliant electronic data capture system. REDCap would facilitate data entry for the research coordinators, lower the risk of errors through the use of data validation, and save the data analyst many hours by allowing export of data in the format of the statistical package.

To truly minimize the risk of data management errors throughout the research process, the new team recognized that it was critical to address the construction of the analysis datasets. The existing process involved multiple decision points around data manipulation that could result in errors, and only the data analyst knew the full process. We therefore expanded the original aim to include working with the data analyst to delineate a step-by-step workflow and assisting in writing a program that would create a reproducible process for creating the analysis datasets. At the time of writing this chapter, the construction of the REDCap database is underway, the workflow analysis has been completed, and the data analyst has mapped the old variable names to the new variable names for the existing data.

The final specific aim for this project was to develop a tool to share this data with the research community. Originally the library team considered building a website to host the data, where data requestors would be asked to provide information about themselves and reasons why they were interested in using the dataset. However, planning for the website stopped when Dr. Galvin left NYU, as the funding would not cover work at another institution. As an alternative, we recommended that the researcher use the popular data sharing service Figshare, where the PIs can make their data private to control who can use them, as well as receive a DOI so that other researchers can cite them.

SYNAPTIC BASIS OF PERCEPTUAL LEARNING IN PRIMARY AUDITORY CORTEX

Dr. Froemke's lab collected a number of different types of data—electrophysiological, behavioral, anatomical, immunohistochemical—from mice and rats and has received numerous requests for data. Responding to these requests could be challenging and time consuming due to a lack of data organization. Conversations with members of Dr. Froemke's lab revealed a number of workflow and organization issues, including lack of uniformity in metadata collection, difficulty of locating information in paper lab notebooks, lack of standardization of animal identifiers, and metadata and data being stored in a mix of locations and formats.

The original aims of the project were to develop an online system to link and download data from published figures, to construct processes to allow researchers to upload results upon publication, and to build a consortium of PIs from multiple institutions to compile similar results across labs. As for the Galvin supplement, there was a discussion with the researcher of the original study issues and broad goals of the specific aims in order to develop a plan that would meet the researcher's needs through the skill set and approach of the new study team.

Further exploration of the aim of attaching downloadable data to each figure in lab publications revealed that the needs of the researcher were best met with a very simple solution. It was determined that it was best to have a link that would download one spreadsheet with data for the entire paper, which eliminated the need for integrating the data downloads with the post-peer review manuscript. Because Dr. Froemke wanted to facilitate, but not require, information about who was downloading the data and why, inclusion of a link to his e-mail address in the download form was sufficient to meet his needs. The simplification of this aim also addressed the issue of sustainability; datasets would have to be added after the informationist supplement ended, so it was important that the system for doing so be simple enough that a member of the Froemke lab could take over this function.

For the second aim, the main impediment to researchers uploading data was the workflow issues we had identified in the lab. The library has been developing a Lab Organization Tool (described in detail below) that would serve as a way to collect centralized, structured metadata across the lab, with that metadata being drawn from discipline standards where possible. For Dr. Froemke's lab, this would facilitate data sharing by ensuring that certain key metadata elements were available for each dataset, and that the data location, date, and researcher for each dataset could be easily found. Dr. Froemke agreed that this tool would provide a good solution to the problems in his lab, and work to implement that system in his lab is ongoing.

The final aim of building a consortium of researchers to compile similar results across labs seemed to be best achieved through a centralized site, rather than any one researcher's institutional website. Fortunately, we discovered the site Collaborative Research in Computational Neuroscience—Data Sharing.[9] This site, with both NIH and NSF funding, was formed as a place for sharing experimental neuroscience data. The primary "customers" for this data were computational neuroscientists, which is the community from which Dr. Froemke received data sharing requests. The site hosted data for sharing, provided information for researchers about who was downloading their data, and had a forum and a number of other resources. Dr. Froemke agreed that uploading data to this site was the optimal way to achieve the third aim.

Data Catalog (2013–present)

The Data Catalog is a key piece of the NYUHSL's data services. It is a discovery tool, not a repository, so it contains only descriptions of datasets. It indexes both large external datasets commonly used for research such as U.S. Census or national health survey data, and datasets generated by NYU researchers.

The Early Stages

As mentioned earlier, integration with the research community has been a key to providing successful data management services. By being in places where researchers talk about their problems around data, we put ourselves in a position to offer solutions, and our Data Catalog grew out of just such a situation. As the liaison to the NYU-HHC CTSI, Alisa attends monthly executive committee meetings, which are attended by researchers and administrators from across the medical school and CTSI partner institutions. These meetings involve a large number of high-level people from a number of different research areas who are rarely all together in one meeting, so discussions often develop around research barriers and possible solutions.

In a CTSI meeting in early 2013, the chair of the Department of Population Health (DPH), along with others, identified a problem in knowing about large external datasets that were heavily used for research. There were concerns that multiple people were paying for licensing of these datasets, some of which could be shared, creating inefficiencies. Alisa suggested that a catalog of these datasets could provide a solution to this problem, which led to a collaboration between the library and the DPH to build a Data Catalog.[10] The catalog would be an effective way to disseminate information about institutional licenses, as well as provide information about what datasets were available and how to access them. Another feature that was incorporated into the Data Catalog was a list of institutional researchers ("local experts") who had worked with a dataset and were willing to answer questions from other researchers about how to access and/or use the dataset.

The initial scope of the project was large external datasets, but the idea of eventually including internal datasets—that is, those datasets created by researchers at NYU—was considered from the earliest stages of the project. The initial iteration of the Data Catalog drew on both the interface and metadata of the large dataset inventory created by the UCSF CTSI.[11] An initial version of the Data Catalog was built in Drupal with limited functionality and metadata only slightly adapted from the UCSF catalog. Population health researchers were shown this initial version for the purposes of getting their feedback before making the Data Catalog live.

The Second Phase

STRATEGY

For the second phase of the creation of our Data Catalog, there was a major focus on improving the metadata gathered from the UCSF model, and building a tool that would be able to evolve with the needs of the Data Catalog. We were enthusiastic at the prospect of cataloging datasets created by researchers across the institution, but fortunately took a step back to consider the most strategic approach and to explore the perspectives of our researchers. One of the factors in our strategy was the result of a series of data interviews[12] we did with investigators from across the biomedical research spectrum (described below in detail).

The data interviews revealed that population health researchers were the most willing to share their data and the most interested in using data from others, while many of the other researchers we talked to expressed reservations around data sharing. Based on these findings and on our own limited resources, we felt that our energies were best concentrated on datasets, both external and internal, that would be of greatest interest to population health researchers. By expanding the scope of the Data Catalog incrementally, we could concentrate on building up the user base in targeted areas, and slowly expand outreach to related areas.

THE TECHNOLOGY

The library decided to move away from the Drupal instance of the Data Catalog, which had significant limitations in functionality, and build a redesigned instance using PHP with an Apache Solr search. This path provided additional flexibility so that it would be easier to make changes to the interface, and the overall structure of the Data Catalog when necessary. Working in close collaboration with our developer Ian Lamb, we provided a blueprint for the look and feel and the functionality we wanted for the Data Catalog. Rebuilding the Data Catalog in PHP also served to facilitate the sharing of the code used to build it.

THE METADATA

Kevin has extensive experience developing metadata schemas for scientific research from his time spent at the NIH,[13] and provided a strategic approach to creating a metadata schema for the Data

Catalog. We took into account the information gained from the data interviews, and then compared a number of existing schemas to identify metadata elements for inclusion. The schemas we included were the NIH Common Metadata Elements created by Kevin at the NIH, DataCite, Dryad, Nature's Scientific Data, and the W3C's Data Catalog Vocabulary. Relevant metadata elements were then presented to members of the DPH, who provided additional insight into their suitability. The intended use of the Data Catalog for both internal and external datasets at times led to metadata elements that were solely or primarily of use for either internal or external users. While this resulted in a less-than-pristine metadata schema, our priority was to adopt a strategy that would maximize Data Catalog use, rather than one that privileged the purity of the metadata.

LOCAL EXPERTS

We felt that the addition of lists of local experts for each external dataset to the Data Catalog would add a great deal of value, and so devoted significant effort to identifying and reaching out to potential local experts. We searched literature and grant databases to identify NYU researchers who had published on or had grants for the analysis of the external datasets we were indexing. Our DPH collaborator reached out to those researchers to request their participation as local experts, with an opt-in approach. This outreach included the entire institution, not just the medical center, both to increase our pool of local experts and to facilitate cross-campus collaboration. As new external datasets are added to the Data Catalog, we identify additional potential local experts based on literature searches, and request their participation via e-mail.

CURRENT STATUS AND FUTURE DIRECTIONS

As of November 2015, the Data Catalog had received over 7,532 unique page views. The Data Catalog currently describes thirty-six external datasets, with additional datasets in a queue to be entered. The library has just begun to include internal datasets described by two researchers within our DPH, and has started to invite additional DPH researchers to contribute.

We hope to expand the scope of the Data Catalog through collaborations with DataCore, the NYUSoM's centralized clinical data services unit, and with the data librarians at the main NYU library. DataCore's plans include working with clinical researchers to manage and store analysis datasets generated from either clinical research or from data pulls from our electronic health record (EHR), and the plan is for the Data Catalog to serve as the discovery layer for this data. This collaboration provides the library with an opportunity to play a key role in the workflow for discovering clinical research datasets generated at our institution, and ensures that the Data Catalog will remain a valuable tool going forward. Discussions with the data librarians from our main campus have included plans to ingest datasets from related researchers at the main campus, such as those in the NYU Global Institute of Public Health, through collaborations with librarians there.

The Data Catalog represents an enormous effort spanning over two years. The process to create a metadata schema, generate researcher and institutional interest, build the Data Catalog, and continue to ingest new datasets is iterative and ongoing. Our hope is that libraries interested in developing their own catalogs will use our code so that these catalogs will be interoperable across institutions. This would significantly increase the discoverability of research datasets in any area of research that chooses to support a data catalog effort of this kind.

Data Interviews (2013-2014)

To gain a better understanding of data management needs at our institution, the library conducted data interviews with a range of researchers from basic science to clinical to population health researchers.[14]

Starting a conversation with these researchers provided us with an opportunity to learn more about their research, understand the challenges they face when collecting and managing data, and identify potential data contributors for the Data Catalog (in other words, those who were most willing to share their data).

Our approach to the interviews was to take the library out of the equation. Before meeting with each researcher, our team reviewed the researcher's publications to familiarize themselves with the research, so that they would be prepared to engage the researcher in his or her own language. Librarians interviewing researchers were careful to refrain from using library jargon (such as Dublin Core, e-Science). The interview questions focused on the research process and data management needs of the investigator, and did not mention the library. Questions were open ended to foster a conversational tone and to minimize bias on the part of librarians as to what the issues of researchers were likely to be. This approach was key to gaining the trust of the researchers and shifting their attitudes about the potential role of the library in data. As librarians, it is up to us to find ways to fit into the researcher's workflow, not the other way around, and we wanted to ensure that our interview process reflected this goal.

In total, thirty researchers were interviewed—eleven from the basic sciences and nineteen from clinical and population health research. Based on these discussions, the library was able to identify a number of major themes that they could act upon. First, we found that basic science researchers were having difficulties managing the data collected by their postdoctoral researchers and graduate students. Postdocs spend a limited amount of time, typically three years, in a lab before moving on to other research ventures, and often do not document their data collection processes effectively. After postdocs leave the institution, the PI often cannot understand their data, and has no way of knowing how the postdocs collected the data at the time of study without contacting them directly. This issue creates inefficiencies within the lab and leaves the PIs with data they cannot use.

On the clinical side, researchers expressed concern about their data quality. There are often many study personnel participating in one clinical research study, and our interviewees stated that frequently those responsible for collecting data fail to do so uniformly (for example, recording weight measured in kilograms as opposed to pounds). These discrepancies in data collection can lead to data that require a great deal of time to sort out or, at worst, may be unusable. The repercussions of not being able to analyze data that were expensive and time consuming to collect can have devastating effects on the study outcomes.

The data interviews also allowed us to identify researchers and departments at the institution that were most willing to share their data for our Data Catalog. Based on the thirty interviews conducted, we found that researchers from our DPH were most interested in sharing their data, as well as locating and using data created by other researchers. This finding contributed to our outreach strategy for describing internal datasets for the Data Catalog.

The data interviews also provided a way for the library to learn more about the challenges researchers face when collecting and managing their data and to identify researchers most interested in sharing their data. They also served to raise the profile and enhance the credibility of the library in the realm of research data management. Finally, these conversations served to identify data management gaps that could be filled in with new library services, such as the lab organization tool described below.

Lab Organization Tool (2014–Present)

One clear theme that emerged from the data interviews was that most bench scientists had lab organization schemes that ranged from minimal to nonexistent. Identifying this need presented a huge potential opportunity for the library. There were, however, significant barriers to addressing an issue of this magnitude. Our data services team was small, so there was a limit to how much individual attention we could afford to give any individual lab. Introducing major changes into lab practices and workflow would likely be met with resistance; a PI would likely need a convincing cost/benefit argument to institute changes, and graduate students and postdocs would likely be very resistant to any changes in their workflow that they saw as burdensome.

Based on the interviews, we believed that there would be great value to the PI in something as simple as having centrally located, searchable information about which researcher in a lab had done an experiment, what the experiment was, on what date(s) the experiment was done, and where the data were stored. The next level of organization would be to supplement those basic parameters with additional metadata elements specific to an investigator's experiments. Ideally those elements would be drawn from existing discipline standards to facilitate interoperability of shared data. Our goal was to develop a system that could be implemented in such a way as to require a relatively small time commitment from the library and cause only a minor disruption in the workflow of the researchers within the lab.

We decided to implement this tool using REDCap, a tool designed for clinical electronic data capture. REDCap is a browser-based database that allows for centralized storage and searching. REDCap is designed to allow different levels of permission, to easily change permissions for users, and to store an audit trail—all important features in a lab environment where lab personnel enter and leave the lab frequently. Building data entry forms is very simple and can be done online or through upload of a formatted spreadsheet, and this flexibility and ease of use was deemed important for minimizing the burden on the data services team. REDCap includes features such as branching logic and calculated fields, which would allow the data entry forms to be designed in such a way as to minimize the burden on the individual researchers in a lab.

The initial outreach to find labs in which to pilot this tool was done through an e-mail blast to the Neuroscience Institute. This initial avenue was chosen both because Alisa is the liaison to that community and because she had a research background in that area. We believed that her additional background knowledge would facilitate vetting discipline standards and discussions with the PI and lab personnel about individual metadata elements. A second pilot came as part of the informationist supplement for Dr. Robert Froemke's neuroscience study, as described above. Finally, a third pilot was found through outreach to researchers to test the waters for another potential informationist supplement application.

In discussing the particular needs of all of these labs, we found that another of the REDCap features was particularly useful for our purposes. REDCap allows for longitudinal data collection, an important feature for clinical electronic data capture. In each of our pilot labs, experiments could consist of multiple recordings with the same or similar parameters, and the longitudinal feature of REDCap could be used for this purpose. These pilots are all in progress, and upon completion, our plan is to do more intensive marketing across the neuroscience labs at our institution, with the idea that having implemented the lab organization tool in three neuroscience labs, each future neuroscience lab should require fewer and fewer modifications. We plan to focus our efforts on neuroscience labs for the immediate future, though eventually broaden our scope.

Discussion

Our approach to building data management services has been piecemeal, driven by opportunity rather than a strategic plan. After four years, this entrepreneurial approach has begun to coalesce into a fairly coherent set of data services. A number of factors contributed to the successes we have had in this area. First, we engaged in a combination of integration with the research community and broad outreach. Second, to combat the credibility issue for librarians in research data management, we took great care to prepare for interactions with researchers, and to speak their language. Finally, we were sensitive to the perspective of researchers and how that impacted the acceptable cost/benefit ratio of services.

Our broad outreach was invaluable for identifying service gaps that the library could fill and for building an association between the library and research data management in the minds of researchers. The informationist supplements provided an excellent opportunity to contact researchers and ask about their data management challenges. For the data interviews, there was no potential funding attached, and we were very pleased to find that most researchers were still quite willing to take the time to meet with us to discuss their workflows and data management issues.

Liaison work was another important piece of the puzzle. Alisa's integration with the CTSI led to opportunities like the Data Catalog, while Kevin's liaison work with Skirball basic science researchers led to new educational opportunities. The importance of these connections was apparent when comparing the disappointing attendance at our data management classes for postdocs to the packed house when we taught the same material for the Skirball Institute.

Outreach to a community is only effective when you have credibility with that community. Our work with our liaison communities gave us credibility with those groups. Our review of researchers' articles for data interviews and informationist meetings allowed us to engage the researchers more effectively and so establish credibility. The Data Management Snafu video strongly resonated with researchers and demonstrated that we understood their issues. Our extensive preparation for the classes we taught researchers paid off in our being able to effectively communicate important data management issues in language that the researchers could relate to.

Providing services that fulfill the needs of researchers *as seen by the researchers* has been a key strategy. The Data Catalog was created in response to a need expressed by the chair of the DPH and the idea for the lab organization tool grew directly out of problems identified by basic science researchers in the data interviews. Our awareness of the growing importance of data sharing and standards then shaped our strategy around the development of these tools. Rather than wait for researchers to document and preserve their data before describing it in the Data Catalog, we set a low bar for inclusion; we believe that requests for data from other researchers will be the most effective motivator for improving data documentation and preservation. The lab organization tool requires changes to the researcher's workflow, but using metadata elements from discipline standards in the tool do not place any additional burden on the researcher.

In designing the Data Catalog and the lab organization tool, we were careful to consider the cost/benefit ratio for the researcher. Consideration of the cost/benefit ratio for the library was something we learned to weigh carefully as well. Informationist projects can serve as a means for librarians to gain greater insight into the research process, pilot new services, and gain credibility with the research community. However, in our informationist work for Dr. Svirsky, we learned the hard lesson that when a labor-intensive collaboration with a researcher involves providing a service that is not scalable, the benefit to the library is likely not worth the cost.

We would be remiss if we did not acknowledge other libraries that were providing data services at the time we were implementing our own. From the beginning, we took the time to look at what services other libraries were providing to identify their challenges and successes. Where it was possible to draw on the work of others and adapt it to our environment, we did so. Now that we have seen success in the tools and services we are providing to our research community like our Data Catalog and Lab Organization Tool, we hope that other medical libraries will be able to adapt some of what we have learned and built to facilitate the growth of their own data management services.

Pearls

- Don't expect researchers to come to you looking for data services—you need to get the message out, and then you need to get the message out again (and again, and again).
- Keep up with the rapidly changing landscape of data management and data sharing—it will give you credibility with researchers, and may present new service opportunities.

- Meet the researchers where they live—familiarize yourself with their language, process, and needs—this is critical in overcoming the perceptions researchers have of librarians.
- Researchers want to be doing research, not data management—if they don't see the immediate benefit of doing something (or repercussions of not doing it), they won't do it.
- Just because it involves data management doesn't mean you have to do it—avoid time-consuming one-off projects that don't help you develop your library's overall service strategy.

Notes

1. Association of Research Libraries, "Overview of the ARL E-Science Institute," 2011, accessed September 15, 2012, http://www.arl.org/storage/documents/publications/arl-dlf-escience-inst-overview-apr11.pdf.
2. "Research Data Lifecycle," UK Data Archive, 2010, accessed September 30, 2015, http://www.data-archive.ac.uk/create-manage/life-cycle; Christine Borgman, "*Scholarship in the Digital Age: Information, Infrastructure and the Internet*" (Cambridge, MA: MIT Press, 2007), accessed November 20, 2015, http://www.ncbi.nlm.nih.gov/entrez/query.fcgi?db=pubmed&cmd=Retrieve&dopt=AbstractPlus&list_uids=5335346543788160500related:MjKc_fB-ZwcJ\npapers2://publication/uuid/7B157C34-AC00-4E3C-89F6-64EFA2C6A13F; Dorothea Salo, "Save the Cows! Cyberinfrastructure for the Rest of Us," *Slideshare*, June 4, 2009, accessed October 10, 2011, http://www.slideshare.net/cavlec/save-the-cows-data-curation-for-the-rest-of-us-1533252.
3. Karen Hanson et al., "Data Sharing SNAFU in 3 Short Acts," YouTube, 2011, accessed December 21, 2014, https://youtu.be/N2zK3sAtr-4.
4. *PLOS ONE*, "Sharing of Data, Materials, and Software," *PLOS* Editorial and Publishing Policies, 2014, accessed February 27, 2015, http://journals.plos.org/plosone/s/data-availability#loc-acceptable-data-sharing-methods.
5. National Institutes of Health, "NIH Genomic Data Sharing Policy," 2014, accessed April 30, 2015, http://gds.nih.gov/03policy2.html.
6. National Institutes of Health, *National Institutes of Health Plan for Increasing Access to Scientific Publications and Digital Scientific Data from NIH Funded Scientific Research*, 2015, accessed July 15, 2015, http://grants.nih.gov/grants/NIH-Public-Access-Plan.pdf.
7. H. E. Jones, "Acceptance of Naltrexone by Pregnant Women Enrolled in Comprehensive Drug Addiction Treatment: An Initial Survey," *American Journal of Addiction* 21, no. 3 (2012), accessed May 2, 2015, doi:10.1111/j.1521-0391.2012.00229.x
8. Jeff Williams and Neil Rambo, "An Extensible and Successful Method of Identifying Collaborators for National Library of Medicine Informationist Projects," *Journal of Medical Library Association* 103, no. 3 (2015): 145.
9. "CRCNS Data Sharing Website," Collaborative Research in Computational Neuroscience, 2000, accessed July 15, 2015, https://crcns.org/.
10. Kevin Read et al., "Promoting Data Reuse and Collaboration at an Academic Medical Center," *International Journal of Digital Curation* 10, no. 1 (2015): 262, accessed March 1, 2015, doi:10.2218/ijdc.v10i1.366.
11. "Large Dataset Inventory," University of California, San Francisco, 2015, accessed June 10, 2015, https://accelerate.ucsf.edu/research/celdac.
12. Kevin Read et al., "Starting the Data Conversation: Informing Data Services at an Academic Health Sciences Library," *JMLA* 103, no. 3 (2015): 132, accessed July 15, 2015, http://www.ncbi.nlm.nih.gov/pmc/articles/PMC4511052/.
13. Kevin Read, "Common Metadata Elements for Cataloging Biomedical Datasets" Figshare, accessed July 15, 2015, doi:10.6084/m9.figshare.1496573.
14. Read et al., "Starting the Data Conversation," 134.

Bibliography

Association of Research Libraries. Overview of the ARL E-Science Institute, 2011. http://www.arl.org/storage/documents/publications/arl-dlf-escience-inst-overview-apr11.pdf.

Borgman, C. *Scholarship in the Digital Age: Information, Infrastructure, and the Internet*. Cambridge, MA: MIT Press, 2007. http://www.ncbi.nlm.nih.gov/entrez/query.fcgi?db=pubmed&cmd=Retrieve&dopt=AbstractPlus&list_uids=5335346543788160500related:MjKc_fB-ZwcJ\npapers2://publication/uuid/7B157C34-AC00-4E3C-89F6-64EFA2C6A13F.

CRCNS Data Sharing Website. Collaborative Research in Computational Neuroscience, 2000. https://crcns.org/

Hanson, Karen, Alisa Surkis, and Karen Yacobucci. *Data Sharing and Management Snafu in 3 Short Acts*. New York, 2012. https://youtu.be/N2zK3sAtr-4.

Jones, H. E. "Acceptance of Naltrexone by Pregnant Women Enrolled in Comprehensive Drug Addiction Treatment: An Initial Survey." *Am J Addict* 21, no. 3 (2012): 199–201. doi:10.1111/j.1521-0391.2012.00229.x.

"Large Dataset Inventory." University of California, San Francisco, 2015. https://accelerate.ucsf.edu/research/celdac.

National Institutes of Health. *National Institutes of Health Plan for Increasing Access to Scientific Publications and Digital Scientific Data from NIH Funded Scientific Research*, February 2015. http://grants.nih.gov/grants/NIH-Public-Access-Plan.pdf.

———. "NIH Genomic Data Sharing Policy." 2014. http://gds.nih.gov/03policy2.html.

PLOS ONE. "Sharing of Data, Materials, and Software." PLOS Editorial and Publishing Policies, 2014. http://journals.plos.org/plosone/s/data-availability#loc-acceptable-data-sharing-methods.

Read, Kevin. "Common Metadata Elements for Cataloging Biomedical Datasets." *Figshare*, 2015. doi:10.6084/m9.figshare.1496573.

Read, Kevin, Jessica Athens, Ian Lamb, Joey Nicholson, Sushan Chin, Junchuan Xu, Neil Rambo, and Alisa Surkis. "Promoting Data Reuse and Collaboration at an Academic Medical Center." *International Journal of Digital Curation* 10, no. 1 (February 18, 2015): 260–67. doi:10.2218/ijdc.v10i1.366.

Read, Kevin, Alisa Surkis, Catherine Larson, Aileen Mccrillis, Alice Graff, Joseph Nicholson, and Juanchan Xu. "Starting the Data Conversation: Informing Data Services at an Academic Health Sciences Library." *JMLA* 103, no. 3 (2015): 131–35. http://www.ncbi.nlm.nih.gov/pmc/articles/PMC4511052/.

"Research Data Lifecycle." UK Data Archive, 2010. http://www.data-archive.ac.uk/create-manage/life-cycle.

Salo, Dorothea. "Save the Cows! Cyberinfrastructure for the Rest of Us," *Slideshare*, June 4, 2009. http://www.slideshare.net/cavlec/save-the-cows-data-curation-for-the-rest-of-us-1533252.

Williams, Jeff D., and Neil H. Rambo. "An Extensible and Successful Method of Identifying Collaborators for National Library of Medicine Informationist Projects" *JMLA* 103, no. 3 (July 2015): 145–47.

Chapter 14

Data Management in the Lab

Caitlin Bakker, Health Sciences Libraries, University of Minnesota

The importance of data management for academic libraries has been well established, with the ACRL Research Planning and Review Committee proclaiming data management and curation to be top trends in academic libraries in both 2012 and 2014.[1] With their experience facilitating connections between departments and campus units, information discovery and dissemination, and instruction, librarians are well-positioned to leverage these existing skills and further expand into data management services, including data management education. The incorporation of data management into the libraries' established information literacy programs "provides a logical entry point into increasing the role of libraries in supporting e-research,"[2] and maintains the relevance of library services while enhancing the overall quality of research.[3]

Much of the conversation surrounding data management services in academic libraries has been focused on funding agency mandates, and library services are often structured around the creation of a data management plan that would meet these requirements.[4] However, while requirements may be one motivating factor for conversations regarding data management, they are not universal, and the benefits of effectively managing research data are not limited to the completion of a successful grant application. Researchers understand the importance of data management in the research process, and surveys have found health sciences faculty to be very interested in libraries' data management services.[5] Although funder requirements could frame these conversations, an approach that is tailored to identify and respond to the unique needs of a group may resonate in a similar way. The sessions described in this chapter focused on the practical considerations of managing data within an active lab, including labs that are and are not subject to data management requirements from funding agencies.

Instruction in a lab poses unique challenges for librarians. Librarians may be accustomed to working with "a constantly revolving community of students . . . [with] uneven skills in data management."[6] However, participants in the lab may be an even more varied group, often including postdoctoral associates, junior scientists, graduate students, and undergraduate students, in addition to the principal investigator (PI). The unifying feature of this population is that they are focused on the practical activities of research within a specific context.

Studies have shown that in such a diverse setting, social interaction and practical application of skills may facilitate a greater understanding of disciplinary norms and practices.[7] General library workshops, whether a series or a one-shot session, may not be suitable for this audience. In a workshop series, which offers an opportunity for a more thorough discussion of data management issues, retention may prove challenging; the one-shot session, although less of a time commitment for participants, may not explore data management practices in depth.[8] In both cases, discipline-specific issues may not be addressed. Particularly when considering postdoctoral scholars, a group known for their high productivity, research-intensive positions, and heavy workloads,[9] neither a large time commitment nor a general conversation would likely prove appealing.

The sessions described here attempted to emphasize the positive aspects of both the workshop series and the one-shot session, while mitigating for the potential drawbacks. Here, two sessions were customized to focus on the pragmatic aspects of research data management within a specific lab.

In developing these sessions, the focus was not on pedagogy but instead on andragogy: the development of teaching and learning strategies for adults. There are six core assumptions of andragogy, four of which are particularly relevant to data management education in a lab setting: (1) adult learners must understand and acknowledge why it is necessary to learn something before doing so;[10] (2) adults are motivated to learn "those things that they need to know and be able to do in order to cope effectively with their real-life situations;"[11] (3) adult learners are more drawn to experiential learning techniques such as group discussion, problem solving activities, and simulation exercises rather than a didactic approach;[12] and (4) adults have "a deep psychological need to be seen by others and treated by others as being capable of self-direction."[13]

Andragogy has faced criticism for these broad assumptions, as they construct a unified vision of the adult learner that does not recognize the impact of culture,[14] gender,[15] and societal forces[16] in the educational setting. These criticisms are acknowledged. However, this is a well-established model within medical education and seems to align with anecdotal observations of labs. Rather than being a complete theory of education, andragogy provides some general guidance in developing an approach to data management education.

Drawing on these four assumptions, the sessions intentionally focused on the everyday work of the participants, meaning that they were immediately practical. These sessions centered on active learning with the use of activities and group discussion to identify areas of concern and brainstorm possible solutions. The responses and workflows of participants were the focal point of the sessions, positioning those individuals as the experts in their own areas of research and recognizing their ability to identify potential data management challenges.

Setting

The University of Minnesota is ranked in the top ten public research universities in the United States and in the top thirty worldwide. The University has five campuses throughout the state, with the largest being the Twin Cities campus in Minneapolis–St. Paul with approximately three thousand seven hundred full-time faculty and over fifty-one thousand students. Six colleges and schools—the School of Medicine, College of Pharmacy, College of Veterinary Medicine, School of Nursing, School of Public Health, and School of Dentistry—make up the Academic Health Center (AHC). At the time of writing, the AHC included over six thousand graduate and professional students and fifteen hundred full- and part-time faculty members.

The University of Minnesota Libraries have identified a number of strategic initiatives and areas in support of research, including data management and curation. A data repository was launched in early 2015, further enhancing the Libraries' data management education activities, which have been formally underway since 2007. These activities include data management plan consultations, workshops for graduate students, access to the DMPTool, and data management plan templates.

In fall 2014, the Health Sciences Libraries hired both a pharmacy liaison and a research services liaison. The former acts as the liaison to the College of Pharmacy, which includes over ninety full-time faculty members in five departments, all of which have PhD programs. The latter serves to support the needs of researchers across the AHC, including grant funding, scholarly communication, data management, and research impact services. Although this chapter is written from the perspective of the research services liaison, the approach to data management education services described here is a collaboration between these two individuals, both of whom were interested in building relationships with researchers and in providing data management education in a style that would be both practical and palatable in a busy lab setting.

Description of the Service

Identifying Opportunities

To identify researchers, I used the NIH RePORTER tool[17] to find those individuals who had current R01 grants within their first five years of funding. R01 is NIH's most established grant mechanism and is arguably the most prestigious and highly sought after of the NIH awards, with the average R01 grant being over $400,000 per year.[18] R01 recipients were selected not only because of their active research portfolios, but also because I assumed that they would have access to larger labs and would more likely be subject to the NIH data sharing policy, which at the time of writing applies to grants of $500,000 or more annually in direct costs. As the Libraries had established data management education and data sharing services, identifying researchers who would have an opportunity to take advantage of those targeted services was a means of ascertaining current levels of awareness and interest. Through these conversations, I confirmed that data management education for graduate students, postdoctoral associates, and other lab members was an area of interest for many researchers.

Between January and June 2015, I independently and collaboratively taught fourteen data management sessions with approximately one hundred forty-five participants. The initial sessions were relatively traditional in their format, focusing more on the didactic approach and describing general best practices of data management. Often, I gave these sessions in a limited time as a portion of a lab meeting. While there was a positive response from participants, these sessions were generally more informational than practical, and it seemed that there were few immediate and meaningful activities in which labs could engage as a result of the sessions. Due in part to these limitations, I began collaborating with the pharmacy liaison to establish a tailored active-learning approach that combined my knowledge of data management with the liaison's subject expertise and understanding of the college.

Goals and Objectives

The purpose of these sessions was not to provide a comprehensive overview of all aspects of data management. We aimed to be pragmatic, highlighting those areas that would be of most relevance or interest to a particular group, in this case an active lab, and conceptualized these lessons as having three separate topics: documentation and metadata, organization and file names, and storage, including access and intellectual property concerns. This is obviously only a small subset of research data management, a fact that we emphasized to the group at the outset of the sessions.

Ideally, the training would be divided into two fifty-minute sessions. However, scheduling two sessions can be challenging, particularly as it is important for the same group members to attend both. The content can be covered in as little as one ninety-minute session, although two hours is preferable to offer more time for discussion. In the two fifty-minute sessions, Session 1 covered the educational component, while Session 2 focused on the practical. In the single, longer session, the two would be combined, with greater emphasis being placed on one or the other, depending on the needs of the group. For the purposes of this chapter, the two-session format will be described.

While scheduling two sessions can often be influenced by factors beyond a librarian's control, it is best to have the two in relatively quick succession, preferably no more than two weeks apart.

Significant delays may mean that more time in the second session will need to be devoted to reintroducing the concepts discussed in the first session rather than building upon them. Moreover, the enthusiasm that may be generated by a successful initial session may wane over time.

We designed the training to be flexible, recognizing that not every lab will have the same level of data management awareness. For some groups, it may be vital to spend more time on the theoretical content in the first session in order to introduce and practice the core concepts of data management. For others who are more familiar with these topics, emphasis may be on the guided discussion in the first session or the practical components of the second session. My objective in this project was not to establish a lesson plan that I would replicate exactly in multiple labs, but rather to have flexible mini-modules that I could select, expand upon, or limit as necessary.

Structure and Content

SESSION 1: THE EDUCATIONAL COMPONENT

Session 1 introduced participants to core concepts in data management and provided some experience applying these concepts in hypothetical scenarios. By the end of the session, our aim was that participants would be able to (1) define documentation and metadata, (2) recognize errors and omissions within example documentation and organizational schemes, (3) express some of the benefits and drawbacks of storage options, and (4) consider some of these points in the context of their own research.

Although labeled the Educational Component, this was not a purely didactic approach to teaching. Each of the elements within the session—metadata and documentation, file naming and organization, and storage—were introduced very briefly in approximately three to five minutes before moving into the activities. The session moved from brief introduction to the activity to sharing and group discussion of one element before moving on to the next element. While certain parts of the introductions were somewhat generic, such as describing best practices regarding backups, we tailored the content to be more relevant to the group. For example, when discussing documentation in a Medicinal Chemistry lab, the introduction was framed using the FDA's ALCOA standard—attributable, legible, contemporaneous, original, and accurate[19]—to reinforce the importance of these practices within that discipline.

The activities were based on those first developed for the Libraries' data management workshop series for graduate students,[20] which we adjusted for working labs in the health sciences. Participants worked with small amounts of fictitious data with obvious errors to give them the opportunity to practice identifying challenges and applying concepts, which was a useful starting point for discussion as participants did not feel that their own practices were being examined or critiqued. Two to three minutes were spent working on the activity, either in pairs or in small groups, before coming back together as a larger group to share.

In the first activity, metadata and documentation, participants studied a table with incomplete, missing, or inconsistent data. They identified the discrepancies and described what information would be necessary in order to understand this work. The purpose of this activity was not only to emphasize the importance of effectively capturing data for analysis, but also to begin a broader conversation about description throughout the research process and to discuss how methods and decisions can be recorded and transmitted. Discussion questions focused on the importance of documentation for verification and in reuse, either by the individual at a later time, by other members of the lab, or by a broader audience if the data were more widely shared.

In Activity 2, participants worked with a screenshot of a directory structure that included ineffective file naming conventions and poor organization. We asked them to name the elements they felt would be necessary or useful to accurately describe the data and to discuss how those files could be organized. In the introduction prefacing the activity, I emphasized best practices, including the need for files to sort properly and be identifiable even if relocated. The conversation focused on how elements of the data can be reflected in the file names and the importance of shared terminology to assist in identification and retrieval.

In these activities, we referenced both the short-term and long-term utility of best practices, emphasizing the lifespan of data and its potential usefulness even once the initial project has been completed. While we did not discuss issues such as proprietary formats until Session 2, the attempt to extend the participants' understanding of the timespan involved was meant to lay the groundwork for that later conversation.

In the final activity, which focused on storage options, we gave participants a list of some of the different university-provided options for their data, such as local desktop storage, storage on a university server, and cloud storage. We assigned each small group two or three different options and asked them to name some of the benefits and drawbacks of each and if there are any considerations to take into account, such as whether some storage options may not be appropriate for data that must be compliant with the Health Insurance Portability and Accountability Act (HIPAA). Although we did not extensively discuss every aspect of all possible concerns, we asked participants to think about the importance of the data to the overall project, including the uniqueness of the data and how difficult the data would be to recreate, as well as general security concerns. Best practices, such as multiple backup locations including remote backup, were included in the introduction to the activity.

In practice, this topic has generated the most discussion from the groups. The primary theme within the guided discussion is that no one storage option is ideal and that the solutions ultimately chosen should be a result of careful consideration of the specific project and any associated restrictions or limitations. This activity focused on storage locations rather than activities to ensure ongoing access, but a discussion of the frequency of backups primed the group for Session 2's greater emphasis on preservation activities.

SESSION 2: THE PRACTICAL COMPONENT

Unlike Session 1, which focused on discrete activities associated with each of the three elements, we structured Session 2 around a single introductory activity in which participants drew their workflows, followed by a guided discussion. In the more theoretical Educational Component, activities were useful to ground the discussion and apply what may be abstract concepts. However, using the participants' workflows as represented in the flowcharts contextualized these concepts within participants' own daily activities and to raise questions surrounding those activities. Our learning objectives were that the participants would be able to (1) explain how they create, manipulate, use and store data; (2) identify key areas for concern regarding data management concepts within their workflows; and (3) discuss possible strategies to overcome these data management challenges.

At the outset of the session, participants drew their workflows on whiteboards and visualized files, instruments, processes, and other actions. These drawings served as the basis of the discussions to follow. As different lab members performed different actions, this activity produced multiple flowcharts. Individuals engaging in similar activities should work together to produce a single flowchart in order to have a more manageable number of workflows for discussion. The flowchart was an attempt to represent the life cycle of data in a way that is meaningful in the lab setting. The goal is that "[b]y articulating and diagramming the stages of a research project, project personnel can describe and account for the activities that need to take place, when they need to take place, and who will carry out these activities."[21]

We established criteria to identify those areas of the flowchart that may be suitable for discussion. When selecting an area for discussion, we chose those places where participants are actively making decisions, such as points where files from multiple lab personnel are being merged, where multiple individuals are using the same file, or where decisions are made about what information is captured and how to capture it. These criteria would likely be applicable in many lab settings in a variety of disciplines and would be easily identifiable on a flowchart.

The guided discussion incorporated questions from a number of publicly available data management checklists, most notably from the UK Data Archive.[22] While many data management checklists cover similar materials, this resource also has a focus on the active processes of collecting and managing data, including relocating data from one device to another and converting data across formats. The visual representation of the diverse hardware, software, and file formats that may be present throughout multiple workflows introduced an opportunity to discuss long-term access and preservation strategies in a way that was immediately applicable to the participants.

Discussion

Developing and Assessing the Activities

The activities have gone through multiple iterations. They are, in essence, a perpetual work in progress born of our previous instruction experience, as well as the work of colleagues within the institution and elsewhere. One effective strategy is to schedule a debriefing shortly after each session to discuss which activities were more or less effective and why. The purpose of these conversations may not be to permanently change the activity, but rather to note that, within a certain context or with a particular group, an approach was less effective.

One lab provided feedback that they found the discussion portion of Session 1 to be more helpful than the activities. Unfortunately, this feedback was not received until the completion of both sessions. A more immediate feedback mechanism would have allowed for adjustments in Session 2, perhaps with more focus on explicitly returning to points of discussion in the previous session. However, after we reviewed the flow and content, we adjusted the timing of Session 1; previously, the time had been equally split between introduction, activity and group discussion, but we decided to increase the time devoted to group discussion, spending approximately half of the session on group discussion.

We discussed eliminating the Session 1 activities entirely, but felt that they were necessary to provide a baseline of knowledge for participants in the practical application of data management skills. However, this baseline may already be present in certain labs. For those labs that are already familiar with data management best practices, activities may be more briefly touched upon as a refresher to the concepts rather than an introduction. It is particularly helpful to have a sense of the data management needs and level of knowledge of the lab prior to planning the session and a conversation with the PI is essential in establishing this. Questions about standardized practices for backups and file names are a simple way to estimate how formalized or well developed these procedures are within the lab.

A very early version of Session 2 did not include the flowchart activity, but instead was a guided discussion that used the data life cycle as a visual to focus the conversation. The data life cycle, while useful when discussing data management with librarians and some faculty, was not effective in this case. Several participants noted that the life cycle did not seem directly applicable to their daily activities. The life cycle is generalized rather than specific to a project and focuses on the complete life cycle of the data, including long-term issues such as preservation and continued access. As lab personnel may have only a short tenure with that project, an activity and visual focusing on the immediate and practical may be more appropriate.

The flowchart activity itself has gone through iterations. Initially, we did not give participants instructions regarding specific shapes or colors to use in the design. While the flow charts were still a useful discussion point, the lack of consistency posed challenges in terms of quickly scanning to identify points of conversation, even with the established criteria in mind. We developed a more structured activity as a result, including designating particular shapes for processes, files, and instruments to be consistently used in all flowcharts. By prefacing the activity with these instructions, the participants had an opportunity to consider what elements should be included and were reminded that files, processes, and instruments are all important components of the workflow.

Positioning Yourself and Anticipating Challenges

While my intention was to develop data management education that would appeal to labs due to its practical nature, nevertheless these are data management best practices from a librarian's perspective, with consideration of documentation, metadata, storage, access control, intellectual property, and data preservation and sharing. While having some understanding of the research being conducted is essential to effectively identify and discuss data management issues, librarians may not have subject expertise in every discipline with which they would be working. Furthermore, it would not be reasonable to expect that a librarian could develop such in-depth knowledge of a wide variety of disciplines, in addition to expertise in librarianship, in a timely fashion. Thus, one key tenet at the outset of this project was that we would not attempt to emulate the expertise of the lab members, but instead would explicitly bring a complementary but distinct set of skills to the conversation. The objective was to highlight the Libraries' value-added services by emphasizing aspects and best practices of data management that may not have previously occurred to subject experts.

However, practical obstacles exist when speaking with labs about detailed workflows. Without a researcher's level of understanding of the research topic, encountering a flowchart outlining procedures and practices may be intimidating to librarians. One of the most significant challenges for a librarian with this approach is changing the mental model and moving from being an instructor who provides solutions to instead being a colleague who asks and encourages others to ask challenging questions.

Anticipating challenges and potential points of discomfort for the librarian, which will be unique to each individual, is an important component of this process. In the case of a complicated workflow representing in-depth practices unique to a discipline, having well-thought-out questions and discussion points; structuring the flow chart activity with the use of colors, shapes, or symbols to ease identification of elements; and doing some background research, including close listening during the first session, can be a means of lessening these barriers.

Rather than attempting to understand the workflow immediately and in its entirety, librarians should ask participants to briefly summarize their processes. In a sense, this can be approached as a group data management plan consultation in which the librarian leverages his or her expertise to pose questions rather than to produce answers. This is not the transmission of information but rather the collaborative development of that information.

Facilitating the Conversation

The learning objectives of these sessions were intentionally low barrier, echoing Van Tuyl's call for librarians to "drop the baseline"[23] of what we are trying to accomplish in data management education. Often, the goals are very robust and rarely met in practice. Reiterating the need to position the librarian as a colleague in a conversation rather than an instructor transmitting a lesson, the role here is to move the discussion to those places that will be most fruitful for the lab.

Timing may be a challenge in any session that incorporates a large amount of audience participation. Participants have a natural tendency to discuss their own data management practices, and if sessions are to be practical, this should be encouraged. However, the librarian needs to have a mechanism to move the conversation forward, particularly if the group discussion is becoming focused on a smaller subset of the participants rather than something more broadly applicable to the group. A "parking lot" approach, in which ideas and points for further discussion are noted on the whiteboard either in a distinct color or on a sticky note, allows a librarian to both verbally and visually recognize the idea while at the same time indicating the need to proceed in the discussion.

This technique can also be useful at those points in the discussion where discord or disagreement arises. The librarian should be attuned to the tone of the room, particularly in those cases where it appears that there may be tension. If possible, it can be very useful to have a sense of interpersonal dynamics beforehand, especially in those cases where there may be differing levels of authority within the group. Separate conversations with lab members, even as brief and informal interactions, can provide some insight into the culture of the lab.

As participants present their workflows and strategies, multiple techniques and strategies for managing data will likely emerge. Different naming conventions or strategies for organizing files or documenting experiments are all relatively commonplace in a lab. It is essential to consider what is already in place in the lab and to discuss different individual's preferences regarding methods and workflows. While this may lead to disagreements, it is counterproductive to attempt to either resolve every point or move away from those topics without acknowledging the disconnect. The aforementioned "parking lot" approach may be one means of providing recognition. Redirecting the conversation to include other individuals in the room, noting a limited amount of time, and acknowledging the validity of multiple perspectives and workflows may also be useful strategies. The most effective way of addressing conflict will depend on the group, the point of disagreement, and the librarian's comfort in taking control of that conversation.

Humor can be an important element of presentation, particularly when the intention is to have a high level of audience participation. The tone of the room should be informal and the librarian, as the facilitator, is responsible for setting that tone. It can be useful to remember that data management may seem like a dry topic to some, or perhaps could seem overwhelming or burdensome to others. Sharing personal experiences with data management issues—the challenge of finding which file named "data" is the correct file, for example—can create a shared space for open dialogue and minimizes the possibility that participants will feel that their practices are being judged or assessed.

Conclusion

The scalability and long-term impact of this approach have yet to be assessed. Informal feedback has indicated that these sessions seem to lead to changes in practice in a way that was not seen with the more didactic approach. Participants reported implementing file naming conventions and engaging in further conversations as a result of these sessions. More formalized feedback mechanisms may be considered as a means of measuring impact and further refining the content, structure, and delivery of the sessions.

These sessions are continually evolving and their focus can vary greatly depending on the needs of the group. While the incorporation of active learning strategies into data management education may not in itself be novel, this approach introduces new challenges and opportunities for the librarians involved. The objective is to establish a model that is simultaneously a relatively minimal time commitment on the part of the lab members while being highly customized and immediately applicable. This may seem to be contradictory. However, by creating a flexible structure that heavily incorporates audience participation, we have been able to leverage existing expertise in data management and provide a customized experience without necessarily developing in-depth subject knowledge or tailoring every aspect of a standard course.

Pearls

- Participants are adults and should be treated accordingly. Lab members bring a wealth of expertise and experience to the conversation and have likely developed their own strategies to manage data. Acknowledging this and approaching the session as a colleague with distinct but complementary expertise creates an opportunity for and an openness to discussion.

- Use activities strategically. Activities can be a useful way of giving participants an opportunity to develop an understanding of the concepts before moving into their application or as a starting point for discussion. However, they also take time away from introducing those core concepts and engaging in that discussion. As such, they should be used only when they serve a purpose within the flow of the session. If an activity does not consistently meet its intended purpose, revise or discard it.
- Make (reasonable) demands. Confirm that you will be given sufficient time and space and that you either will be provided with or will be able to bring any necessary materials. If split over two sessions, confirm that participants will attend both in their entirety. While flexibility is important, there are basic elements that are necessary for a successful session, and those should not be compromised.
- Lower the barriers to change. Making recommendations can be problematic in that it is ultimately the responsibility of the lab to devote time and energy to implementing those changes. While this cannot be entirely eliminated, emphasizing available tools, such as on-campus storage and bulk renamers, can minimize potential difficulties.
- Structure your discussion. Before entering the lab, have an idea of what the core takeaway messages will be and ask questions that will reinforce those points. Have an assortment of questions and discussion points ready to respond to the flow of conversation rather than attempting to abruptly redirect it.
- Disagreement will happen. When asking individuals about their workflows and practices, it is inevitable that different people will do things differently. There may be cases in which one person feels very strongly about a particular course while another disagrees. Rather than attempting to resolve every point of discord, instead develop strategies to acknowledge those differences and move forward in the discussion.

Recommended Reading and Resources

Crowe, Ruth M., Greta Elysee, Lindsay Jubelt, Armine Lulejian, Martin Pusic, Mark Schwartz, and Marc Triola. 2014. "Healthcare by the Numbers: Populations, Systems, and Clinically Integrated Data." NYU School of Medicine. http://education.med.nyu.edu/ace/

Henkel, Heather, Viv Hutchison, Carly Strasser, Stacy Rebich Hespanha, Kristin Vanderbilt, and Linda Wayne. 2012. "DataONE Education Modules." *DataONE*. https://www.dataone.org/education-modules.

Johnston, Lisa R., and Jon Jeffryes. 2014. "Instructor Guide to the Flipped Data Management Course." University of Minnesota Libraries. http://z.umn.edu/teachdatamgmt.

Lamar Soutter Library, University of Massachusetts Medical School. "New England Collaborative Data Management Curriculum." http://library.umassmed.edu/necdmc.

Acknowledgment

I gratefully acknowledge the contributions of Franklin Sayre, liaison to the College of Pharmacy at the University of Minnesota Twin Cities, with whom the approach described in this chapter was collaboratively developed.

Notes

1. ACRL Research Planning and Review Committee, "Top Ten Trends in Academic Libraries," *College & Research Libraries News* 73, no. 6 (2012): 312; ACRL Research Planning and Review Committee, "Top Trends in Academic Libraries," *College & Research Libraries News* 75, no. 6 (2014): 294.

2. Jake R. Carlson et al., "Determining Data Information Literacy Needs: A Study of Students and Research Faculty," in *Data Information Literacy: Librarians, Data, and the Education of a New Generation of Researchers*, ed. Jake R. Carlson and Lisa R. Johnston (West Lafayette, IN: Purdue University Press, 2015), 12.
3. Birte Christensen-Dalsgaard et al., *Ten Recommendations for Libraries to Get Started with Research Data Management*, 2012, http://libereurope.eu/wp-content/uploads/The%20research%20data%20group%202012%20v7%20final.pdf.
4. Katherine G. Akers, "Going beyond Data Management Planning: Comprehensive Research Data Services," *College & Research Libraries News* 75, no. 8 (September 1, 2014): 435–36, http://crln.acrl.org/content/75/8/435.
5. Katherine G. Akers and Jennifer Doty, "Disciplinary Differences in Faculty Research Data Management Practices and Perspectives," *International Journal of Digital Curation* 8, no. 2 (2013): 14; Andrew Creamer et al., "An Assessment of Needed Competencies to Promote the Data Curation and Management Librarianship of Health Sciences and Science and Technology Librarians in New England," *Journal of eScience Librarianship* 1, no. 1 (2012): 20.
6. Tracy Gabridge, "The Last Mile: Liaison Roles in Curating Science and Engineering Research Data," *Research Library Issues* 265 (2009): 17.
7. Robert A. Campbell, "Preparing the Next Generation of Scientists: The Social Process of Managing Students," *Social Studies of Science* 33, no. 6 (2003): 922–23; John C. Weidman, Darla J. Twale, and Elizabeth Leahy Stein, *Socialization of Graduate and Professional Students in Higher Education: A Perilous Passage?* ASHE-ERIC Higher Education Report, vol. 28 (San Francisco, CA, 2001), http://files.eric.ed.gov/fulltext/ED457710.pdf. 30; David Streatfield, David Allen, and Tom Wilson, "Information Literacy Training for Postgraduate and Postdoctoral Researchers: A National Survey and Its Implications," *Libri* 60, no. 3 (2010): 238.
8. Jake R. Carlson et al., "Developing an Approach for Data Management Education: A Report from the Data Information Literacy Project," *International Journal of Digital Curation* 8, no. 1 (2013): 206.
9. Tina O'Grady and Pauline S. Beam, "Postdoctoral Scholars: A Forgotten Library Constituency?," *Science & Technology Libraries* 30, no. 1 (2011): 76.
10. Malcolm Shepherd Knowles, *The Adult Learner: A Neglected Species*, 3rd ed. (Houston, TX: Gulf Publishing Company, 1984). 55.
11. Ibid. 59.
12. Ibid. 57.
13. Ibid. 56.
14. Donald A. Misch, "Andragogy and Medical Education: Are Medical Students Internally Motivated to Learn?," *Advances in Health Sciences Education* 7, no. 2 (2002): 159; Daniel D. Pratt, "Conceptions of the Self within China and the United States: Contrasting Foundations for Adult Education," *International Journal of Intercultural Relations* 15 (1991): 303.
15. Alan Bleakley, "Gender Matters in Medical Education," *Medical Education* 47, no. 1 (2013):67.
16. Steven A. Schapiro, "From Andragogy to Collaborative Critical Pedagogy: Learning for Academic, Personal, and Social Empowerment in a Distance-Learning Ph.D. Program," *Journal of Transformative Education* 1, no. 2 (2003): 152.
17. National Institutes of Health, "NIH RePORTER," 2015, https://projectreporter.nih.gov/.
18. National Institutes of Health, "National Institutes of Health (NIH) Data Book: Fiscal Year 2013," 2014, http://report.nih.gov/nihdatabook/pdf/NDB_2013_Final.pdf.
19. 21 CFR 11; Stan W. Woollen, "Data Quality and the Origin of ALCOA," *The Compass*, 2010, http://www.southernsqa.org/newsletters/Summer10.DataQuality.pdf.
20. Lisa R. Johnston and Jon Jeffryes, "Steal This Idea: A Library Instructors' Guide to Educating Students in Data Management Skills," *College & Research Libraries News* 75, no. 8 (2014): 431–34; Lisa R. Johnston and Jon Jeffryes, "Instructor Guide to Flipped Data Management Course," University of Minnesota Libraries, 2014, http://z.umn.edu/teachdatamgmt.

21. Jake R. Carlson, "The Use of Life Cycle Models in Developing and Supporting Data Services," in *Research Data Management: Practical Strategies for Information Professionals*, ed. Joyce M. Ray (West Lafayette, IN: Purdue University Press, 2014), 71.
22. "Data Management Checklist," UK Data Archive, accessed May 27, 2015, http://www.data-archive.ac.uk/create-manage/planning-for-sharing/data-management-checklist.
23. Steve Van Tuyl, "Treating Data like Data: Unifying Data Processing Workflows for Datasets in the IR" (presented at the Research Data Access and Preservation Summit, Minneapolis, MN, 2015).

Bibliography

ACRL Research Planning and Review Committee. "Top Ten Trends in Academic Libraries." *College & Research Libraries News* 73, no. 6 (2012): 311–20. http://crln.acrl.org/content/73/6/311.full

———. "Top Trends in Academic Libraries." *College & Research Libraries News* 75, no. 6 (2014): 294–302. http://crln.acrl.org/content/7/6/294.full

Akers, Katherine G. "Going beyond Data Management Planning: Comprehensive Research Data Services." *College & Research Libraries News* 75, no. 8 (September 1, 2014): 435–36. http://crln.acrl.org/content/75/8/435.

Akers, Katherine G., and Jennifer Doty. "Disciplinary Differences in Faculty Research Data Management Practices and Perspectives." *International Journal of Digital Curation* 8, no. 2 (2013): 5–26. doi:10.2218/ijdc.v8i2.263.

Bleakley, Alan. "Gender Matters in Medical Education." *Medical Education* 47, no. 1 (2013): 59–70. doi:10.1111/j.1365-2923.2012.04351.x.

Campbell, Robert A. "Preparing the Next Generation of Scientists: The Social Process of Managing Students." *Social Studies of Science* 33, no. 6 (2003): 897–927. doi:10.1177/0306312703336004.

Carlson, Jake R. "The Use of Life Cycle Models in Developing and Supporting Data Services." In *Research Data Management: Practical Strategies for Information Professionals*, edited by Joyce M. Ray, 63–86. West Lafayette, IN: Purdue University Press, 2014.

Carlson, Jake R., Michael Fosmire, C. C. Miller, and Megan Sapp Nelson. "Determining Data Information Literacy Needs: A Study of Students and Research Faculty." In *Data Information Literacy: Librarians, Data, and the Education of a New Generation of Researchers*, edited by Jake R. Carlson and Lisa R. Johnston, 11–34. West Lafayette, IN: Purdue University Press, 2015.

Carlson, Jake R., Lisa R. Johnston, Brian Westra, and Mason Nichols. "Developing an Approach for Data Management Education: A Report from the Data Information Literacy Project." *International Journal of Digital Curation* 8, no. 1 (2013): 204–17. doi:10.2218/ijdc.v8i1.254.

Christensen-Dalsgaard, Birte, Marc van den Berg, Rob Grim, Wolfram Horstmann, Dafne Jansen, Tom Pollard, and Annikki Roos. *Ten Recommendations for Libraries to Get Started with Research Data Management*, 2012. http://libereurope.eu/wp-content/uploads/The%20research%20data%20group%202012%20v7%20final.pdf .

Creamer, Andrew, Myrna Morales, Javier Crespo, Donna Kafel, and Elaine Martin. "An Assessment of Needed Competencies to Promote the Data Curation and Management Librarianship of Health Sciences and Science and Technology Librarians in New England." *Journal of eScience Librarianship* 1, no. 1 (2012): 18–26. doi:10.7191/jeslib.2012.1006.

Gabridge, Tracy. "The Last Mile: Liaison Roles in Curating Science and Engineering Research Data." *Research Library Issues* 265 (2009): 15–21. http://old.arl.org/bm~doc/rli-265-gabridge.pdf.

Johnston, Lisa R., and Jon Jeffryes. "Instructor Guide to Flipped Data Management Course," University of Minnesota Libraries, 2014. http://z.umn.edu/teachdatamgmt.

———. "Steal This Idea: A Library Instructors' Guide to Educating Students in Data Management Skills." *College & Research Libraries News* 75, no. 8 (2014): 431–34.

Knowles, Malcolm Shepherd. *The Adult Learner: A Neglected Species*. 3rd ed. Houston, TX: Gulf Publishing Company, 1984.

Misch, Donald A. "Andragogy and Medical Education: Are Medical Students Internally Motivated to Learn?" *Advances in Health Sciences Education* 7, no. 2 (2002): 153–60. doi:10.1023/A:1015790318032.

National Institutes of Health. "National Institutes of Health (NIH) Data Book: Fiscal Year 2013," 2014. http://report.nih.gov/nihdatabook/pdf/NDB_2013_Final.pdf.

———. "NIH RePORTER," 2015. https://projectreporter.nih.gov/.

O'Grady, Tina, and Pauline S. Beam. "Postdoctoral Scholars: A Forgotten Library Constituency?" *Science & Technology Libraries* 30, no. 1 (2011): 76–79. doi:10.1080/0194262X.2011.545680.

Pratt, Daniel D. "Conceptions of the Self within China and the United States: Contrasting Foundations for Adult Education." *International Journal of Intercultural Relations* 15 (1991): 285–310.

Schapiro, Steven A. "From Andragogy to Collaborative Critical Pedagogy: Learning for Academic, Personal, and Social Empowerment in a Distance-Learning Ph.D. Program." *Journal of Transformative Education* 1, no. 2 (2003): 150–66. doi:10.1177/1541344603001002008.

Streatfield, David, David Allen, and Tom Wilson. "Information Literacy Training for Postgraduate and Postdoctoral Researchers: A National Survey and Its Implications." *Libri* 60, no. 3 (2010): 230–40. doi:10.1515/libr.2010.020.

UK Data Archive. "Data Management Checklist." Accessed May 27, 2015. http://www.data-archive.ac.uk/create-manage/planning-for-sharing/data-management-checklist.

Van Tuyl, Steve. "Treating Data like Data: Unifying Data Processing Workflows for Datasets in the IR." Presented at Research Data Access and Preservation Summit, Minneapolis, MN, 2015.

Weidman, John C., Darla J. Twale, and Elizabeth Leahy Stein. *Socialization of Graduate and Professional Students in Higher Education: A Perilous Passage?* ASHE-ERIC Higher Education Report. Vol. 28. San Francisco, CA, 2001. http://files.eric.ed.gov/fulltext/ED457710.pdf.

Woollen, Stan W. "Data Quality and the Origin of ALCOA." *The Compass*, 2010. http://www.southernsqa.org/newsletters/Summer10.DataQuality.pdf.

Chapter 15

Demystifying Data Management

DESIGNING SERVICES FOR HOSPITAL-BASED RESEARCHERS

Jeannine Cyr Gluck, Eastern Connecticut Health Network

Research data management (RDM) has received a great deal of attention among health sciences librarians over the past few years. Employment opportunities are often posted to discussion lists, usually for positions in academic health sciences libraries, seeking individuals with specialized skills and experience. Understandably, hospital librarians may gloss over these position announcements with foreign-sounding jargon, considering them to belong to another realm. We should look deeper. Although it may not rise to the level of sophistication commonly found in larger institutions, there is research activity in many hospitals. A librarian who identifies these needs and adapts the practices of academic colleagues will realize benefits to the researchers themselves, the hospital as a whole, and the library. A description of one such program is presented here.

A broad search of the Library, Information Science and Technology Abstracts (LISTA) database using the terms "data management" and "hospital" retrieved only irrelevant articles. Items of potential interest resulted from a search of the Internet via Google using the same terms. The website of Hartford Hospital's research data management program[1] indicates that it is a component of the Research Administration Department, not connected with the library. Boston Children's Hospital and Massachusetts General Hospital have similar offerings, through departments other than the library. All three are large institutions with strong academic affiliations. Similarly, a search of American hospitals listed as users of REDCap,[2] a data management platform, turned up only those affiliated with academic centers, or those for which no evidence of library involvement in RDM could be found.

Springshare's LibGuides, a Web publishing platform for libraries, can function as a discovery tool. Through it, users can locate web pages created by their colleagues in support of learning on a wide variety of topics. The LibGuides site claims over forty-eight hundred libraries as customers.[3] An exploration of the LibGuides Community pages retrieved many RDM sites, virtually all from universities. Those pages contain a great deal of useful information, but no leads to other hospital-based RDM programs.

Not every program of every institution need be represented on the Web, but the dearth of findings indicates that RDM programs in hospitals are very few. In addition, queries to the MEDLIB-L discussion list, with 1,946 subscribers as of this writing, and the more focused HLS list, from the Medical Library Association's Hospital Libraries Section, resulted in questions from interested colleagues, but none reporting on another hospital-based RDM program.

Setting

Eastern Connecticut Health Network (ECHN) is an affiliation of two community hospitals, Manchester Memorial and Rockville General Hospitals. An affiliation with the University of New England College of Osteopathic Medicine (UNECOM) has been in place since 2011 and ECHN has supported a Graduate Medical Education (GME) program for the past two years.

ECHN has a library staffed by one professional librarian and one support staff. The director of the library is involved with the GME program, teaching students and residents about evidence-based medicine and effective search techniques. In addition to the medical and GME staff, the library's primary user groups include the Eastern Connecticut Cancer Institute, the hospital's quality and safety staff, and administrators, department directors, and managers.

Description

The seeds of the RDM project were sown in early 2014 when the director of the library stopped to greet a former employee who had returned to ECHN as the administrator of the Cancer Center. When asked what he was currently working on, he mentioned that the Center would soon hire a research coordinator. The librarian took that opportunity to tell him that some of her colleagues are involved in teaching researchers about managing their data sets. He was happy to hear this. The need for this support had been identified, but no relevant expertise had been found within the hospital. At his suggestion, the librarian spoke to the chair of the Cancer Committee, a pathologist with whom she works on an ongoing basis. After explaining what she could potentially offer, she made it clear that she did not already have the skills for data management, but was willing to learn. The pathologist's response was "You go, girl."

The librarian quickly contacted staff of the Lamar Soutter Library at the University of Massachusetts Medical School. They were very helpful in pointing out the way to gain that knowledge. The librarian was already familiar with their E-Science Portal[4] and *Journal of e-Science Librarianship*,[5] and she learned of two upcoming educational opportunities. The NN/LM would soon offer "Doing It Your Way: Approaches to Research Data Management for Libraries," a one-and-a-half-day workshop on tailoring an RDM program to fit the needs of one's own institution.[6] The Cancer Center agreed to underwrite expenses for travel and lodging to New York. At that workshop, the ECHN librarian was one of very few people not affiliated with a large research university.

She next attended a one-day ACRL seminar entitled "Teaching Research Data Management with the NECDMC." *The New England Collaborative Data Management Curriculum*[7] offered a framework for the teaching of best practices to researchers. Through it, the Lamar Soutter Library, in partnership with several other institutions, offers a wealth of teaching materials, available for use through a Creative Commons license.

Meanwhile, she sought to learn what other pockets of research might exist within the hospital. From the director of Graduate Medical Education, she learned that our residents would now be required to conduct research as part of their curriculum. Her participation was encouraged by the physician leading the research aspect, and by the chair of the Institutional Review Council. ECHN's vice president of nursing also indicated that she hopes to reinstitute the Nursing Research Council in the not-too-distant future.

In order to learn more about the practical aspects of RDM, the librarian enrolled in a five-week class offered through Coursera,[8] a platform for free online university-based classes. It was taught by the faculty of Vanderbilt University, who had developed a tool called REDCap (Research Electronic Data CAPture).[2] Learning to use this program gave her the knowledge of the practical application of RDM best practices that she felt she had been missing.

As she began to plan services to fit the needs of ECHN, she attempted to license REDCap as a platform for data sets, and to provide for an appropriate data repository. REDCap would not agree to license the product to ECHN, as it will accept only universities or nonprofit institutions, and ECHN was about to be acquired by a for-profit hospital network. Competing products were difficult to use, expensive to implement, or both. ECHN was without a real RDM platform, which could better meet researchers' needs for uniformity and de-identification of data, workflow and collaboration, and much more. Excel was the only viable option at the time. Still, the principles of good data management apply to any platform, and could be taught to our researchers.

The initial one-hour presentation to medical trainees was very short, but a good beginning. It began with a lighthearted animation about how to manage data very badly, created by the NYU Health Sciences Library staff.[9] Another animation provided an outline of the most important steps to cover.[10] Attendees indicated on the evaluations that they enjoyed this approach and appreciated the information. Emphasis was on the beginning stages of research, including the creation of simple data management plans, choice of variables, naming conventions, and workflows. Storage, backup, and security issues were covered by a staff member from IT. The librarian briefly explained that those in her profession were considered to have the skill set most applicable to RDM, as reflected in the ARL/NSF report, *To Stand the Test of Time.*[11] The librarian explained why a dedicated RDM platform was not being used, and promised to continue monitoring the possibilities. She pointed them toward Kristen Briney's blog, *Data ab Initio*,[12] and reiterated that once they had completed the beginning stages of their research, a statistician from UNECOM was available to help them with data analysis.

Since each resident would have different needs, the librarian offered to consult with them individually. An RDM page on the library's LibGuides site is being developed, and the librarian e-mails the residents occasionally when she sees information that may be useful to their RDM efforts. This reminds them of the availability of the library's RDM services.

In the first year of the research program, several residents consulted with the librarian. She helped them to locate previous publications on their topics, reviewed one RDM plan, asked the difficult questions about enrolling a sufficient number of subjects, and connected them to the statistician. The chair of the Cancer Center recruited a few of the residents to conduct oncology-related research, thus closing one loop.

Evaluation

The involvement of the ECHN librarian began with the initial year in which a research component was added to the curriculum. As such, no comparison group existed. General evaluations, given by the GME office after all didactic presentations, indicated the timing was not optimal. Although the expectation for research had been discussed with the residents and students, they felt they had not had sufficient opportunities to choose research topics of their own before attending this presentation on data management. They believed they would have gained more if they already had a firm idea for a project to which they could apply this new knowledge. The scheduling will be more carefully considered in the second year. Still, three-quarters of attendees indicated that they did learn something new as a result of the RDM presentation.

Discussion

One of the first steps in developing a program is assessing the need for RDM services in your hospital. There may be several groups who could benefit from RDM services, perhaps more than you realize. A discussion with the chair of the Institutional Review Board is a good place to begin. Many training programs, including those affiliated with the Accreditation Council for Graduate Medical Education[13] or American Osteopathic Association[14] require or strongly encourage research. The American Nurses Credentialing Center Magnet Recognition Program[15] includes research in its New Knowledge, Innovation and Improvements Component. Cancer centers wishing to earn or retain accreditation through the American College of Surgeons Commission on Cancer now must be involved in research.[16] Employees furthering their education, especially at the graduate level, often must conduct research as part of their curriculum—for example, physical therapists returning to school to earn the DPT degree.[17]

In her MLA webinar *Research versus research: Sometimes the Little r Is All You Need*,[18] Heather Holmes distinguishes between two types. ("Capital R") Research, is a "systematic investigation, including research development, testing and evaluation, designed to develop or contribute to generalizable knowledge." It is more formalized and may be grant-funded. Conversely, ("little r") research, such as a quality improvement investigation, primarily benefits an individual institution. Physicians participating in the ABMS Maintenance of Certification Part 4 must complete a performance improvement activity.[19] Several data-related elements are among those listed in an ABMS blog post, "Quality Thoughts: The Anatomy of a Good Quality Improvement Effort."[20] Some within the hospital may indeed be involved in "capital R" Research, as part of a multi-institution clinical trial, with uniform procedures for all participants worked out by the principal investigator or the primary research site.

At the outset, it is important to ensure that those in charge of the various pockets of research activity understand the contribution the librarian can make. James L. Mullins, relating his own experience at Purdue, writes, "It would fall to me to explain the principles of identification and organization of information; that, traditionally, it had been tangible items, such as books and print journals, but the same principles of cataloging or assigning metadata applied to nontangible data. Using terms such as 'metadata' seemed to resonate with the researchers rather than 'cataloging' of the data. Quite often the researcher would have an 'aha' moment when realizing that librarians were the specialists for whom they had been searching after expecting that computer scientists and information technologists would be their salvation."[21] These words apply equally to research done in any setting.

Be assured that taking on the teaching of best practices in data management in a hospital setting is a worthwhile investment of time and effort, and represents a gain to the employer. As with other endeavors, disorganization wastes a great deal of time. Staff conducting research on behalf of the institution are expected to use their time as wisely as possible. Those working on their own time, such as the staff returning to school, will appreciate the support and guidance they receive, thus increasing employee satisfaction. For example, teaching the nursing staff or a cancer center's personnel to better manage data will help ensure continued accreditation status.

Hospital librarians cannot rely on the usual sources to discover learning opportunities, as most of the activity is outside their own circles. In the case described here, the librarian might never have known of valuable educational activities, as they were primarily sponsored through the Association of College and Research Libraries. Some events came to her attention only because she reached out to staff at the Lamar Soutter Library at UMass. Consider all available sources of learning—reading, websites, workshops, online courses, and personal contacts. The books, journals, and websites mentioned in the resources list, below, are just a small sampling of those available, and they will lead you to other resources. Talk to the people you meet through these channels, pick their brains, and network.

Hospital librarians should adapt the best practices of the academics to their own setting. The basics are not so different: Brian Westra reported on the results of an RDM needs assessment at the University of Oregon:

> The most common issues to be identified were the lack of file organization, insufficient storage and backup procedures, and insubstantial and highly variable documentation/metadata that negatively impacted the primary investigator's ability to later find and retrieve data. These challenges in local practice also were reflective of gaps in infrastructure, data management tools, and the absence or lack of adoption of best practices—all issues that have been identified at other institutions. Concerns about data sharing and preservation were subsumed by these issues that more directly impact organizational issues.[22]

If even investigators in academia are most in need of the basics of RDM, we can assume that teaching these same principles to hospital-based researchers will go a long way.

Educating our users in the best practices related to this subset of issues is fairly straightforward. It is an unfortunate reality that only a very limited amount of time will likely be provided for that teaching. To maximize its use, present an overview of the basics and offer yourself as consultant.

Roadblocks will probably emerge as situations change, as when we learned we cannot license REDCap at this time. Be flexible and find routes around the obstacles.

Conclusion

First and foremost, this project demonstrates the benefits that can be realized by speaking up and being willing to stretch outside of one's comfort zone. It also provides an example of the repurposing of librarians' skills to work that is crucial to the hospital. Data management programs have the potential to positively impact the educational mission, (re)accreditation efforts, time management, and staff satisfaction.

A research data management program in a hospital cannot and need not be as sophisticated as those offered in research institutions. Levels of both the research being conducted and the resources available differ substantially. Learn from our colleagues in academia, and adapt their best practices to create a program appropriate to your own setting.

Pearls

- Determine all the groups in your institution who could benefit from learning about research data management. There may be more demand than you realize.
- Be prepared to educate others on why a librarian is uniquely positioned to teach data management.
- Adapt practices of academic and research libraries to fit the needs of your own institution.
- Even in a short session in which to introduce data management, you can teach the basics and offer one-on-one consults.

Recommended Reading and Resources

Briney, Kristin. *Data ab Initio.* Accessed June 7, 2015. http://dataabinitio.com/.

———. *Data Management for Researchers: Organize, maintain and share your data for research success.* Exeter, UK: Pelagic Publishing, 2015.

Lamar Soutter Library, University of Massachusetts Medical School. *Journal of eScience Librarianship.* Accessed April 1, 2015. http://escholarship.umassmed.edu/jeslib/.

———. *New England Collaborative Data Management Curriculum.* Accessed April 1, 2015. http://library.umassmed.edu/necdmc.

NYU Health Sciences Library. *Data Sharing and Management Snafu in 3 Short Acts.* Accessed April 1, 2015. https://www.youtube.com/watch?v=N2zK3sAtr-4.

———. *How to Avoid a Data Management Nightmare.* Accessed April 1, 2015. https://www.youtube.com/watch?v=nNBiCcBlwRA.

Ray, Joyce M., ed. *Research Data Management: Practical Strategies for Information Professionals* (Charleston Insights in Library, Archival and Information Sciences). West Lafayette, IN: Purdue University Press, 2014.

Notes

1. Hartford Hospital, Clinical Research Center, accessed June 29, 2015, www.harthosp.org/research/CRC/default.aspx.

2. Vanderbilt University, *Project REDCap: Research Electronic Data Capture*, accessed April 1, 2015, http://www.projectredcap.org/.
3. LibGuides Community, accessed June 7, 2015, http://libguides.com/community.php.
4. Lamar Soutter Library, University of Massachusetts Medical School, E-science portal for New England Librarians, Sep 22, 2014, accessed June 29, 2015, http://esciencelibrary.umassmed.edu/.
5. Lamar Soutter Library, University of Massachusetts Medical School, *Journal of eScience Librarianship*, accessed April 1, 2015, http://escholarship.umassmed.edu/jeslib/.
6. National Network of Libraries of Medicine, New England Region, "Highlights of: Network of Libraries of Medicine Symposium: Doing It Your Way: Approaches to Research Data Management for Libraries." *NEReastah: Newsletter of the New England Regional Medical Library*, August 13, 2014, https://nnlm.gov/ner/blog/2014/08/13/.
7. Lamar Soutter Library, University of Massachusetts Medical School, *New England Collaborative Data Management Curriculum*, accessed April 1, 2015, http://library.umassmed.edu/necdmc.
8. Vanderbilt University, *Data Management for Clinical Research*, June 2–July 23, 2014, https://www.coursera.org/course/datamanagement.
9. NYU Health Sciences Library. *Data Sharing and Management Snafu in 3 Short Acts*, accessed April 1, 2015, https://www.youtube.com/watch?v=N2zK3sAtr-4.
10. NYU Health Sciences Library, *How to Avoid a Data Management Nightmare*, accessed April 1, 2015, https://www.youtube.com/watch?v=nNBiCcBlwRA.
11. Association of Research Libraries, *To Stand the Test of Time: Long-Term Stewardship of Data Sets in Science and Engineering. A Report of the ARL/NSF Workshop on Long-Term Stewardship of Digital Data Collections, September 26–27, 2006*. (Washington, DC: Association of Research Libraries, 2006), accessed June 24, 2015, http://files.eric.ed.gov/fulltext/ED528649.pdf.
12. Kristin Briney, *Data ab Initio* (blog), accessed June 7, 2015, http://dataabinitio.com/.
13. Accreditation Council for Graduate Medical Education, accessed June 29, 2015, http://www.acgme.org/acgmeweb/.
14. American Osteopathic Association, Commission on Osteopathic College Accreditation, *The Basic Documents for Postdoctoral Training*, July 1, 2014, http://www.osteopathic.org/inside-aoa/accreditation/opti-approval/Pages/default.aspx.
15. American Nurses Credentialing Center, *2014 Magnet Application Manual* (Silver Spring, MD: ANCC, 2013).
16. American College of Surgeons, Commission on Cancer, *Cancer Program Standards 2012*, accessed June 29, 2015, https://www.facs.org/quality-programs/cancer/coc/standards.
17. Commission on Accreditation in Physical Therapy Education, *Evaluative Criteria PT Programs* (Alexandria, VA: American Physical Therapy Association, 2014), accessed June 22, 2015, http://www.capteonline.org/AccreditationHandbook/.
18. Heather N. Holmes, *Research versus research: Sometimes the Little r Is All You Need.* (recorded webinar) (Chicago, IL: Medical Library Association, 2014), accessed October 5, 2015, https://www.mlanet.org/event/research-versus-research-sometimes-little-r-all-you-need-webinar.
19. American Board of Medical Specialties, *Assessed through a Four-Part Framework*, accessed June 24, 2015, http://www.abms.org/board-certification/a-trusted-credential/assessed-through-a-four-part-framework/.
20. Paul V. Miles, "Quality Thoughts: The Anatomy of a Good Quality Improvement Effort," *American Board of Medical Specialties Multispecialty Portfolio Approval Program*, May 14, 2014, accessed June 24, 2015, http://mocportfolioprogram.org/20140514/.
21. James L. Mullins, "The Policy and Institutional Framework," in *Research Data Management: Practical Strategies for Information Professionals*, ed. Joyce M. Ray (West Lafayette, IN: Purdue University Press, 2014), 37.

22. Brian Westra, "Developing Data Management Services for Researchers at the University of Oregon," in *Research Data Management: Practical Strategies for Information Professionals*, ed. Joyce M. Ray (West Lafayette, IN: Purdue University Press, 2014), 380.

Bibliography

Accreditation Council for Graduate Medical Education. http://www.acgme.org/acgmeweb/. Accessed June 29, 2015.

American Board of Medical Specialties. *Assessed through a Four-Part Framework.* http://www.abms.org/board-certification/a-trusted-credential/assessed-through-a-four-part-framework/. Accessed June 24, 2015.

American College of Surgeons. Commission on Cancer. *Cancer Program Standards 2012*. Accessed June 29, 2015. https://www.facs.org/quality-programs/cancer/coc/standards.

American Nurses Credentialing Center. *2014 Magnet Application Manual*. Silver Spring, MD: ANCC, 2013.

American Osteopathic Association. Commission on Osteopathic College Accreditation. *The Basic Documents for Postdoctoral Training*. July 1, 2014. http://www.osteopathic.org/inside-aoa/accreditation/opti-approval/Pages/default.aspx.

Association of Research Libraries. *To Stand the Test of Time: Long-Term Stewardship of Data Sets in Science and Engineering. A Report of the ARL/NSF Workshop on Long-Term Stewardship of Digital Data Collections, September 26–27, 2006*. Washington, DC: Association of Research Libraries, 2006. Accessed June 24, 2015. http://files.eric.ed.gov/fulltext/ED528649.pdf

Briney, Kristin. *Data ab Initio* (blog). Accessed June 7, 2015. http://dataabinitio.com/.

Commission on Accreditation in Physical Therapy Education. *Evaluative Criteria PT Programs*. Alexandria, VA: American Physical Therapy Association, 2014. Accessed June 22, 2015. http://www.capteonline.org/AccreditationHandbook/.

Hartford Hospital. Clinical Research Center. 2014. Accessed June 29, 2015. www.harthosp.org/research/CRC/default.aspx.

Holmes, Heather N. *Research versus research: Sometimes the Little r is All You Need.* (recorded webinar) Chicago, IL: Medical Library Association, 2014. Accessed October 5, 2015. https://www.mlanet.org/event/research-versus-research-sometimes-little-r-all-you-need-webinar.

Lamar Soutter Library, University of Massachusetts Medical School. E-science portal for New England Librarians, September 22, 2014. Accessed June 29, 2015. http://esciencelibrary.umassmed.edu/.

———. *Journal of eScience Librarianship*. Accessed April 1, 2015. http://escholarship.umassmed.edu/jeslib/.

———. *New England Collaborative Data Management Curriculum.* Accessed April 1, 2015. http://library.umassmed.edu/necdmc.

LibGuides Community. Accessed June 7, 2015. http://libguides.com/community.php.

Miles, Paul V. "Quality Thoughts: The Anatomy of a Good Quality Improvement Effort." *American Board of Medical Specialties Multispecialty Portfolio Approval Program*. May 14, 2014. Accessed June 24, 2015. http://mocportfolioprogram.org/20140514/.

Mullins, James L. "The Policy and Institutional Framework." In *Research Data Management: Practical Strategies for Information Professionals*, edited by Joyce M. Ray, 25–44. West Lafayette, IN: Purdue University Press, 2014.

National Network of Libraries of Medicine, New England Region. "Highlights of: Network of Libraries of Medicine Symposium: Doing It Your Way: Approaches to Research Data Management for Libraries." *NEReastah: Newsletter of the New England Regional Medical Library*, August 13, 2014. https://nnlm.gov/ner/blog/2014/08/13/.

NYU Health Sciences Library. *Data Sharing and Management Snafu in 3 Short Acts.* Accessed April 1, 2015. https://www.youtube.com/watch?v=N2zK3sAtr-4.

———. *How to Avoid a Data Management Nightmare.* Accessed April 1, 2015. https://www.youtube.com/watch?v=nNBiCcBlwRA.

Vanderbilt University. *Data Management for Clinical Research.* June 2–July 23, 2014. https://www.coursera.org/course/datamanagement.

———. *Project REDCap: Research Electronic Data Capture.* Accessed April 1, 2015. http://www.projectredcap.org/.

Westra, Brian. "Developing Data Management Services for Researchers at the University of Oregon." In *Research Data Management: Practical Strategies for Information Professionals*, edited by Joyce M. Ray, 375–91. West Lafayette, IN: Purdue University Press, 2014.

Index

Page references for figures are italicized.

academic library, medium-sized. *See* Rutgers University
academic medical centers. *See* NYU Health Sciences Library
ACC (Animal Care Committee), 117
Accidental Data Scientist (Affelt), 86
ACRL (Association of College and Research Libraries), 82, 84, 85, 203, 216
ADC Working Group on the Future of the NLM, 8
Affelt, Amy, 86
ALA (American Library Association), 83
American Association of Colleges of Nursing, 176
Annals of Oncology, 58
Applied Informatics, 54
archives, 31–39; archival theory, 34–39; terminology, 31–34. *See also* data preservation
ARL (Association of Research Libraries), 84, 187–88
ASIS&T, 86

BD2K (Big Data to Knowledge) initiative, 1, 5–8, 189
Beall, Jeffrey, 54
Beniger, James, 141
"big data," 70–71, 123–26
BioCaddie, 5
BioMed Central, 54, 55, 56, 57, 60
Biomedical Data Journal, 53, 54, 56, 57, 61
BitBucket, 57
bit rot, 20–22
BMC (BioMed Central), 53
BMC Research Notes, 57
BMJ (British Medical Journal), 58
Borgman, Christine, 79
Bourne, Philip, 5, 7
Briney, Kristin, 217
Brockett, Ralph G., 81

California Digital Library, 83, 98
Carlson, Jacob, 99, 101, 102, 112, 173
Carnegie Mellon University Libraries, 116, 157–58, *158*
Cell Press, 58
Chiropractic and Manual Therapies, 54
Clardy, Alan, 81, 83
cloud computing and storage, 20–22, 129, 179
Code Academy, 76
Collins, Francis, 3
Commons, 7–8
computational science *vs.* data science, 69–70
consultations, 99–100, 102, 112, 145–46, 159
continuing education, 82–83, 110–11
Cornell University, 83
Council of Education in Public Health, 176
courses and curricula, 82–83; Code Academy, 76; Coursera (learning platform), 76, 86, 216; Curating and Managing Research Data for Re-use (workshop), 82; Data Carpentry (online course), 76; DataONE Curriculum, 82; Data Scientist Training for Librarians, 111; DigCCurr (Digital Curation Curriculum), 39; EarthCube Summer Institute for Technology Exploration, 165; e-Science Symposium, 82; Library Juice Academy, 83; Lynda (learning platform), 86; MANTRA data management curriculum, 82; MLA CE classes, 191–92; MOOC (Massive Online Open Courses), 7; NECDMC (New England Collaborative Data Management Curriculum), 82, 112, 216; Research Data Access and Preservation conference, 84, 86; Udacity (learning platform), 86; Virginia Data Management Boot Camp, 174
CTSI (Clinical and Translational Science Institute), 100, 101, 188, 194–95, 199
Curating and Managing Research Data for Re-use (workshop), 82

DART project, 100
data analysis, 22–23, 73, 92, 115, 161–62. *See also* visualization of data
Data Carpentry (online course), 76
data citation, 112
data collection, 16–17, *17*, 92, 160–61, 179, 191
data curation, 74, 82, 83, 100, 125, 130–31
Data Curation Profile Toolkit, 99, 112

data destruction, 179-80
Data in Brief, 53, 54, 55, 56, 57, 58, 61
Data Information Literacy Project, 83, 173-77
data interviews, 59, 112, 179, 187, 195-99
Data (journal), 53, 54, 57
data journals, 49-67; features, 53-58; librarian's role, 59-61; lists, 50-53. *See also* data repositories; data sharing
data life cycle, 14, *15*, 35, 91-93, 157, *158*, 208
data loss, 13, 20-22
Data Management Snafu video, 189, 199, 217
DataONE, 14-15, *15*, 82
data papers. *See* data journals
data preservation, 20-22, 91-92; backup, 20-22, 207, 208, 218; storage, 112, 116, 127, 129, 179-80, 198, 207. *See also* archives
data quality, 18, 36, 161
data repositories, 71, 100, 111, 115, 125, 128; in academic libraries, 155-56, 163-64, 190; archives, 37-38. *See also* data journals; data sharing
data retention, 5, 179-80
data science, 69-75; computation and analysis, 69-75; courses and curricula, 76, 81-86; defined, 86; as discipline, 2, 5; ingestion, 72; modeling and application, 69-75; pipeline, 71; reporting and visualization, 69-75; tools, 69-75
Data Scientist Training for Librarians, 111
data security, 116
Dataset Papers in Science, 53, 54, 55, 56, 57
datasets, 18-23, 71-75, 110-12, 114-16, 193-97. *See also* data journals
data sharing, 1-8, 38-39, 75, 92, 163-64, 189-90. *See also* data journals; data repositories
Dataverse, 56
dbGAP (Database of Genotypes and Phenotypes), 3
DigCCurr (Digital Curation Curriculum), 39
digital curation, 31
Digital Media Commons, 143, 144, 146
DigitalPreservationEurope project, 37-38
discovery tools, 5-6, 194-95
DIWG (Data and Informatics Working Group, 3-6
DMCI (Data Management and Curation Institute), 125-26
DMP (data management plans), 84, 91-92, 94-104, 109; approaches, 101-4; defined, 95-97; librarian's role, 97-101; training, 159. *See also* DMPTool
DMP reviews, 100, 102
DMPTool, 83-84, 98-99, 101-2, 174, 178. *See also* data management plans
DOAJ (Directory of Open Access Journals), 54
Doing Data Science (O'Neil and Schutt), 86
Dutch SURFshare project, 36

EarthCube Summer Institute for Technology Exploration, 165
Eastern Connecticut Health Network, 216
electronic lab notebooks, 160-61
embedded librarians, 113
Erdman, Christopher, 111
e-Science, 69-70, 82

file organization and management, 18-23, 55-59, 145, 159-160, 206-10
Florent van Langren, Michael, 140, *141*
F1000 Posters, 54
F1000 Research, 54, 55-56, 57
Fourth Paradigm (Gray), 69
Froemke, Robert, 192-94, 198
Frontiers journals, 54, 56, 57

Galvin, James, 192-94
Garrison's Model of self-directed learning, 81
Garritano, Jeremy R., 99
Genomic Medicine, 54
Genomics Data, 53, 54, 56, 57
GigaDB, 56, 61
GigaScience, 53, 56, 57, 61, 190
Gold, Anna, 80
Gray, Jim, 69
Green, Eric, 5

Halley, Edmund, *140*
Han, Nathan, 69
Hanson, Karen, 188-89
Health and Justice, 54
Henderson, Margaret E., 110
Hiemstra, Roger, 81
Holmes, Heather, 218
hospitals, 215-19

ICPSR (Inter-university Consortium for Political and Social Research), 82
IMLS (Institute of Museum and Library Services), 83, 84, 100
Information Entropy, *19*
Institute for Quantitative Social Sciences (Harvard University), 56
IRB (Institutional Review Board), 117, 176, 177-80, 217

James Madison University, 98, 156, 172-80; IRB (Institutional Review Board), 176, 177-80; liaison librarians, 173-75; research, 175-77

Johns Hopkins University, 178
Johnston, Lisa R., 97, 100, 102, 103, 112
Journal of eScience Librarianship, 216

Knott, Theresa L., 110
Knowles, Malcolm, 80

laboratories, 197-98, 203-11; description of RDM services, 205-8; discussion, 208-10
Lamar Soutter Library. *See* University of Massachusetts
Lamb, Ian, 188
Lancet, 58
Larson, Catherine, 188
learning, self-directed, 80-83, 147-48
librarian's skillset, 1-2, 8-9, 79, 130-31, 164-65
library infrastructure, 123-34; "big data," 123-25; researcher needs, 125-27; sustainability, 127-134
Library Juice Academy, 83
library sizes and types, 152-53
lifecycle models, 91-92
Lynda (learning platform), 86

Maher, William J., 35
Manovich, Lev, 139-40
MANTRA data management curriculum, 82
mapping tools, 162-63
McLure, Merinda, 99
Medical Library Assistance Act, 7
metadata, 5, 18-20, 35, 37, 113, 195-96, 206
MLA (Medical Library Association), 82, 85, 191, 218
Mocker, Donald W., 80
MOOC (Massive Online Open Courses), 7, 86
Mullins, James L, 218
munging and wrangling of data, 72-73

Nature journals, 18, 57
NCBI (National Center for Biotechnology Information), 71
NDAR (National Autism Research Database), 3
NECDMC (New England Collaborative Data Management Curriculum), 82
Neuroinformatics, 53, 54, 56, 57
New York University Health Sciences Library, 187-200, 217; data catalog, 194-96; education, 188-92; Lab Organization Tool, 197-98; NLM Informationist Supplements, 192-94; RDM needs of researchers, 187, 196-97
NIH (National Institutes of Health), 2, 3-9, 96; Common Fund, 5; Data Management Requirements, 190; Data Sharing Repositories website, 190; Genomic Data Sharing Policy, 96, 98, 190; grants, 91, 151; Open Access Policy, 103; Public Access Policy, 79; RePORTER tool, 205
NLM (National Library of Medicine), 7-8, 192-94
NSF (National Science Foundation), 1-2, 79, 83, 96, 110, 171

Office of Research and/or Sponsored Programs, 116-17
Office of Technology Management/Intellectual Property/Business Development, 117
O'Neil, Cathy, 86
Open Health Data, 53, 54, 56, 57, 61
OpenScienceLink, 56
OSTP (US Office of Science and Technology Policy), 1, 79, 96, 103, 110

partners, campus, 116-17, 146-47, 165
peer review, 57-58, 60
PHI (protected health information), 56-57, 60
Pinfield, S., 99
PLoS (Public Library of Science), 49, 53, 54, 55, 57, 189
policies, 1-2, 79-81, 91-92, 96-98, 114, 131-33
poor RDM, 13-23; analysis phase, 22-23; data collection stage, 16-17; documentation phase, 18-20; planning stage, 14-15; preservation phase, 20-22; quality assurance phase, 17-18
PPC (Person Process Context) model, 81
predatory journals, 54
PRO (Personal Responsibility Orientation) model, 81
Purdue University, 83, 99, 115, 173, 218

Raboin, Regina, 110
Rambo, Neil, 188
RDA (Research Data Alliance), 86
RDM needs of researchers, 6-7, 93, 124-31, 133-34, 151-52, 164-67, 217
RDM policy, 79-80, 131-33
RDM services beyond DMP, 109-18; collaborative, 114-18; internal preparation, 110-11; offered by librarians, 111-14
Read, Kevin, 188-190, 199
REDCap, 193, 198, 215, 216
Research Data Access and Preservation conference, 84, 86
retractions of articles, 13, 18
Robyn, Dorothy, 141
Roche, Ellen, 178
roles for librarians, 59-61, 74-75, 97-98; in data management, 6-7; RDM plans, 97-104; In visualization, 143-47
R (programming language), 22, 76, 144
Rutgers University, 155-67, *158*; discussion, 164-67; services, 157-64; setting, 156-57

Sage Publications, 58
Salo, Dorothea, 80
scalability. *See* library infrastructure
Schellenberg, T.R., 39
scholarly communication, 2
Scholarship in the Digital Age (Borgman), 79
Science (journal), 58
Scientific Data, 53, 54, 55, 56, 57, 61, 190
self-directed learning, 79-86, 165
Skirball Institute of Biomolecular Medicine, 190
SLA (Special Libraries Association), 83, 84, 85
Snow, John, 140-41
social media, 84
SourceForge, 57
Spear, George E., 80
spreadsheets, 16-7, *17*, 21
Springer Open, 53, 54, 55, 57, 60
staffing, 103, 117-18, 151
Strategic Agenda for Research Data Services, 110
Surkis, Alisa, 188-89
sustainability, 127-34
Svirsky, Mario, 192
SWOT analysis, 187

Tenopir, Carol, 110
To Stand the Test of Time (ARL/NSF), 217
Tough, Allan, 80
training for librarians, 7-9, 165, 190-92
Tufte, Edward, 139, 141
Tufts University, 156

UCSF (University of California at San Francisco), 195
Udacity (learning platform), 86
UK Data Archive, 208
undergraduates. *See* James Madison University
University of Massachusetts Medical School, 59, 82, 156, 216, 218
University of Michigan, 82, 99, 101, 143-48
University of Minnesota, 83, 97, 100, 125-33, 204-11. *See also* laboratories
University of North Carolina, Chapel Hill, 39
University of Oregon, 99, 100, 102, 218
University of Pittsburgh, 97-102, 116
University of Rochester, 60
University of Wisconsin, 156

VCU (Virginia Commonwealth University), 98-99
version control, 22-23
Virginia Data Management Boot Camp, 174
visualization of data, 18, 86, 115-16, 139-48, *140*, *141*; context, 139-41; librarian's role, 142-47. *See also* data analysis
volume, velocity, variety, 70, 124
VO SDLP (vocationally oriented SDL projects), 81, 83

WebCite, 55
Web of Science, 54
Westra, Brian, 110, 218
Worcester Polytechnic Institute, 59

About the Authors

Katherine G. Akers, PhD, is a biomedical research and data specialist in the Shiffman Medical Library at Wayne State University in Detroit, Michigan. In her current position, Katherine provides support for research data management and sharing, scholarly publishing, compliance with funding agency policies, and systematic reviews. Katherine was originally trained as a researcher in behavioral neuroscience focused on studying the connections between the brain and behavior. She started her career in libraries through Council on Library and Information Resources (CLIR) postdoctoral fellowships at Emory University Libraries and the University of Michigan Library.

Caitlin Bakker is the biomedical/research services liaison at the University of Minnesota, Twin Cities. Her focus is on developing and providing research support services for faculty in the Academic Health Center, including data management, scholarly communication, and research impact assessment. Previously, she held positions at the University of Northern British Columbia and Wilfrid Laurier University.

Marci Brandenburg is the bioinformationist at the University of Michigan's Taubman Health Sciences Library. She works closely with the Department of Computational Medicine and Bioinformatics and the Bioinformatics Core, in addition to supporting other bioinformatics research on campus. In addition to offering instruction on a variety of visualization tools, she helps with tool documentation and coordinates a weekly Tools and Technology seminar. Before coming to the University of Michigan in November 2010, she was the biosciences informationist at the National Cancer Institute–Frederick. In addition to getting an MS in biology from Ohio University and an MSI from the University of Michigan, Marci has worked for the National Wildlife Federation, the USDA Wildlife Services, and as a lab technician at the University of Michigan's Medical School.

Steven Braun is the data analytics and visualization specialist in the Northeastern University Libraries (Boston), providing support to students, faculty, and staff engaged in digital scholarship across all disciplines. Prior to joining Northeastern, Steven served as the informatics specialist in the University of Minnesota Libraries, where he was actively involved in data management and curation efforts. Steven has a background in biophysics (MS, Yale University, 2013) as well as chemistry and Asian studies (BA, St. Olaf College, 2011), and he sustains highly interdisciplinary interests in his work and research.

Kristin Briney, PhD, is the data services librarian at the University of Wisconsin–Milwaukee, where she advises researchers on data management plans and data best practices. She has a PhD in chemistry and a master's degree in library and information studies. Kristin is the author of the book *Data Management for Researchers* and blogs about how to manage research data at http://www.dataabinitio.com.

Christopher Eaker is data curation librarian at the University of Tennessee, Knoxville (UTK), Libraries. He is interested in scientific data curation and in integrating sound data stewardship skills into science and engineering curricula. Christopher helps UTK's researchers navigate federal requirements for data management and sharing and educates researchers in the skills needed to manage data well. He holds a bachelor's degree in civil engineering from Georgia Institute of Technology and a master's degree in information science from UTK.

Lisa Federer is research data informationist at the National Institutes of Health (NIH) Library, where she provides training and support in the management, organization, and reuse of biomedical research data for researchers in the NIH's Intramural Research Program. She received her master's of library and information studies from the University of California, Los Angeles in 2011 and also holds an MA in English. She has also completed graduate certifications in data visualization from New York University and data science from Georgetown University.

Valerie Florance, PhD, is an associate director of the National Library of Medicine, NIH. There, she directs the Extramural Programs Division, which has overall responsibility for NLM's research and resource grant programs in biomedical informatics and information sciences, and for NLM's highly regarded university-based informatics training program. Before coming to NLM in February 2001, she spent three years as project director for *better_health @ here.now*, a visioning project undertaken at the Association of American Medical Colleges (AAMC) to help the association's members understand the power of computers and networks for managing health information. She has graduate degrees in medical anthropology and library and information sciences, and was elected to the American College of Medical Informatics in 2005.

Bonnie L. Fong is the physical sciences librarian and head of Emerging Technologies at the John Cotton Dana Library on the Rutgers University-Newark campus. She teaches information literacy and data management skills, provides reference service, performs collection management, organizes graduate student workshops, and oversees technology in the library. Her research focuses on the needs of graduate students—especially those in the sciences.

Jeannine Cyr Gluck, AHIP, is the director of the library at Eastern Connecticut Health Network. She works closely with the Graduate Medical Education program, presenting to the students and residents on the many ways that the library can support their research projects. She has also worked extensively with the Cancer Committee for many years.

Abigail Goben is an information services and liaison librarian at the University of Illinois at Chicago Library of the Health Sciences. She is liaison to the College of Dentistry and collaborates with health science researchers on research data management. Her research focuses on institutional data policy, self-education in research data management, and open access. She blogs at http://www.hedgehog librarian.com.

Carrie L. Iwema, PhD, AHIP, is an information specialist in molecular biology for the Health Sciences Library System, University of Pittsburgh. She provides bioinformatics support and training for researchers, is a member of the Data Management Services group, coordinates a workshop series for postdocs, and teaches workshops and webinars on personal genomics and precision medicine. Prior to her library degree, Carrie earned a PhD in Neuroscience.

Justin Joque, PhD, is the visualization librarian at the University of Michigan. There he assists users in finding, manipulating, analyzing, and visualizing diverse types of data. Before becoming the visualization librarian, Justin was a spatial and numeric data librarian, also at the University of Michigan. He completed a master's of science of information at the University of Michigan, School of Information with a focus on information analysis and retrieval and his PhD in communications at the European Graduate School.

Andrea M. Ketchum, AHIP, is a reference librarian at the Health Sciences Library System, University of Pittsburgh, where she is lead librarian for scholarly communication as well as a member of the

Systematic Review Workshop faculty and Data Management Services group. She is currently serving a three-year term on the MLA Scholarly Communications Committee, and is cochair of the MLA Ad Hoc Committee to Review Core Clinical Journals.

Bethany Myers, AHIP, is a research informationist at the Louise M. Darling Biomedical Library at the University of California, Los Angeles. She serves as a liaison librarian for several departments and also provides support for researchers regarding data management, scholarly communications, and systematic searching. Before coming to UCLA, Bethany interned at the University of Pennsylvania Biomedical Library and worked at the University of Pennsylvania Barbara Bates Center for the Study of the History of Nursing. Bethany holds an MSLIS from Florida State University and a BA in Digital Media from the University of Central Florida.

Rebecca Raszewski, AHIP, is associate professor and information services and liaison librarian at the Library for the Health Sciences at the University of Illinois at Chicago. She has been the library liaison for the UIC nursing community in Chicago for over seven years. Her research interests include the intersection of nursing and librarianship within collections and collaborations and library science education. Rebecca received her bachelor's degree in English writing from La Salle University and her master's in information science from Drexel University.

Melissa A. Ratajeski, AHIP, is the coordinator of Data Management Services and liaison to the Institutional Animal Care and Use Committee at the Health Sciences Library System, University of Pittsburgh. In this role, she provides support and training for researchers at each stage of the data life cycle. Before receiving her master's in library and information science, Melissa was a research coordinator within the Department of Neurobiology/Center for the Neural Basis of Cognition, at the University of Pittsburgh School of Medicine.

Kevin Read is a member of NYU Health Sciences Library's Data Services Team, where he provides research data management support to faculty, postdocs, and students. In this role, Kevin teaches research data management, is the cocreator of an institutional data catalog, and provides individualized data support to the academic community. Kevin is co-PI for an NIH Big Data to Knowledge training grant designed to teach librarians to both understand and teach data management. He is also a member of the NIH BioCADDIE initiative, where he is working to develop a metadata schema for the new NIH Data Discovery Index. He has published a number of articles about how librarians can engage with researchers around the topic of data, the impact and scope of federally funded biomedical research data, and what common metadata elements should be used to describe research data.

Carolyn Schubert is the nursing and health sciences librarian at James Madison University; her work as the Libraries and Educational Technologies representative to the Institutional Review Board and her participation in the Institute for Research Design in Librarianship inform her relationship with teaching and consulting on data management. Her previous publications include a chapter in *Curriculum-Based Library Instruction: From Cultivating Faculty Relationships to Assessment*, a *Nurse Educator* article, and several *Charleston Advisor* reviews. Her research interests include information-seeking behavior in clinical practice, health informatics, collection assessment, and team-based liaison programs.

Yasmeen Shorish is the scholarly communication and data service coordinator at James Madison University (JMU). Previous to 2016, she was the physical and life sciences librarian at JMU. Her previous publication topics include data management and curation, chemical and data information literacy instruction, and research into scholarly publishing models, and she is a regular contributor to the

ACRL *TechConnect* blog. Her research interests include the changing nature of scholarly communication, the evolution of library services to support learning and research, and increasing the dissemination of, and access to, information.

Alisa Surkis, PhD, is the translational science librarian at the NYU Langone Medical Center, where she serves as a member of the NYU Health Science Library's Data Services Team and as the director of Team Science for the NYU-HHC Clinical and Translational Science Institute. Through these roles she teaches research data management, provides direct data management support to researchers, is involved in the development of an institutional data catalog and supports and develops a number of other programs and systems to promote and support collaboration. She also provides education in research data management to the broader medical library community through continuing education courses for the Medical Library Association and an NIH Big Data to Knowledge-funded project to create curricula to teach librarians to both understand and teach research data management.

Minglu Wang is the data services librarian at Dana Library and liaison to the Department of Sociology and Anthropology as well as the Office of Research. She teaches workshops to undergraduates and graduate students on the use of different statistical software packages as well as NVivo and Census-mapping data software. Minglu helps individual professors and students to solve their data analysis problems and provides consulting on data management. She also conducts data analysis and visualization for faculty members, research centers, and other departments in Rutgers University-Newark.

Ann Vreeland Watkins is life sciences librarian at Dana Library, where she provides research support to undergraduate, master's, and doctoral students, as well as faculty in the biological sciences, neuroscience, nursing, and psychology. Her delivery of information services takes place in multiple reference venues including individual consultations and instruction. As collection development coordinator, Ann collaborates with selectors on the growth of Dana's collections and works with the technical services librarian on collection management.

Lisa D. Zilinski is the research data consultant at Carnegie Mellon University. As part of the Research Curation Division, she consults and collaborates with faculty, staff, and students to identify data literacy opportunities, develops learning plans and tools for data education, and investigates and develops programmatic and sustainable data services for the Libraries. Her research interests include data-informed learning, data management principles, data policy, and information dissemination/access practices.